Orthopaedics and Fractures

T. DUCKWORTH

BSc, MB, ChB, FRCS
Professor and Head of
the Department of Orthopaedic Surgery
University of Sheffield

Third Edition

b

Blackwell
Science

© 1980, 1984, 1995 by
Blackwell Science Ltd
Editorial Offices:
Osney Mead, Oxford OX2 0EL
25 John Street, London WC1N 2BL
23 Ainslie Place, Edinburgh EH3 6AJ
238 Main Street, Cambridge
  Massachusetts 02142, USA
54 University Street, Carlton
  Victoria 3053, Australia

Other Editorial Offices:
Arnette Blackwell SA
  1, rue de Lille, 75007 Paris
  France

Blackwell Wissenschafts-Verlag GmbH
  Kurfürstendamm 57
  10707 Berlin, Germany

  Feldgasse 13, A-1238 Wien
  ·Austria

First published 1980
Reprinted 1981, 1982, 1983
Portuguese translation 1980
Second edition 1984
Reprinted 1986, 1988 (twice) and 1991
German translation 1984
Arabic translation 1988
Third edition 1995
Four Dragons edition 1995

Set by Excel Typesetters Company, Hong Kong
Printed and bound in Great Britain
at the Alden Press Ltd, Oxford and Northampton

DISTRIBUTORS

  Marston Book Services Ltd
  PO Box 87
  Oxford OX2 0DT
  (Orders: Tel: 01865 791155
          Fax: 01865 791927
          Telex: 837515)

North America
  Blackwell Science, Inc.
  238 Main Street
  Cambridge, MA 02142
  (Orders: Tel: 800 215-1000
           617 876-7000
          Fax: 617 492-5263)

Australia
  Blackwell Science Pty Ltd
  54 University Street
  Carlton, Victoria 3053
  (Orders: Tel: 03 347-0300)
          Fax: 03 349-3016)

A catalogue record for this title
is available from the British Library

ISBN 0-632-02781-9 (BSL)
ISBN 0-86542-983-9 (Four Dragons)

Library of Congress
Cataloging-in-Publication Data

Duckworth, T.
  Lecture notes on orthopaedics and fractures/
  T. Duckworth.—3rd ed.
      p.   cm.
  Includes bibliographical references
  and index.
  ISBN 0-632-02781-9
  1. Orthopedics—Handbooks, manuals, etc.
  2. Fractures—Handbooks, manuals, etc.
  I. Title.
  [DNLM: 1. Orthopedics—handbooks.
  2. Fractures—handbooks. WE 39 D836L 1995]
  RD732.5.D83 1995
  617.3—dc20
  DNLM/DLC
  for Library of Congress
                                    94-23689
                                        CIP

Orthopaedics and
Fractures

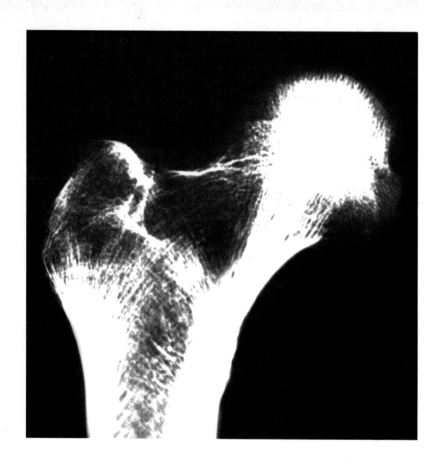

Contents

Preface to the third edition

There are fashions in medical education, as in most things. Rote learning is now regarded with suspicion. The grim certainties of the traditional undergraduate courses have given way to the diffuse educational concepts of the new. Many medical schools now have the stated aim of producing 'educated doctors', unburdened by factual knowledge, but well-versed in the techniques of self instruction and information technology. The old divisions between pre-clinical and clinical subjects and between specialties are being steadily broken down.

Curiously, in the postgraduate world the move is towards more structured, defined and condensed vocational courses with a strong instructional content. 'Training' is the fashion here. Would it be heresy to suggest that this latter trend has become a necessity because of the deficiencies of the former?

It is an unfortunate fact that the practice of medicine requires the acquisition of a great deal of knowledge and it is inefficient and impractical to have to seek out this knowledge at the time when it is needed. Regrettably, however, a knowledge of anatomy, physiology and pathology is no longer second nature to the qualifying doctor. Practical procedures are not being taught. The building blocks are not secure.

The trends in the UK are similar to those elsewhere, but some traditions die hard. The concept of a period of General Professional Training (GPT), common to all clinicians and preceding specialization, is gaining ground. In surgery, the British Royal Colleges continue to support the idea of Basic Surgical Training (BST), designed to give all surgical trainees a grounding in the principles of surgery and an overview of the surgical specialties. This is to be followed by Higher Surgical Training (HST) in the chosen surgical specialty. Many of the subjects previously covered at undergraduate level are now having to be fitted into these postgraduate courses, sometimes at a very late stage.

These developments have been taken into account in compiling this third edition. The basic science content now seems even more important than before. For the undergraduate, principles are still stressed, but it is hoped that the book will also prove to be a useful and reliable reference source. The information is presented in a form which should continue to serve the needs of the same student when he/she progresses through General Professional Training and becomes a general practitioner. For the Basic Surgical Trainee the book should more than cover the syllabus for the relevant examinations and, hopefully, will also serve as a useful introduction to Higher Surgical Training in orthopaedics and traumatology. With the latter in mind, a chapter on the management of major trauma, based on the American Advanced Trauma and Life Support courses has been added and the sections on surgical techniques have been updated.

ACKNOWLEDGEMENTS

It is a pleasure to acknowledge the help of my secretary, Mrs Ann McArthur and the staff of Blackwell Science, particularly Andrew Robinson and Jonathan Rowley. I have also been greatly helped by the Medical Illustration Department of the Central Sheffield Universities Hospital Trust.

I am indebted to Mr R. Grimer and Dr M. Snaith for their advice on the subjects of neoplastic conditions and inflammatory rheumatic conditions, respectively, and to Mr M. Saleh for Fig. 11.5.

I am grateful to Mr M. J. M. Sharrard for allowing me to reproduce Figs 22.1, 23.1, 23.2, 23.3, 23.6, 24.1, 24.2, 26.1, 27.3, 28.6, 30.2 and 50.11 taken from *Paediatric Orthopaedics and Fractures* (2nd edition) published by Blackwell Scientific Publications. Manufacturers supplying illustrations of their products are acknowledged in the text.

Preface to the first edition

At first sight there would appear to be little difficulty in compiling a short textbook of orthopaedics and fractures to meet the needs of medical students, general practitioners and others with a non-specialist interest in the subject. They are all likely to require a quick and reliable source of reference and some practical advice on management. But how much material, how much detail, and how much practical advice?

Many medical schools have reduced the time available for the study of disorders of the musculo-skeletal system. The medical student is now lucky if he can gain experience in the techniques of clinical examination, let alone become familiar with those common orthopaedic conditions which occupy so much of the average general practitioner's time and encroach on every branch of medicine.

It would be a short textbook indeed which covered only the contents of this type of course. Students often complain that they are given no guidance as to how far their reading should take them beyond the confines of their limited clinical experience. They often ask in desperation for a syllabus or a list of reading material: how much do we need to know? Unfortunately, although examiners may be prepared to confine themselves within pre-determined limits, patients rarely do so. They present with obscure problems, or, worse still, common problems in unfamiliar guises. No matter how well he has been taught and has understood the principles of diagnosis and management no textbook can provide the new doctor with what will become his most valuable asset — experience. It can however provide him with other peoples' experience and also with something almost equally valuable — an awareness of what are the possibilities. Without this awareness, a diagnosis can rarely be made.

In the absence of clear guidance from the medical faculties about what their end-product, the newly qualified doctor, is supposed to be, it seemed reasonable to try to produce a book which would attempt to provide answers, albeit often brief and incomplete ones, to most of the questions the interested and intelligent student and post-graduate would be likely to ask about the subject.

In doing so, emphasis has been placed on the principles of diagnosis and management and on classification. It is hoped that the latter will be an aid to understanding relationships and also perhaps to memory. Common conditions have been allocated relatively more space, and some details of the management of such conditions, which might be of value to junior staff, are included, with short sections on orthopaedic and operative procedures. Rarities are either excluded or simply receive a brief mention to make the student aware of their existence. Inevitably, some sections will appear too condensed and others too detailed. The section on ankle fractures, for example, is perhaps more appropriate for a trainee orthopaedic surgeon than a student, but here, as in other places, it was felt that the subject could become almost meaningless if less detail were included.

The layout of the book may be found convenient by some readers, irrational and perhaps irritating by others. This particular arrangement has been chosen so that answers will be easy to find, embedded in related information which will make the subject more of a whole. The regional chapters provide an alternative approach to the same information, and cross-references have been provided to avoid repetition.

The content is, of course, the author's choice, based on experience of what has been found useful and of interest to students. Orthopaedics is a strongly clinical subject with a high visual content. This is reflected in the relatively large number of illustrations. X-rays are so much a part of the world of orthopaedics, that it is difficult to imagine the specialty without them, and wherever possible these have been used to illustrate the various conditions. Nevertheless, some experience is required in their interpretation, and where this could be a problem diagrams have been substituted for their extra clarity.

Finally, and in response to suggestions from students, an appendix has been added, giving useful pathological and clinical data for rapid reference.

If this volume proves useful on the wards and in the clinics, and stimulates an interest in a fascinating subject, it may justify adding to the rising tide of published material which threatens to overwhelm students and practising doctors alike.

ACKNOWLEDGEMENTS

I would like to thank my secretary, Mrs Margaret Chapman, for her unfailing patience and skill in interpreting my often revised notes. My thanks must also go to Mr A. Tunstill and the staff of the Photographic Department of the Sheffield Area Health Authority for the photographs; to Mrs Debbie Davies of Oxford Illustrators Ltd for the line diagrams; and to Dr G. Owen for supplying pathological data.

I am grateful to Mr W.J.W. Sharrard for allowing me to reproduce Figures 21.1, 22.1, 22.2, 22.3, 22.6, 23.1, 23.2, 23.3, 25.1, 26.3, 27.6, 29.2 and 50.11 from *Paediatric Orthopaedics and Fractures* published by Blackwell Scientific Publications.

SECTION I

General principles

CHAPTER I

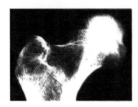

The skeletal structures

Modern orthopaedics is concerned with the diagnosis and management of disorders of the musculo-skeletal system, that is the skeleton and the soft tissues associated with it. The skull is usually excluded, being the province of several other specialties, and there is an overlap of interest in the spine between the orthopaedic surgeon and the neurosurgeon. In many countries orthopaedic surgeons deal with injuries of the musculo-skeletal system, particularly fractures, as well as non-traumatic conditions, but sub-specialization is increasingly occurring and it is becoming more and more difficult for one individual to encompass the whole field. Sub-specialization has tended to be disorderly, occurring sometimes by age of the patient, as for example with paediatric orthopaedics; by region of the body, as with knee or hand surgery; or by condition as, for example, with scoliosis.

It is still possible, however, to define the speciality in terms of the structures with which it is primarily concerned and a knowledge of the anatomy, physiology and pathology of these structures and tissues forms a logical starting point for studying the clinical aspects of the subject.

BONES

A long bone is characteristically tubular with expanded ends and is remarkably strong for its weight. The shaft is often called the *diaphysis* and the zone adjacent to the epiphyseal line is the *metaphysis*. This is the part of the developing bone most likely to be the seat of disease, probably because it is the most metabolically active area and has the greatest blood supply. Damage to, or abnormal development of the epiphyseal plate itself is likely to result in growth disturbance.

Growth does not occur equally at the two ends of a long bone. It is more active, for example, at the ends farthest from the elbow and nearest to the knee. Diseases such as osteomyelitis and tumours are noticeably more common at these sites. The spongy ends of the bone have a complex architecture and it is here that the trabeculae can be seen to follow the lines of greatest stress (Fig. 1.1).

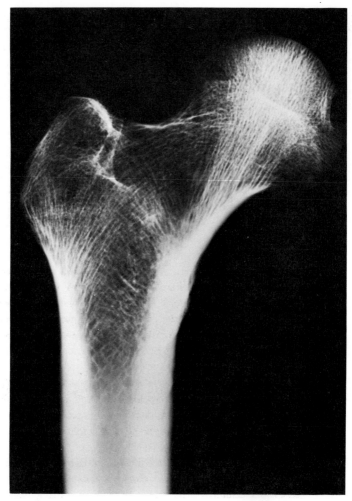

Fig. 1.1 X-ray of femur.

A normal bone can resist large compressive forces and considerable bending stresses and only breaks when subjected to considerable violence. It may, however, be weakened by disease and can then fracture as a result of minimal trauma. Such *pathological fractures* are often orientated transversely across the bone.

The short bones consist of a cancellous core surrounded by a layer of cortical bone, partly covered by articular cartilage. They contain red marrow in their trabecular spaces and the vertebral bodies are important sites of blood formation throughout life.

The bones form fixed points for muscle attachments and their periosteal sheaths blend with the collagen of the tendons and ligaments.

REMODELLING AFTER A FRACTURE

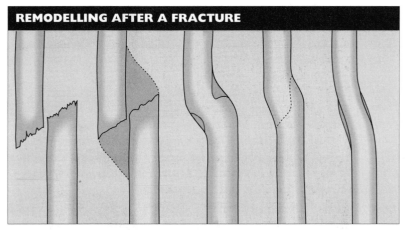

Fig. 1.2

Remodelling of bone continues throughout life, but particularly during growth and after fracture healing. In children, even severe residual deformities can be corrected fully, with the possible exception of rotational deformities; this capacity for remodelling is less in the adult and, although the bone smoothes itself out, it is usually possible to spot the site of a fracture many years later (Fig. 1.2).

JOINTS

The function of a limb is heavily dependent on the smooth working of the joints, and joint diseases are common and troublesome.

Three types of joint are usually recognized.

1 *Fibrous joints or syndesmoses.* As the name suggests, in this type of joint the bones are connected by a continuous band of fibrous tissue, as is the case with the sutures of the skull. These joints are strong and not readily disrupted, but they allow little movement.

2 *Cartilaginous joints or synchondroses.* These consist of a cartilaginous band joining the bones. This may be hyaline, as between some of the skull bones, in which case ossification usually occurs at maturity. Secondary cartilaginous joints consist of a mass of fibro-cartilage lying between two thin plates of hyaline growth cartilage. The intervertebral discs and symphyses are of this type and all are midline structures.

3 *Synovial joints.* This type of joint allows the greatest mobility. The joint surfaces are covered with hyaline cartilage and the joint is enclosed by a fibrous capsule which is usually attached close to the edge of the articular surface. It is lined by a vascular synovial membrane which secretes the synovial fluid. This latter is a remarkable substance which performs a nutritive function and has important lubricating properties.

Articular cartilage, apart from its deepest layer, derives most of its nutrition from the synovial fluid which must, therefore, have access to the whole articular surface. There is some evidence that degenerative joint disease may be, at least partly, due to an interruption in the free flow of this fluid.

Some joints contain fibro-cartilaginous discs partly separating the joint surfaces. The menisci of the knee are examples of this and they have been shown to have an important stress-distributing function.

Articular cartilage, normally smooth and elastic, may be pitted or eroded by disease or completely worn away to reveal the underlying bony cortex. The earliest stages of this process are known as 'fibrillation'. The articular cartilage becomes irregular and tends to fray and split. To some extent, this phenomenon is age-related, but it does not occur uniformly throughout the joints and varies in its extent from individual to individual. It is essentially a focal change, and there are certain sites where it is common, particularly those areas which rarely contact the opposing articular surface. In certain circumstances, this condition progresses to fully developed osteoarthritis (Chapter 39).

LIGAMENTS

These may be either discrete structures or thickenings of the joint capsule. Being necessary for joint stability, they are strong and are orientated to resist specific stresses. They are, however, occasionally ruptured, either completely or partially, and are difficult to restore when damaged. A partial rupture is known as a *sprain* or *strain*, and usually heals completely.

BLOOD SUPPLY AND INNERVATION OF JOINTS

All joints have a free blood supply with many anastomosing arteries. An operation on a major joint without a tourniquet provides a good demonstration of joint vascularity. There is a fine plexus of lymphatics within the synovial membranes.

The nerve supply of a joint is the same as that of the overlying muscles moving the joint and the skin over their insertions (Hilton's Law). Most of the nerve end-organs lie in the joint capsule, but muscle and tendon end-organs are equally important for proprioception. Autonomic nerves also reach the joint, mainly with the blood vessels, and control the blood supply and perhaps the formation of synovial fluid.

The protective and proprioceptive functions of spinal nerves are vital to the normal functioning of a joint, which rapidly disintegrates if this protection is lost (Charcot's joint).

MUSCLES

The functions of joints and muscles are closely interrelated. Not only are muscles important for moving the joints, but their coordinated action is essential for joint stability. This is very evident in paralytic conditions where the lack of stability may have to be compensated by the use of external splints.

Skeletal muscle is composed of fibres whose length varies from a few millimetres to about 30 centimetres. Each fibre contains many nuclei embedded in its syncytium and the fibre itself is built up of many myofibrils, each of which consists of units of the proteins actin and myosin. These are arranged in interlocking bands. They give the fibre its characteristic cross-sections, and are the contractile elements of the muscle.

The form of a muscle determines its power and contractility. If the fibres are arranged parallel to the line of pull, the contractility is greatest: where there are many fibres arranged obliquely to the line of pull the power is greater but the ability to shorten is less.

Nerve supply

The nerve enters the muscle at the motor point which is usually fairly constant and is the point at which electrical stimulation is most effective. The smaller branches of each nerve fibre supply a variable number of muscle fibres, each junction being called a *motor end-plate*. Where fine control is needed, as with the small muscles of the hand, the number of muscle fibres supplied by each nerve fibre is small, whereas more coarsely innervated muscles may have one nerve fibre dividing to supply over a hundred motor end-plates. Afferent fibres derive from muscle spindles and are essential for the feedback mechanisms controlling contraction.

Muscles have many actions, sometimes functioning as prime movers, at other times as coordinating antagonists, synergists and cooperating muscles. Many of their so-called 'voluntary' activities are concerned with posture and are essentially unconscious.

TENDONS AND BURSAE

Most muscles are attached to the bone ends by a tendon which may be a few millimetres or many centimetres long. Many of the larger tendons move within a fibrous sheath, which has a synovial lining (Fig. 1.3a).

Tendons do not resist pressure very well and are frequently separated or protected from their underlying bones by thin-walled cavities

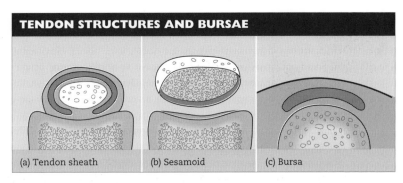

TENDON STRUCTURES AND BURSAE

(a) Tendon sheath (b) Sesamoid (c) Bursa

Fig. 1.3

containing synovial fluid. Some of the larger tendons contain a bone within their substance at the place where they cross a joint and have to bear considerable stresses. These are known as *sesamoid bones*. Examples are the patella and the sesamoids under the first metatarsal head. They have articular cartilage on their deep surfaces (Fig. 1.3b).

Small sacs or *bursae* are often found overlying bony prominences. They may be fairly constant anatomical structures, like those overlying the ischial tuberosity or olecranon, or they may be produced as a response to external pressure when they are called 'adventitious' bursae, as for example the one which develops over the patellar tendon in occupations involving continuous kneeling, or the first metatarsal head from pressure on the shoe (Fig. 1.3c). Certain anatomical bursae communicate with the nearby joint and may become distended or diseased if pathology develops in the underlying joint.

CHAPTER 2

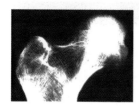

The connective tissues

STRUCTURE

The connective tissues of the body are composed of cells embodied in a matrix which varies in its quantity and composition. The cells can be categorized by the nature of the intercellular material, of which there are three types:
- collagenous tissue (produced by fibroblasts);
- chondroid (produced by chondroblasts);
- osteoid (produced by osteoblasts).

In each case the matrix is mainly composed of a complex mixture of proteoglycans and glycoproteins, forming a ground substance in which is embedded a meshwork of fibrils, mostly of collagen, a protein. At least four genetically different types of collagen are now recognized—bone contains Type I and hyaline cartilage Type II. Skin contains Types I and III and, being a convenient tissue for biopsy, is used for the study of certain collagen-related bone diseases. Elastin, a prominent constituent of one type of cartilage is also thought to be a component of collagen.

Matrix disorders, which may be genetically determined or acquired, cause a variety of clinical manifestations. In the so-called 'mucopoly-saccharoidoses' (see page 208), an enzyme deficiency interferes with the breakdown of large mucopolysaccharide molecules, which accumulate in the tissues causing widespread abnormalities.

Bone

Bone consists of osteoid which is resilient, but is heavily infiltrated with calcium salts giving it hardness and strength. The mechanism of mineraliz-ation is not well understood. The mineral is mainly deposited in crystal-line form as hydroxyapatite, but there is also an amorphous phase which is found particularly in newly formed bone. It is worth noting that various ions such as strontium, fluoride and lead can enter the crystal lattice of bone mineral.

BONE STRUCTURE

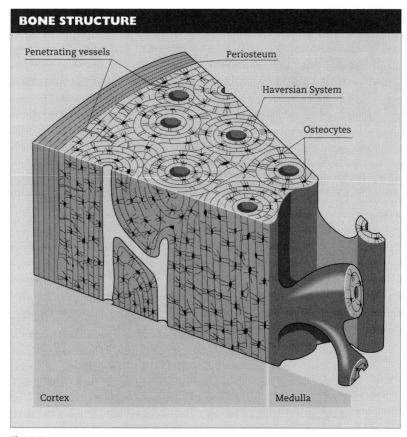

Penetrating vessels

Periosteum

Haversian System

Osteocytes

Cortex

Medulla

Fig. 2.1

A normal bone is composed of concentric cylinders of matrix with cells lying in lacunae between the layers, the whole forming a 'Haversian System'. In the hard cortex the Haversian systems are packed tightly together; in the spongy or cancellous bone they are more loosely arranged (Fig. 2.1). The bony trabeculae are structured and orientated to withstand the stresses of weight-bearing and muscle activity, obeying Wolff's Law. The interstices of the cancellous bone and the hollow centres of the shafts of long bones are filled with marrow. Haemopoiesis occurs in the marrow throughout the bones in the child, but in the adult is confined to the short bones, particularly the vertebral bodies, and to the ends of the long bones.

Each bone is ensheathed by fibrous periosteum with an underlying layer of osteoblasts, and is vascularized from the periosteum and by one or more nutrient arteries penetrating the cortex.

Cartilage

This varies in its appearance and physical characteristics depending on the predominant type of fibril and the density of the matrix. Two types of fibril, collagen and elastin, are found in varying proportions. Three types of cartilage are normally recognized.

1 Hyaline cartilage. The pre-ossified epiphyses and the articular surfaces both consist of hyaline cartilage which is indistinguishable by ordinary histological techniques, but has different properties and, of course, different functions in the two tissues.

2 White fibro-cartilage is found mainly in midline structures such as intervertebral discs and symphyses. The collagen content is much greater than in hyaline cartilage and the fibres are much more obvious. This type of cartilage has the ability to withstand strong tension and bear heavy compressive loads.

3 Yellow or elastic fibro-cartilage is found in the nasal and aural cartilages and contains the highest proportion of elastin.

Collagenous tissue

Fibrous tissue is widespread throughout the body and consists mainly of collagen fibres with relatively little matrix.

Disorders of collagen metabolism are being extensively studied because of their dramatic effects on body structure and development. These conditions are sometimes called 'true collagen diseases', as opposed to the non-developmental diseases of collagen, such as rheumatoid arthritis. Osteogenesis imperfecta (see page 209), is an example of an inherited disorder of collagen metabolism, mainly affecting the structure and strength of bone.

GROWTH AND DEVELOPMENT

Connective tissues grow by cell proliferation and deposition of intercellular material.

Bones

These develop initially in early intrauterine life as condensations of mesenchymal tissue in the axis of the limb (Fig. 2.2a), and by the 6th week the connective tissue cells have started to lay down cartilage to form the shape of the future bone (Fig. 2.2b). At the centre of the cartilage mass the cells hypertrophy and apparently die and with the ingrowth of vascular connective tissue, the matrix calcifies and eventually ossifies (Fig.

BONE GROWTH AND DEVELOPMENT

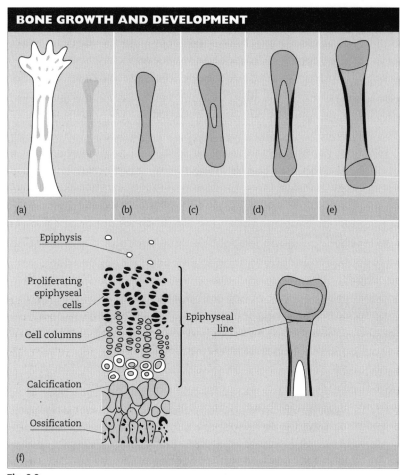

(a)   (b)   (c)   (d)   (e)

Epiphysis

Proliferating
epiphyseal
cells

Cell columns

Epiphyseal
line

Calcification

Ossification

(f)

Fig. 2.2

2.2c). This process spreads along the bone (Fig. 2.2d) so that it eventually consists of a bony shaft with cartilaginous ends (Fig. 2.2e) which become the sites of secondary ossification centres (Fig. 2.2f). The intervening or epiphyseal cartilage remains until maturity as the growth point for bone length, the proliferating cartilage cells on the diaphyseal side forming into columns and undergoing a series of changes, eventually 'ballooning' as the zone of vascularization reaches them and ossification of the matrix begins. This results in gradual growth of the epiphysis away from the centre of the shaft. Growth in width occurs by deposition of non-cartilaginous sub-periosteal bone and the whole bone is constantly re-modelled as the child grows.

The earliest bone to be laid down is often called 'woven bone' because its histological structure shows the fibrils to be randomly distributed, unlike the regular lamellar structure of mature bone. Some bones develop entirely by intramembranous ossification, with no intermediate cartilage stage, the clavicle and bones of the calvarium being examples.

Cartilage

This grows by direct proliferation of the cells with peri-cellular deposition of matrix, but even during rapid active growth relatively few cells can be seen dividing. The capacity of hyaline cartilage to regenerate and repair itself is strictly limited, which means that damage to an articular surface can have long-lasting consequences. There is some evidence that intrinsic mechanisms of repair can be supplemented by ingrowth and metaplasia of peri-articular collagenous tissue, but repair of any but the smallest defect is seldom complete.

Collagen

Collagen growth is an important aspect of general body development and fibroblasts are frequently to be seen proliferating and laying down collagen fibres. This is particularly the case in any situation where repair of tissues is required. The usual end-result of repair, the scar, consists almost entirely of collagenous material. In situations where there is continuing damage to the tissues, with concomitant repair, the scar tissue formed can be extremely dense. As it matures, collagenous scar tissue tends to contract, sometimes producing distortion and obstruction of internal structures or contractures of skin and joints. Occasionally, the healing of a skin wound may be complicated by the formation of over-exuberant scar tissue, producing a wide and thickened scar known as 'keloid'. This is more common in Negroid races.

PHYSIOLOGY

Connective tissues are by no means inert and play an important role in biochemical processes in the body.

Ground substance is an important water-binding agent and acts as an ion-exchange resin in controlling the passage of electrolytes. Its deposition is influenced by many factors such as hormones and vitamins, and its composition reflects abnormalities in the supply of these factors.

Cartilage 'turnover' is relatively little understood, but balanced synthesis and degradation of the ground substance has been shown to continue throughout life.

Bone is known to play a vital role in metabolism, mainly because of its calcium and phosphate content. These minerals enter into the formation of crystals of hydroxyapatite and their deposition is sensitive to many influences. There is some evidence that bone surfaces are bathed in a special type of extracellular fluid which is different from that of the rest of the body. Diseases such as rickets, osteomalacia and hyper-parathyroidism are associated with dramatic changes in bone develop-ment (Chapter 40).

Demineralization of bone results in loss of strength and may be caused by diminished matrix formation, inadequate calcification or bone resorption. The latter occurs as a result of the activity of special cells—*osteoclasts*—which remove both the organic and inorganic com-ponents. The radiographic appearances of loss of density are similar whatever the cause of the demineralization and these appearances give rise to the term 'osteoporosis'.

CHAPTER 3

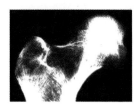

Examination of the musculo-skeletal system

HISTORY TAKING

The art of taking a good history lies in eliciting as much relevant information as possible in the shortest possible time. Most patients need help to describe their complaints and it is usually best to go through the history in chronological order. It is important to establish what the patient's immediate complaint is and the extent to which the symptoms are causing disability. Pain is by far the commonest symptom, but the patient may complain more of the effect the pain has on his daily activities than of the pain itself. Symptoms other than pain may predominate. Joint stiffness or instability may be a problem and neurological disorders may result in characteristic functional difficulties. Many orthopaedic conditions are chronic and may result in the patient being unable to dress, manage normal toilet functions or go out of doors. The exact nature of the patient's work should be ascertained and some estimate should be made of how much working time is being lost because of illness. Financial worries may complicate the situation and may influence eventual decisions about treatment. It is helpful to get into the habit of making a provisional shortlist of possible diagnoses on the basis of the symptoms alone, as this helps to direct the history taking.

Pain

This is the commonest orthopaedic complaint. Its exact site should be determined and it should be remembered that referred pain is common, for example, along the sciatic nerve from lesions in the lumbo-sacral spine, or into the arm from disease of the cervical spine.

The duration of the pain and its quality, e.g. aching, sharp, burning, etc., should be noted and also the degree to which it is aggravated by external factors such as walking or straining as well as its response to analgesics. Pain is a *symptom* and is not the same as *tenderness*, which is a *physical sign*.

Stiffness

Stiffness of joints or inability to carry out a specific activity may also be a symptom, but it is surprisingly seldom that patients complain of this in the absence of pain.

Deformity or swelling

These may be the prevailing symptoms and it is important to ask the patient to point out, or describe, the abnormality. Where a swelling may be due to a neoplasm, the duration of symptoms can be all-important and the patient should be asked if the swelling has increased or fluctuated in size.

Weakness

This or similar loss of function may suggest a neurological abnormality. A full and detailed neurological history will then be required. Many neurological conditions present as disturbances of musculo-skeletal function and many orthopaedic conditions may, in turn, produce neurological loss.

As a routine, enquiry should always be made as to whether there is any history of trauma, and details of previous surgical or other treatment should be sought. The history should always end with a general systematic enquiry which need only take a few seconds.

EXAMINATION

Much can be learnt from the patient's general appearance—does he/she look well or ill, haggard, wasted, feverish, etc.? Does he/she appear nervous or over-anxious? Are his/her movements normal or is there a general or local abnormality of gait or in the use of their arms and hands? Height, weight and build may be relevant, and in children, abnormalities of growth and development need to be considered, with due regard to the normal range of variation at any given age.

The local examination

The patient is more likely to feel at ease if the initial examination is directed to the part of the body of which he/she complains. A suggested scheme of examination is given below. *Both limbs should always be compared.*

INSPECTION

Attitude of the trunk and limbs

This includes the gait and stance. The patient should be watched as he walks, climbs on the examination couch, crouches or kneels, and uses his arms and hands. With practice, inspection of the gait may give a useful clue to the underlying disorder. It is usually easy to decide if the problem lies with the hip, knee or foot. Typical examples of common gait abnormalities include the Trendelenberg or 'dipping hip' gait, the stiff-legged gait of knee disease, and the gait associated with a painful foot, where the patient looks as though he is walking on hard pebbles. Many neurological disorders produce characteristic gait abnormalities, such as the tendency to 'back-knee' because of quadriceps weakness or to catch the toe of the shoe as a result of a 'drop foot' gait associated with weakness of the ankle dorsiflexors.

Wasting

Localized or generalized muscle wasting may be an important and sometimes the only physical sign. It should always be searched for specifically and may not always be obvious when the patient is lying down.

Surface abnormalities

The whole skin surface should be inspected carefully for discoloration, scars, ulceration, bruising, rashes, etc.

Abnormalities of contour

The shape of the limb should be inspected for swelling, deformities, hollows, etc.

PALPATION

Certain important physical signs can be elicited only by careful palpation. The whole area should be lightly but firmly palpated, and then attention directed to certain key diagnostic points.

Landmarks

A limb or joint may be grossly distorted by trauma or disease, and palpation should always begin by identifying the characteristic bony landmarks of the part, e.g. the anterior superior spine, greater trochanter, ischial tuberosity and symphysis pubis for the hip; for the elbow, the two epicondyles and the olecranon. The relationships between them should be carefully considered.

Tenderness

This is frequently the most important physical sign and must be localized accurately, e.g. is it maximal over the shaft, epiphysis, joint line, muscle, tendon, etc.? It should be remembered that certain anatomical sites are quite tender in normal circumstances and it is always advisable to compare sides carefully.

Temperature

Comparison with the normal side is necessary and discrepancies caused by clothing or dressings must be avoided. Minor differences of temperature are more easily distinguished by palpating with the back of the hand.

Swelling

Any swelling must be careully palpated and a note made of its size, position, shape, consistency, fluctuation, etc. Its position in relation to the various tissue planes and its attachments are particularly important. Is it attached to bone, muscle, tendon, skin, etc.?

MOVEMENTS

The main function of a joint is to allow movement, so that disturbances of movement are a usual accompaniment of joint disease.

Normal movements (i.e. movement within the normal planes.)

Active movements

The patient should be asked to move the joint and the range of movements noted. In assessing joint ranges the anatomical position is usually taken as the reference point of 0 degrees (Fig. 3.1).

Passive movements

The examiner attempts to put the joint through a range of movements and notes the range and quality of the movements, i.e. is it smooth and progressive, or rough and crepitant, or is there a 'catch' at some point in the range? Occasionally the range is increased beyond the normal.

Abnormal movements

Joints rely for their stability mainly on ligaments, aided by muscle activity. When a ligament is ruptured it may be possible to move a joint in an abnormal direction. These movements should be tested specifically. Muscle relaxation is always essential for accurate ligament testing. An acute strain is likely to cause pain in the ligament when the latter is put on the stretch. Occasionally, an acute ligament rupture may have to be

JOINT RANGES

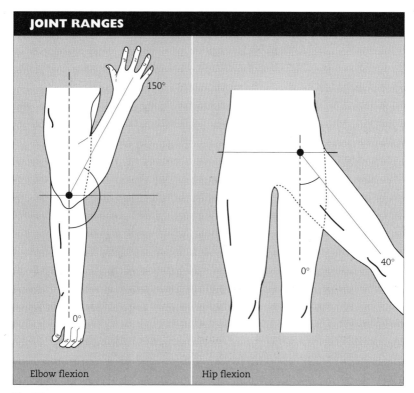

Elbow flexion

Hip flexion

Fig. 3.1

diagnosed by passively stressing the joint under X-ray control with local or general anaesthesia.

Causes of restriction of movements include:
- mechanical block, e.g. loose body, torn meniscus, etc.;
- soft-tissue contracture;
- effusion;
- paralysis;
- spasm (and pain); and
- spasticity.

Definition of deformity

The word is used in two senses.

1 Deformity of a bone means the bone is of abnormal shape or length, e.g. following a mal-united fracture.

2 Deformity of a joint means that the joint *cannot be put into the anatomical position*. The deformity is named according to the direction in

JOINT DEFORMITIES

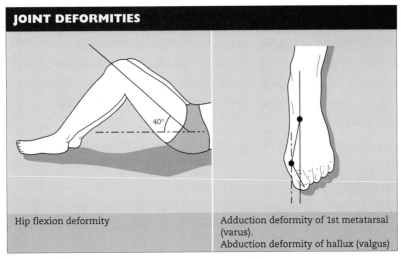

| Hip flexion deformity | Adduction deformity of 1st metatarsal (varus). Abduction deformity of hallux (valgus) |

Fig. 3.2

which the joint is bent, e.g. (Fig. 3.2) flexion deformity, adduction deformity, etc. The word 'contracture' is often used in the same sense as deformity. A deformity essentially means a loss of range, but the converse is not necessarily true. The expression 'mobile deformity' is to some extent a contradiction in terms, but is used in the situation where the joint is held constantly in a deformed position, but can, in the appropriate circumstances, be put into the anatomical position. This is commonly the case with spastic conditions such as cerebral palsy, or following a stroke.

MEASUREMENTS

Limb girth may be important in the assessment of wasting or swelling. The girth should always be compared with the normal side at a fixed distance from a bony landmark. Limb length may be measured as required, using a tape measure and again measuring between recognizable bony landmarks. It is difficult to achieve an accuracy of more than 1 cm.

NEUROLOGICAL SYSTEM

Many orthopaedic conditions are associated with neurological problems and examination of the musculo-skeletal system should *always* include a quick neurological assessment, which may be made more detailed if any abnormality is suspected.

The main points to be tested are:

1 muscle power using the Medical Research Council (MRC) grading scale (Table 3.1) where relevant;

2 sensitivity to pinprick and cotton wool; and

3 reflexes.

MRC SCALE	
0	No muscle power
1	Flicker of activity
2	Movement with effect of gravity eliminated i.e. in a plane at right angles to gravity but not against resistance
3	Movement against gravity but not against applied resistance
4	Movement against applied resistance but less than full power
5	Normal power

Table 3.1 MRC scale for recording muscle power

CIRCULATION

The colour and state of the limbs should be observed and pulses palpated. The presence or absence of hairs on the digits is often a useful test of circulatory insufficiency.

Both neurological and circulatory examinations are particularly important in assessing the injured limb.

LYMPHATIC SYSTEM

Where relevant, the lymphatic channels and nodes should be inspected and palpated. This is particularly important with tumours and acute infections.

Extent of examination

The above scheme can be applied to any part of the musculo-skeletal system, but each area may require one or more specific tests which do not apply generally.

When examining a limb, it is usually necessary to split up movements and concentrate on each joint in turn. To examine the foot, for example, it is best to examine first the ankle, then the subtalar and midtarsal joints, then the forefoot and finally the toes. The examination should, at the very least, include an assessment of all possible sources of disease relevant to the complaint; an examination of the abdomen and breasts should, for example, be considered routine for anyone complaining of low back pain; and pain in the hand normally warrants an examination of the neck.

If a careful history is taken and the examination is carried out as described above, it should be possible to arrive at a shortlist of differential diagnoses. It must, however, be admitted that in clinical practice many conditions are diagnosed on the basis of past experience—with the clinician employing a process of pattern recognition leading to a 'spot-diagnosis'.

CHAPTER 4

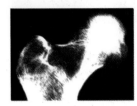

Wound healing

Many tissues do not regenerate when damaged and are repaired by collagenous scar tissue. Some tissues such as bone, mucous membrane, liver, the superficial layers of skin, are capable of complete repair.

WOUND HEALING PROCESSES

The basic processes are seen best in the healing of a clean incised wound.

1 The wound bleeds and fills with clot.

2 The inflammatory process is initiated and there is dilatation of capillaries, exudation of fluid and white cells, and the process of capillary budding begins.

3 Dead tissue and clot are removed by phagocytes, and capillaries and fibroblasts migrate into the damaged area. The new tissue is known as *granulation tissue* and is highly vascular (2–3 days).

4 The skin surface begins to heal by the proliferation and migration of epithelial cells from the edges of the wound to cover the defect.

5 The cellular reaction diminishes and the fibroblasts start to lay down collagen fibres (3rd day onwards).

6 Vascularity diminishes and the collagen increases.

7 Scar contraction makes the defect much smaller. This effect is more marked in some areas than others, e.g. in the midline of the body, particularly over the back (2 weeks onwards).

8 Scar consolidation and further shrinkage occurs, and the scar becomes almost avascular.

The tensile strength of a wound increases to a safe functional level in 15 days and is back to normal in about 3 months, depending on the tissue.

FRACTURE REPAIR

This follows the same steps, except that the migrating cells have osteogenic potential and lay down osteoid which eventually ossifies forming bone, sometimes laying down cartilage as an intermediate stage (Fig. 4.1).

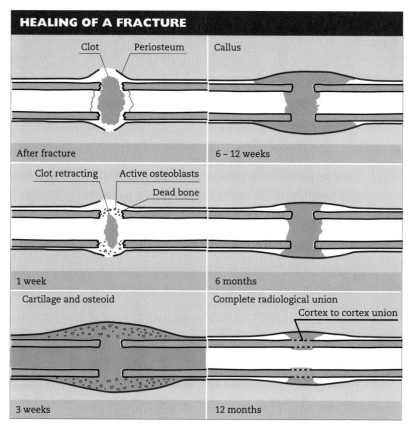

HEALING OF A FRACTURE

Clot   Periosteum   Callus

After fracture   6 – 12 weeks

Clot retracting   Active osteoblasts   Dead bone

1 week   6 months

Cartilage and osteoid   Complete radiological union   Cortex to cortex union

3 weeks   12 months

Fig. 4.1

There is no general agreement about the source of these cells. One theory is that they derive from specialized cells which are to be found on all free bone surfaces and particularly on the deep surface of the fibrous periosteum. These are morphologically indistinguishable from fibroblasts but are thought to give rise to osteoblasts, which then lose the capacity to divide. The alternative theory is that the active cells are derived from non-specialized fibroblasts in the surrounding soft tissues and that these cells can develop the power to lay down bone, given the necessary stimulus. It has also been suggested that the osteogenic cells may be derived from marrow cells or even from vascular endothelium.

The ultimate aim of fracture healing may be considered to be what is called 'cortex-to-cortex' union, with bone directly joining the fracture surfaces, but this is esentially a slow process and requires the fracture to be immobilized in some way before it can occur. Many fractures are joined initially and rapidly by a cuff of provisional woven bone known as *callus*. This varies in amount and is greatest when the fracture is allowed to move. If the fracture is rigidly fixed, virtually no callus is seen and direct union across the fracture gap may eventually occur without a callus stage. In these circumstances the rigid fixation takes the place of the callus. In the first case the callus allows early return to some function; in the second case the artificial fixation often allows even better early function. In both cases cortex-to-cortex union then occurs slowly over a period of several months.

Fracture healing may involve several interlinked processes contributing in varying degrees to the healing of any individual fracture. It has been suggested that in the first few days and weeks there is a primary callus response occurring as a fundamental reaction to bone injury. This response is thought to be short-lived and peters out if it fails to provide satisfactory bridging between the fragments. In that case, a second mechanism may come into play called 'bridging external callus', possibly derived from a process of bone induction in surrounding soft-tissue cells and very dependent on blood vessels from these tissues. If this succeeds in providing a bridge, then end-to-end union can occur, with remodelling and the gradual replacement of dead bone. Whether or not temporary bone bridging is achieved, a third process of bone union may become important in the later stages. This has been called late medullary callus and appears to be responsible for the slow growth of new bone across the fracture gap, and even, given a sufficient degree of stability, across a fibrous tissue barrier. It is very dependent on the bone circulation and may be inhibited by intramedullary internal fixation.

Rigid internal fixation may suppress or even replace the first two processes of fracture healing, and may cause the final stage of cortex-to-cortex union to be long delayed, because the fixation device takes most of the stresses. There is, therefore, interest in fixation systems which are capable of providing satisfactory mechanical stability, but can allow a controlled degree of movement. The hope is that these will utilize the natural processes of fracture healing rather than tending to inhibit them. This principle has already been used with some success for intero-external fixation frames (p. 71) and non-rigid resin plates reinforced with carbon fibres are currently being assessed.

Clinical union of a long bone in an adult normally takes about 3–4 months. There is then a gradual process of remodelling to produce cancellous and cortical bone with normal trabecular orientation.

CLOSURE OF WOUNDS

With all wounds, particularly those communicating with a fracture or a joint, a decision has to be made as soon as possible about closure. This

TECHNIQUES OF CLOSURE

SUTURE
Or apposition by adhesive dressings (e.g. butterfly sutures).

SKIN GRAFTING

1 Partial thickness or split-skin grafting
This is the easiest and most reliable technique and uses split skin taken from a convenient donor site. It may be used as a primary or secondary technique. It utilizes only part of the thickness of the epidermis and, if it is correctly taken, the donor site should bleed from the skin papillae only and will re-epithelialize spontaneously.

The graft may be held in place with dressings or suture. 'Superglue' has also been used with success to hold grafts in place during healing.

2 Full thickness detached grafts
Until recently these have been rarely used except for small areas such as defects on the fingers. When used as free grafts they are much less likely than split skin to 'take' adequately. With the development of techniques for micro-vascular anastomosis, there is now much more interest in using various types of 'free' full-thickness grafts, either of skin alone or using thicker grafts of skin, subcutaneous tissue and muscle. It is also possible, for special requirements, to transfer composite grafts of skin, soft tissues and bone, a technique which is being increasingly used for the management of difficult open fractures, particularly of the tibia.

3 Attached skin flaps
These are the more conventional types of full-thickness grafts which may be rotated or swung, taken from one limb to another, or from chest or abdomen to limb. Considerable skill is needed to obtain good results. They provide much more satisfactory skin cover, but leave a defect elsewhere, which has to be closed by split skin. They resist pressure better and are essential for certain areas. They are usually detached from the donor site in 10–15 days and may require further adjustment later.

4 Foreign skin
Taken either from animal or human, this is occasionally used as a temporary dressing for large areas of loss, e.g. after burns. It is eventually rejected and secondary grafting may then be needed.

decision will normally depend on the degree of contamination of the wound, the extent of surrounding soft-tissue damage, the condition of the surrounding skin and the time which has elapsed since the injury. The decision may be altered by the circumstances of follow-up. Where the patient can be kept under observation, primary wound closure may be attempted in circumstances which might be considered too risky if close follow-up were not possible as, for example, in wartime conditions. If the decision has been made to close the wound this should be done as soon as possible. Closure is best achieved with skin, either by direct suture or, for larger defects, by skin-grafting.

1 *Primary closure* is usually safe if carried out in the first 6 hours after injury, provided all foreign material and dead tissue is removed and there is little surrounding soft-tissue damage. A clean incised wound may be safely sutured up to 8 hours after injury. After this time, contamination is almost unavoidable and the risk of infection is much greater. It is then usually safer to leave the wound open and, after 24 hours, if it remains clean, perform:

2 *Delayed primary closure.*

3 *Secondary closure* means closure after the wound has been allowed to granulate, having overcome any sepsis. This may be 4–5 days and up to several weeks after the injury. Suture may still be possible at this late stage, but frequently, skin-grafting will be necessary.

Large defects fill initially with granulation tissue which is very resistant to infection. An area of clean granulation tissue is the best bed for a skin-graft when primary grafting is not possible. Grafting in the presence of severe infection is usually unsuccessful, and tendons, ligaments, and particularly articular cartilage, do not usually form suitable beds for non-vascularized grafts, although bone often takes skin-grafts without difficulty.

Following burns, areas of skin slough may need to be excised when demarcation has occurred, and the defect may then be covered by a suitable graft.

SECTION 2

Trauma

CHAPTER 5

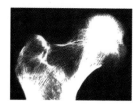

Trauma to the soft tissues: 1

SUPERFICIAL WOUNDS

Abrasions

These are caused by trauma to the superficial skin layers, usually by friction. They heal with little scarring, but any foreign material should be removed by scrubbing or scraping, otherwise 'tattooing' will result.

TREATMENT

A simple protective dressing is usually all that is required.

Incised wounds

These are usually relatively uncontaminated and heal well with little scarring.

Lacerations

These may be clean and very similar to incised wounds, but are caused by blunt trauma and may be associated with crushing and haematoma formation in the surrounding tissues.

TREATMENT

All dead and foreign material should be excised and the wound closed by one of the methods described in Chapter 4. If there is any possibility of a foreign body, an X-ray is essential. Most foreign bodies such as metal, stone or glass are radio-opaque to some extent, but some materials, notably wood, are not visible on ordinary X-rays.

Burns

These may be partial thickness, that is within the epidermis, or full thickness — through the whole skin and into the subcutaneous or deeper tissues. The distinction is not always clear at the time of injury, but loss of sensation in the area is suggestive of full thickness loss.

TREATMENT

Partial thickness burns usually heal rapidly and completely; if full thickness, the damaged tissue will slough and eventually separate or may need to be excised. The resulting wound is then closed by suture or more usually by skin grafting. Extensive burns are best dealt with in special units where facilities exist for the control of fluid loss, sepsis and later reconstruction.

DEEP WOUNDS

These may be extensions of lacerations or burns, or caused by a stabbing type of injury, when they may be much more widespread than is apparent from the surface.

TREATMENT

Any penetrating wound where there is the possibility of important soft-tissue damage should be explored. This is particularly important with stab wounds of the chest and abdomen, where extensive internal injury may be associated with a minor skin wound. In these circumstances a laparotomy or thoracotomy may be necessary to achieve an adequate exploration.

HAEMATOMA

This is a collection of blood in the tissues. If small, it will usually resolve and be replaced by scar tissue. If larger, it may fail to resolve completely, leaving a cyst which occasionally may expand and destroy surrounding tissues. This is particularly likely to happen in bleeding disorders such as haemophilia.

TREATMENT

Large haematomata, particularly in confined spaces, may need decompression or evacuation to prevent necrosis of overlying tissues. Resorption can be speeded by active use of the limb, and occasionally by the use of hyaluronidase, short-wave diathermy or ultrasound. Secondary infection of a haematoma is not uncommon.

CONTUSION

This is the same as a bruise and consists of tissue damaged by a blow or crush. It is usually swollen and infiltrated with blood.

FOREIGN BODIES

If sterile or non-irritative, these may cause little trouble, or may not be recognized. They frequently do cause a local reaction or abscess and may be the cause of a continually draining sinus.

TREATMENT

Removal is not always necessary, but if it is considered desirable, it should be carried out in good theatre conditions, with a tourniquet if possible, and with X-ray facilities available in case of difficulty.

GUNSHOT WOUNDS

Missile injuries are usually classified as being of low-velocity or high-velocity types. In civilian practice the former are commoner since these are usually caused by revolvers or hand guns which deliver a heavy bullet at relatively low velocity—around 200 m/s. The bullets from rifles, particularly the Armalite rifle, travel at much higher velocities—up to 1000 m/s, or even higher. Though they may be smaller bullets, the energy released in the tissues, being derived from the high kinetic energy of the projectile, is much greater, causing more widespread and serious damage. The fragments thrown out of an exploding bomb or shell similarly behave as high-velocity missiles, causing correspondingly serious wounds.

Low-velocity gunshot wounds

The extent of this type of wound depends on how much the bullet is slowed and whether it is brought to rest in the tissues. This is influenced by the stability of the bullet. A stable perforating bullet may only release a small proportion of its available energy and cause relatively little damage.

In general, low-velocity wounds tend to be well circumscribed, with the tissues surrounding the track being damaged for a few millimetres only. The injury may not, therefore, be serious provided no important structure is directly hit.

TREATMENT

This consists essentially of excising foreign, necrotic and contaminated material. The extent of this excision may be quite small and the trend is to keep the surgery to a minimum. Fractures can usually be managed by standard techniques, wounds being left open with a view to secondary closure.

High-velocity gunshot wounds

Here, although the projectile and the entry wound may be small and innocent-looking, the amount of damage sustained by the internal tissues is often very extensive, due mainly to the phenomenon known as cavitation. This is caused by the violent acceleration of the tissues around the path of the missile, producing a large cavity which subsequently collapses, leaving necrotic tissue extending over a wide area around the track. During cavity formation, air and debris are sucked in through the entry and exit wounds so that in addition to widespread necrosis there may be much contamination. These effects may be particularly severe in the case of wounds of the chest, abdomen and head, causing widespread and often fatal damage. Fractures can be very severe with gross comminution.

TREATMENT

The management of this type of wound can present many surgical problems but, in principle, wounds should be opened widely, and extensive debridement and decompression carried out. All foreign and non-viable tissue must be removed and the wound left open. Wounds of the abdomen and chest will normally require exploration, and tissues such as bowel and liver can be expected to be much more severely damaged than they appear at first sight.

INJURIES TO ORGANS

These are common and not necessarily associated with superficial damage. Particularly vulnerable are the lungs, liver, spleen and genito-urinary tract.

Cerebral damage often follows head injury, whether the skull is fractured or not.

INJURIES TO LIGAMENTS

Joint injuries frequently involve complete rupture or partial tearing of ligaments. The latter is usually called a *sprain* or *strain*. Commonly injured are the ligaments of knee and ankle. Adequate diagnosis may require stress X-rays taken under anaesthesia (Fig. 5.1).

LATERAL LIGAMENT RUPTURE

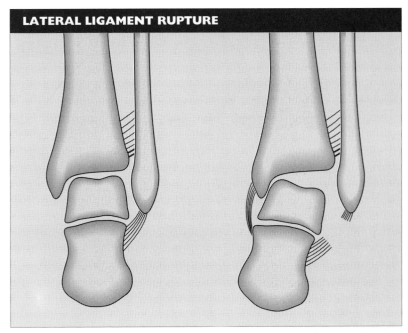

Fig. 5.1

TREATMENT

Strains or partial tears usually heal with minimal treatment. They are usually painful in the acute stage and respond to immobilization with Elastoplast strapping or, in more severe cases, a plaster-cast. During the first 24 hours the symptoms can be helped by the use of ice or cold water compresses applied repeatedly, evaporation from the surface helping to maintain the cooling effect. As the pain settles the joint should be mobilized to avoid stiffness. Recovery is usual in 2–3 weeks.

A complete ligament rupture requires apposition of the divided ends followed by a period of protection if satisfactory healing is to be obtained. Depending on the situation, the injury may be treated conservatively by immobilization in a plaster-cast or, preferably, in a functional brace designed to allow joint movement whilst restricting the stresses on the healing ligament. If there is reason to doubt whether the torn ends are in apposition, surgical suture may be advisable. Three weeks' protection is usually sufficient to secure healing and mobilization can then be gradually increased.

The widespread use of pain-relieving injections into the damaged ligaments of athletes and sportsmen is to be deplored, since further damage can occur without the patient being aware of it.

TENDON SUTURE

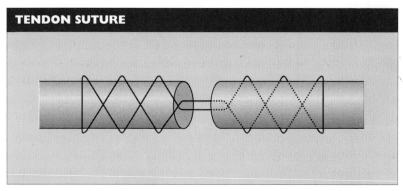

Fig. 5.2

NO MAN'S LAND

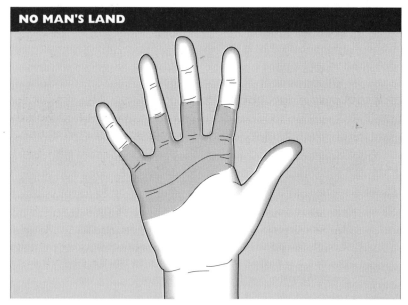

Fig. 5.3

INJURIES TO TENDONS

Tendons are frequently divided by injury. When the injury is recognized, suture may be possible at the time the wound is closed. This is usually done with a wire monofilament Kessler's suture and protecting the repair by splintage for a period of 3–6 weeks (Fig. 5.2).

In the case of the finger flexor tendons in the zone between the distal palmar crease and the proximal interphalangeal joint—usually called 'no-man's land'—(Fig. 5.3) primary suture of both tendons is indicated whenever possible, but in this area the tendons run within the flexor tendon sheaths and skill is required to achieve good results because of the tendency for adhesions to form in the sheath. In less skilled hands it is safer to close the skin and perform a tendon repair or grafting operation later. Protected movement by careful splintage is an important part of the overall treatment. The 'Belfast' system, which involves splinting the finger in partial flexion but allowing some degree of active flexion, has become popular in the UK.

The usual secondary procedure if both flexor tendons are severed in this area is to excise the flexor digitorum superficialis and to repair the flexor digitorum profundus with a free tendon graft, usually taken from the palmaris longus, plantaris or one of the toe extensors, suturing this to the tendon stumps in such a way that the sutures are outside the flexor sheaths. This helps to avoid adhesion formation. Sometimes a silastic 'former' is placed in the finger to form a track or tunnel prior to the insertion of the tendon graft. The finger must be mobile before the grafting procedure and vigorous physiotherapy is usually necessary afterwards.

INJURIES TO VESSELS

Any injured limb should be examined for evidence of ischaemia. Excessive swelling, especially if it is increasing, should arouse suspicion, and failure to secure return of circulation when a fracture is reduced should be an indication for exploration and, if necessary, repair of vessels. Commonly injured are the femoral artery and the arteries of the lower leg. The aorta is occasionally ruptured in multiple injuries and this may be difficult to differentiate from other causes of shock. Occasionally, if a damaged vessel has not been repaired or ligated, a false aneurysm may develop at the point of rupture and this may expand or possibly rupture in its turn, causing delayed ischaemic or pressure effects.

TREATMENT

If time allows, it is usual to assess the situation before surgery by angiography. With major vessels, suture may be possible or the vessel may have to be repaired with a vein patch or a graft, usually taken from a vein. Fasciotomy is often necessary (see below).

COMPARTMENTAL SYNDROMES

Occasionally, following trauma to a limb, particularly a closed fracture, the venous outflow from a fascial compartment may become obstructed, causing the pressure to rise gradually within the compartment. When the pressure reaches a critical level any nerves passing through the compartment cease to function, causing paraesthesiae initially, followed by loss of sensation in the area supplied by the nerve. As the pressure continues to rise, tissue perfusion may cease, particularly in the muscles, and, rarely, a point can be reached when the pressure rises above arterial level and all structures within the compartment become ischaemic. If the pressure is not relieved, muscle necrosis may occur and the eventual replacement of the muscle by fibrous tissue may result in contracture of the muscle and deformity of the associated joints (*Volkmann's ischaemic contracture*).

Clinical features

The condition occurs most commonly following closed fractures of the tibia and fibula, but can arise in any of the fascial compartments of the upper or lower limbs and may follow open fractures or more proximal vascular injuries. The syndrome usually develops during the 24–48 hours after injury, but occasionally later. Pain at the site of the affected compartment is usually the earliest and most important feature, with paraesthesiae, numbness and muscular weakness developing later. The pain is typically made worse by stretching the affected muscles which are also tender. Swelling of the ankle, foot or hand is not necessarily a feature. Neurological signs eventually develop if the pressure is not released and in the late case the peripheral pulses may become impalpable. Presence or absence of the pulses is *not*, however, a good guide to the diagnosis.

TREATMENT

The most important aspect of management is an awareness that the condition may develop. If any of the above features appear, the condition should be suspected. It is possible to measure the intracompartmental pressures using a simple manometric device and pressures higher than 30 mmHg are usually regarded as an indication for decompression. This is carried out by splitting the deep fascia over most of the length of the compartment (*fasciotomy*). The skin is also often left open. In the lower leg it may be necessary to decompress all four muscle compartments. If the equipment is not available for measuring the pressures, decompression should be carried out on clinical suspicion. Provided the pressure does not rise above 40 mmHg, decompression within 24 hours of symptoms developing will usually avoid significant muscle necrosis.

PRESSURE SORES

These arise from continued pressure, usually over a bony prominence. They are essentially ischaemic and more likely to occur if there is loss of sensation. They are preventable by avoiding long periods of continuous pressure. Three to four hours may be sufficient to cause skin necrosis. The sacrum and heels are the most vulnerable sites for true bed sores and these can usually be avoided by moving or turning the patient every 2 hours. Pressure sores from splints and plasters are also common.

TREATMENT

It is better to go to considerable trouble to prevent pressure sores than to have to treat them, because they are difficult to heal. Small sores will often heal with simple dressings, after removal of sloughs if necessary. The most important factor in successful treatment is to avoid further pressure. Large sores may require wide surgical excision and skin grafting, often by the rotation of thick flaps of skin and subcutaneous tissue. Chronic peripheral ulcers, caused by pressure and usually associated with sensory loss, can often be healed by enclosing the limb in a series of 'skin-tight' plaster-casts and avoiding weight-bearing until healing has occurred.

SELF-INFLICTED INJURIES

Any recurrent haematoma or recurrent bleeding which is apparently inexplicable should arouse suspicion of self-infliction. The dorsum of the hand and wrist is a particularly common site. A period in a plaster-cast will usually allow healing, but the damage may recur when the plaster is removed. These injuries often cease when their cause has been discovered.

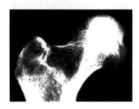

CHAPTER 6

Trauma to the
soft tissues: 2

PERIPHERAL NERVE INJURIES

Because of their importance these merit separate discussion. Peripheral nerve injuries may be caused by one of the conditions listed below.

1 Direct trauma e.g. lacerations, gunshot wounds, penetrating injuries, burns, etc.

2 Indirect trauma e.g. fracture fragments may stretch or tear a nerve. A fracture may also produce delayed effects on a nerve. A good example is the palsy caused by the ulnar nerve being stretched around the medial side of an elbow which has grown into valgus as a result of damage to the lateral epicondylar epiphysis (Fig. 6.1).

3 Chronic or acute entrapment e.g. the median nerve may be trapped within the carpal tunnel as a result of fracture, or disease of the wrist or tendon sheaths—as seen, for example, in rheumatoid arthritis. There are a number of such 'tunnel syndromes', often with no obvious cause, but producing characteristic clinical pictures.

Carpal tunnel syndrome

This condition tends to occur in young to middle-aged women and is particularly likely to occur during pregnancy. It is occasionally an early manifestation of rheumatoid arthritis.

CLINICAL FEATURES

The presenting symptom is usually pain or paraesthesiae in the thumb, index and middle fingers, often occurring at night and sometimes relieved by hanging the arm out of bed. Some patients complain of numbness or clumsiness when carrying out fine manipulations.

There may be obvious wasting of the thenar muscles, lack of sweating over the median nerve distribution and occasionally objective sensory loss. Pressure over the carpal tunnel may reproduce the symptoms. Nerve conduction studies may be needed to confirm the diagnosis.

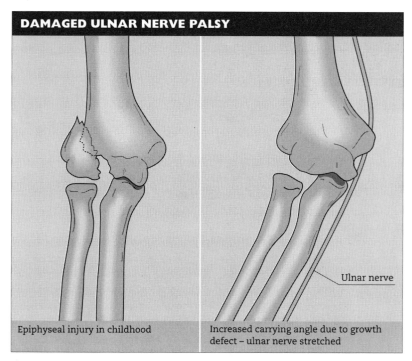

DAMAGED ULNAR NERVE PALSY

Epiphyseal injury in childhood | Increased carrying angle due to growth defect – ulnar nerve stretched

Ulnar nerve

Fig. 6.1

TREATMENT

Those cases developing during pregnancy often settle after delivery. A trial of a plaster back-slab to immobilize the wrist is often useful. An injection of a steroid preparation into the carpal tunnel is often helpful, but persistent cases can be relieved quickly by operative decompression of the carpal tunnel.

Acute peripheral nerve injuries

Nerves may be injured at root, plexus or trunk level, and severe injuries to the major plexuses may result in avulsion of the roots from the spinal cord.

DIAGNOSIS

Nerve injuries can usually be accurately diagnosed by a careful consideration of the detailed neurological anatomy. A systematic examination should be carried out, recording the power of all muscle groups, the distribution of sensory loss to various modalities, and the presence or absence of reflexes. In the difficult case, electromyography or conduction studies and occasionally myelography may help to clarify the diagnosis and the prognosis. These tests are also valuable in following the progress of denervation and recovery.

RECOVERY FROM TRAUMA

Peripheral nerves are capable of repair after injury. Three types of damage are theoretically possible.

1 Neurapraxia

This is usually due to blunt trauma or compression. The axons remain in continuity and usually recover quickly over minutes, hours or occasionally longer. The condition is analogous to cerebral concussion.

2 Axonotmesis

This involves damage to individual axons but within intact sheaths. It may be caused by direct trauma or by stretching. In the latter case the prognosis is usually worse. Axons regenerate from the central end, provided the cell body remains alive, and recovery should be good if the fibres are able to grow down their original neurilemmal sheaths. Recovery depends on axons reaching appropriate end-organs and may take months in the case of the longer nerves such as the sciatic.

3 Neurotmesis

In this condition the nerve is completely divided or irreparably damaged over part of its length. Each divided axon tends to die back to the next Node of Ranvier or even further, and there are usually retrograde changes in the motor cell body. The peripheral axon disintegrates, the myelin sheath breaks up and the neurilemmal cells become disorganized. Recovery follows in the same way as after axonotmesis, but the reconnections of fibres and end-organs are likely to be much less satisfactory. Regeneration rarely occurs unless the nerve ends are opposed. At best, recovery tends to be incomplete, although the prognosis is much better in children. Clean divisions, with little trauma on either side of the lesion have the best prognosis, and the more peripheral the lesion, the better the outlook.

NERVE SUTURE

1 Primary suture

This is possible with clean wounds and cleanly divided nerves. It is usually necessary to cut back the nerve ends to remove nerve tissue damaged by bleeding within the sheath. If much cutting back or excision of a length has been necessary, the nerve will have to be mobilized up and down the limb and perhaps the joints flexed to allow apposition. Suture is carried out using very fine sutures passed through the nerve sheath. Modern techniques involve suturing individual nerve bundles, under microscopic vision. If primary repair is not thought possible, the ends should be loosely labelled with a suture and tacked together, and the wound then closed.

2 Secondary suture

This can be carried out when the skin wound is healed and up to 6 months after the injury. The scarred and thickened junction is excised and again the nerve is mobilized and the sheath sutured. Secondary suture may require more excision of the nerve, but operative conditions and expertise may be more favourable. After both methods of suture the repair is protected by immobilizing the joints for several weeks. If the gap is too great for suturing, grafting is possible, using a sensory nerve such as the sural which can be sacrificed without too much functional loss. Results tend to be indifferent. An interesting experimental technique involves the use of strips of muscle as a nerve graft.

TIME OF RECOVERY

Axons are capable of regenerating at the rate of 1 mm per day. It is, therefore, possible to calculate roughly how long will be necessary before functional recovery can be expected.

Tinel's sign

This is a useful sign for following recovery. Gentle tapping with the finger-tip along the course of the nerve will result in the patient feeling pins and needles in the distribution of the nerve when the point of regeneration is reached. This point will gradually move more distally as recovery proceeds.

BRACHIAL PLEXUS INJURIES

These produce complex neurological pictures. Some common patterns can be discerned.

I Erb's palsy

This is produced by damage to the 5th and 6th cervical roots, e.g. during difficult forceps deliveries in which the upper part of the brachial plexus

ERB'S PALSY

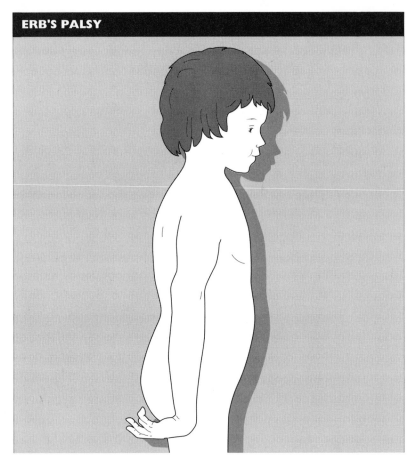

Fig. 6.2

is stretched. The paralysis affects the deltoid, shoulder girdle muscles (except part of pectoralis major), the elbow flexors, wrist extensors and supinators. The limb assumes the position said to be characteristic of a waiter asking for a tip (Fig. 6.2).

2 Klumpke's palsy

This is caused by damage to the 8th cervical and 1st thoracic nerve roots, usually by traction on the arm in full abduction, and produces signs similar to those of an ulnar nerve lesion, i.e. mainly paralysis of the small muscles of the hand, but in this case with more extended sensory loss along the inner border of the forearm, and with weakness of flexor carpi ulnaris.

Both of these so-called 'obstetrical palsies' have a variable prognosis. Some recovery occurs in at least fifty per cent of cases of Erb's palsy, but the lower plexus injuries carry a worse prognosis.

TREATMENT

This consists simply in maintaining passive joint movements by physiotherapy, in anticipation of recovery.

3 Other and mixed patterns

These are fairly common following road accidents, especially motorcycling, where the neck may be violently flexed laterally and the shoulder depressed.

Plexus injuries, in general, have a poor prognosis, particularly if the injury is proximal to the dorsal root ganglia. This is an important prognostic point. With injuries to the higher roots the exact site of damage may be obscure, but if the injury is proximal, myelography may reveal the damage to the root sleeves. If the first thoracic root is injured proximally to its ganglion, Horner's syndrome will be present because the sympathetic outflow from the spinal cord to the pupil of the eye passes through this root. Horner's syndrome is characterized by pupillary constriction, enophthalmos and ptosis, with some degree of loss of sweating on the affected side of the face. If a root is torn proximally to the dorsal root ganglion, the triple response to histamine injection into the skin theoretically ought to be preserved, even though there will be sensory loss in the skin area supplied by that nerve.

Recovery and treatment

Attempts at reconstruction of the plexus are rarely successful, although better results are claimed for early exploration and suture performed in specialist centres. Some recovery may occur over the first one or even two years following a severe brachial plexus injury. When this has reached its maximum, reconstructive procedures on the arm may be considered. Unfortunately, chronic pain is often a disabling feature and may prevent satisfactory rehabilitation. Severe plexus injuries may eventually require amputation of the limb becuase of persistent pain, but unfortunately, even this drastic step does not always succeed in relieving the pain.

INJURIES TO NERVE TRUNKS

1 MEDIAN NERVE

This is most commonly damaged at the wrist, occasionally in the forearm, or at the elbow. The neurological loss is mainly sensory, producing anaesthesia over the thumb, index, middle and, occasionally, ring fingers. Its effects on hand function are considerable. Lesions at wrist level produce paralysis and wasting of the thenar muscles, with the exception of the adductor pollicis which is supplied by the ulnar nerve. Higher lesions may paralyse flexor digitorum profundus to the index and middle fingers, and usually the whole of flexor digitorum superficialis, so that the index finger cannot be actively flexed at either interphalangeal joint.

2 ULNAR NERVE

The loss here is mainly motor. Damage may occur at any level, but is commonest at the wrist or elbow. The intrinsic muscles in the hand, when working normally, put the fingers into a position of flexion at the metacarpophalangeal joints and extension at the interphalangeal joints. When these muscles are paralysed by an ulnar nerve lesion, the fingers take up the opposite position ('clawing') due to the unopposed long flexors (see Fig. 45.5). This effect is less in the index because the first two lumbricals are innervated by the median nerve. Thumb adduction is lost (but may be disguised). The long flexors to the ring and little fingers and the ulnar wrist flexors may be lost in high lesions in which case clawing does not occur. Sensation is lost over the little, part of the ring and possibly middle fingers.

3 RADIAL NERVE

This is usually damaged at the level of the mid-humerus by fractures or pressure e.g. going to sleep with the arm over the back of a chair. The lesion results in paralysis of wrist, finger and thumb extensors, and a characteristic 'drop wrist'. The motor branch to the triceps is often spared. There is usually little sensory loss.

4 SCIATIC NERVE

This is occasionally damaged in association with a dislocated hip. Division of the sciatic nerve is a serious injury producing complete loss of function and total anaesthesia below the knee.

5 FEMORAL NERVE

Femoral nerve palsy is often caused by penetrating injuries e.g. by a butcher's knife. Its main effect is loss of quadriceps function, making standing and walking difficult. Stairs are particularly difficult to manage. The patient may learn to brace his knee back by using his hand.

6 COMMON PERONEAL NERVE

This is commonly injured, often following splintage, because the nerve is vulnerable where it winds round the neck of the fibula. Its loss produces a drop foot with anaesthesia over the dorsum. This often fails to recover and a toe-raising appliance may eventually be needed to correct the tendency to catch the toe when walking (Chapter 50).

CHAPTER 7

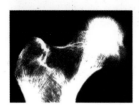

Fractures

A fracture is a break in continuity of a bone. A *comminuted* fracture is one with more than two fragments. Gross comminution is usually caused by severe violence and in such cases union is often delayed or difficult to achieve.

The type of fracture which occurs depends on the magnitude and direction of the force causing it.

1 A *transverse* fracture is usually caused by a force applied directly to the site at which the fracture occurs. This often represents a three-point force system (Fig. 7.1).

2 A *spiral* or oblique fracture is usually caused by violence transmitted through the limb from a distance (Fig. 7.2).

3 A *greenstick* fracture occurs in children, whose bones are soft and yielding. The bone bends without fracturing across completely, the cortex on the concave side usually remaining intact (Fig. 7.3).

4 A *crush* fracture occurs in cancellous bone as a result of a compression force (Fig. 7.4).

5 A *burst* fracture usually occurs in a short bone such as a vertebra from strong direct pressure; in the vertebrae this usually occurs as a result of impaction of the disc (Fig. 7.5).

6 An *avulsion* fracture is caused by traction, a bony fragment usually being torn off by a tendon or ligament (Fig. 7.6).

7 A *fracture dislocation* or *subluxation* is a fracture which involves a joint and results in mal-alignment of the joint surfaces (Figs. 7.6, 7.7).

A surface wound may communicate with a fracture. This is known as an *open* or *compound* fracture. A compound fracture sometimes communicates with an internal body surface, e.g. a pelvic fracture may communicate with a rupture of the rectum or a rib fracture may penetrate a lung. Open fractures are potentially infected and need urgent treatment.

All fractures involve some soft-tissue damage, but when there is important soft-tissue damage to nerves, vessels or internal organs then the fracture is termed *complicated*. Occasionally, the bone ends may be separated by soft tissue such as muscle and this may delay union.

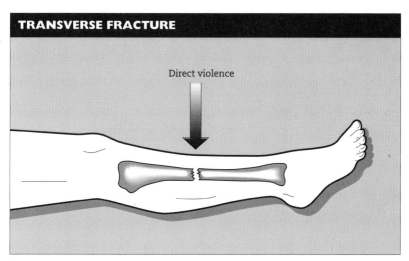

TRANSVERSE FRACTURE

Direct violence

Fig. 7.1

A fracture is *impacted* when the fragments are driven into one another. Such a fracture is usually *stable*, as also is a fracture which is held firmly by soft-tissue attachments, usually periosteum. An *unstable* fracture is one which is displaced or has the potential to displace. Occasionally, when a fracture is realigned or *reduced*, the fragments lock together and the fracture then becomes stable. More usually, following reduction, the fracture will re-displace if not held in some way. If the periosteum is intact on one side this may be used to help secure stability.

Displacement may mean shortening, rotation, sideways-shift or tilt, and reduction of the fracture will usually involve reversing these various displacements.

A *dislocation* is a complete loss of congruity of the joint surfaces.

A *subluxation* is a partial loss of contact of the joint surfaces.

Either may be associated with a fracture and may, of course, be open or compound.

Epiphyseal injuries occur in children. In certain circumstances they may interfere with growth. The Salter and Harris classification is usually used for these injuries (Fig. 7.8; p. 51). The fracture line normally runs through the calcifying layer of the epiphysis on the side away from the germinal layer. The first three types have a good prognosis and are usually easy to replace, provided they are treated early by manipulation. The third type tends to occur in older children and adolescents and, since it is intra-articular and involves the joint surface, may require open reduction and pinning in position.

SPIRAL FRACTURE

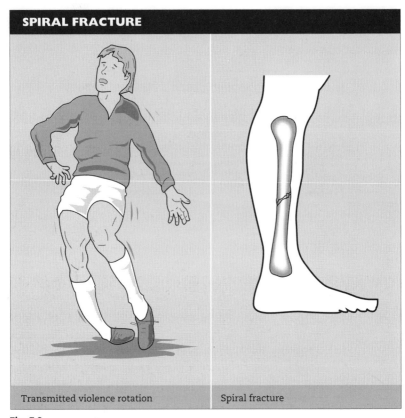

| Transmitted violence rotation | Spiral fracture |

Fig. 7.2

GREENSTICK FRACTURE

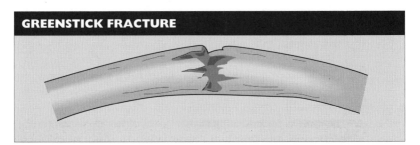

Fig. 7.3

CRUSH FRACTURE

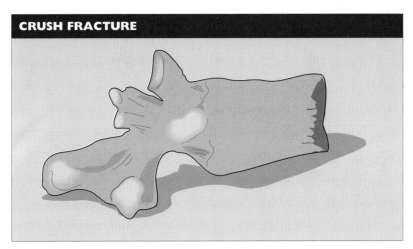

Fig. 7.4

BURST FRACTURE

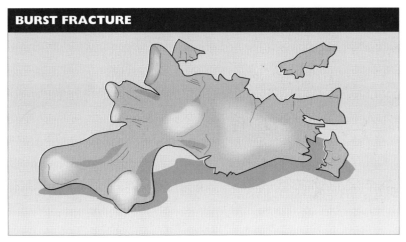

Fig. 7.5

FRACTURES—DIAGNOSIS

Many fractures can be readily diagnosed from the history or from the fact that the limb is mal-aligned.

History

A brief history is essential in order to assess the mechanism of injury and to raise suspicion of other, less apparent, injuries. If the violence has been

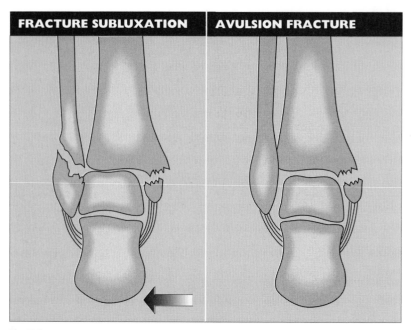

Fig. 7.6

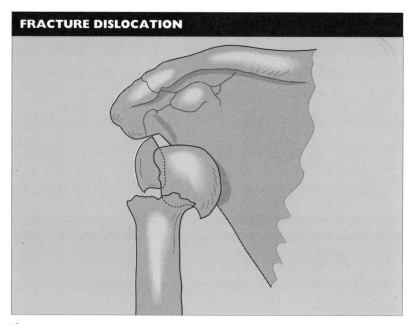

Fig. 7.7

SALTER AND HARRIS CLASSIFICATION

Type I: The fracture line passes cleanly along the epiphyseal line with no metaphyseal fragment. This type tends to occur in young children or babies and in pathological conditions such as spina bifida or scurvy

Type II: The commonest type, in which the fracture line runs across the epiphyseal line and then obliquely, shearing off a small triangle of metaphysis

Type III: The epiphysis may be split vertically and a fragment displaced along the epiphyseal line

Type IV: The fracture extends through the epiphyseal line from the metaphysis into the epiphysis. This type may interfere with growth because union may take place across the growth plate

Type V: Severe crushing of the epiphysis may occur from longitudinal compression and this is very likely to result in growth arrest and deformity

minimal and hardly sufficient to have caused a fracture then this may arouse a suspicion that the fractured bone has been weakened by disease or previous damage—a so-called *pathological* fracture.

1 *Pain.* This is the commonest symptom, but varies with the site and instability of the fracture. Individuals also vary greatly in their response to pain.

2 *Loss of function.* There is almost always some impairment of function in the injured area, so that the patient may be unable to move the limb at all, or may use it with difficulty. Some degree of function may be retained. Following a femoral neck fracture, for example, the patient may manage to walk, but always limps and there is always some functional impairment.

3 *Loss of sensation or motor power.* This is a particularly important symptom, suggesting nerve or vascular complications. The time of injury should be ascertained as accurately as possible, especially with a compound fracture or where there are signs of ischaemia.

Physical signs

The classical signs of a fracture may or may not be present (see p. 53).

Having diagnosed a fracture or joint injury, the presence and extent of any wound should be noted, and the area examined for evidence of

EPIPHYSEAL INJURIES

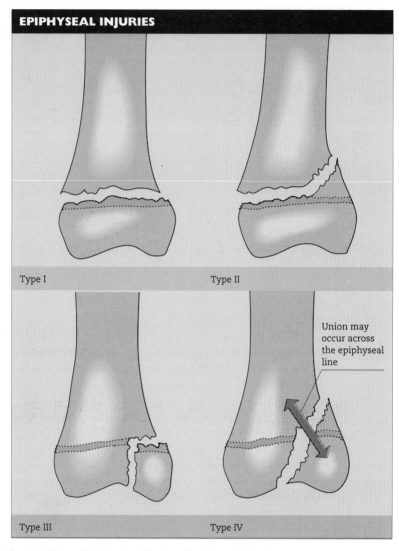

Type I

Type II

Union may
occur across
the epiphyseal
line

Type III

Type IV

Fig. 7.8 Salter and Harris classification of epiphyseal injuries.

EPIPHYSEAL INJURIES (CONTINUED)

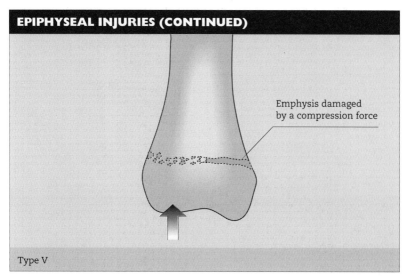

Emphysis damaged by a compression force

Type V

Fig. 7.8 (Continued)

ischaemia and nerve or other important soft-tissue damage. This is essential routine in examining any injury of the musculo-skeletal system. Other injuries should also be suspected and sought.

CLASSICAL SIGNS OF A FRACTURE

1 *Tenderness* is almost invariable with a recent fracture, assuming the patient is conscious. Its exact distribution should be determined.
2 *Deformity* may or may not be evident. The limb may be bent or shortened, or there may be a step in the alignment of the bone or joint.
3 *Swelling* is usual when the fracture is fairly superficial; gross swelling usually implies a vascular rupture. Swelling takes some time to appear and may increase over the first 12–24 hours. It is sometimes associated with blistering of the skin. Swelling is partly due to haematoma, partly due to inflammatory exudation. There may be obvious bruising. A joint which is fractured may fill with blood—a *haemarthrosis*.
4 *Local temperature increase* is essentially part of the inflammatory response which rapidly follows the injury and may be evident even if the damage is confined to the soft tissues.
5 *Abnormal mobility* or *crepitus* i.e. grating of the fracture ends, may be noticed. Vigorous attempts to elicit it should be avoided.
6 *Loss of function* is almost always found to some extent. The patient usually has difficulty in moving the adjacent joints.

FUNCTIONS OF THE X-RAY EXAMINATION

The X-ray examination:
1 localizes the fracture accurately and determines the number of fragments;
2 indicates the degree and direction of displacement;
3 provides evidence of pre-existing disease in the bone;
4 may show a foreign body;
5 may reveal an unsuspected fracture and for this reason the film should always include the whole bone and the joint at either end;
6 may show air in the tissues, suggesting a penetrating injury, e.g. of the knee joint; and
7 may require special techniques to reveal soft-tissue damage, e.g. IVP, cystogram, arteriogram, etc.

Radiological examination

The X-ray examination is designed to give information additional to that obtained by clinical judgement.

X-rays in at least two planes, usually at right angles, are essential. A fracture may be missed if only one film is taken.

Some fractures may elude both clinical and radiological diagnosis and treatment may have to rest on suspicion initially, with X-ray changes occurring later as bone resorption occurs.

Computed tomography (CT) scanning has become a useful aid in diagnosing the more difficult injuries, particularly fractures of the pelvis and spine. It can be useful for planning the details of surgery when open reduction is contemplated.

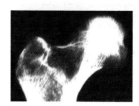

CHAPTER 8

Fractures – principles of management

Having diagnosed the fracture accurately and carried out any resuscitation which may have been necessary, several decisions have to be made.

COMPOUND OR OPEN FRACTURES

The most important consideration when dealing with an open fracture is to reduce the risks of infection. The development of chronic osteomyelitis at the fracture site is a catastrophe which may lead to delayed or non-union, requiring months or even years of treatment and sometimes leading to loss of the limb. There is general agreement that sepsis is best prevented by early and aggressive cleaning of the wound with excision of dead tissue and all foreign material. In order to achieve this, the wound may have to be extended. Large, loose fragments of bone may need to be retained to act as a bone-graft.

There are two schools of thought about the wisdom of closing wounds which communicate with a fracture or dislocation. One argues that primary closure always carries too much risk and that all communicating wounds should be left open and covered with a sterile dressing, with a view to later closure when infection has been avoided or overcome. The other school argues that primary closure is desirable if it can be achieved safely and would advocate closure if the degree of contamination and soft-tissue damage is minimal and if the time from the accident is not too great, usually less than 6 hours. To this must be added the proviso that the patient should be kept under observation, preferably in hospital. If this philosophy is followed, then each case is judged on its merits, but if closure is decided upon then it should be done as quickly as possible. *Antibiotics* should always be given. There is general agreement that in wartime conditions, where transportation may be necessary, communicating wounds are usually better left open. If primary closure is not considered appropriate, every attempt should be made to close the wound within 72 hours.

Open fractures are emergencies

Closure may be by suture or by one of the usual methods of skin-grafting (Chapter 4). The precise method of closure may depend on the method of treating the fracture itself, so these decisions must be made together.

Does the fracture need reduction?

Fractures are reduced for several reasons.

1 Usually because function will be impaired if the fracture is left to unite in the displaced position.

2 The appearance of the limb may be unsatisfactory even though function may be reasonable, for example, a fracture through the tibia may function perfectly well if left overlapping, but it is likely to look ugly.

3 Some fractures unite with difficulty, usually because of impaired blood supply. In these cases union may be helped by accurate reduction, which should give any remaining blood vessels a chance to function. A subcapital fracture of the femur is a good example.

4 There may be impacted soft tissues distorted by the fracture or trapped between the bone ends and these may need to be extracted by reducing the fracture.

If none of these criteria apply then the fracture may be left to unite in the displaced position.

The degree of accuracy of reduction required varies from fracture to fracture, and some types of displacement matter more than others. Many fractures do not need anatomical reduction, e.g. slight overlap of a femoral shaft fracture will not normally prejudice function, healing or appearance, whereas with fractures of the shafts of the radius and ulna, any mal-alignment is likely to cause restriction of pronation and supination.

In general, fractures involving joints require anatomical reduction if possible because of the need for the surfaces to glide accurately and because of the risks of later degeneration if the joint is left mal-aligned.

TECHNIQUE OF REDUCTION

If reduction is necessary, how will it be achieved?

1 *Manipulation*, usually with anaesthesia, either local, regional or general. This is the method adopted for most fractures and dislocations.

2 *Traction*. Some fractures and dislocations may be reduced slowly by traction—this is usually used when manipulation is inappropriate, perhaps because an anaesthetic would be dangerous. Examples are: reduction of a subcapital fracture (which may later be fixed internally) or a subluxation of the cervical spine.

3 *Open reduction.* This has the advantage of allowing very accurate reduction, but carries the risk of infection. Usually, open reduction is reserved for those cases where closed methods will not give the desired reduction, or where internal fixation is going to be needed for some other reason (see below). Open reduction does not necessarily imply internal fixation.

HOLDING THE REDUCTION

Once reduction has been achieved how will it be held?

1 *Intrinsic stability.* Some fractures require no additional stabilization.

2 *External fixation*
   (a) Splintage (Chapter 9).
   (b) Traction (Chapter 9).

3 *Internal fixation.*

See Chapter 9.

MAINTAINING FIXATION

How long should fixation be maintained?

Fractures vary in the length of time needed for union. Most fractures of the shafts of long bones in adults take at least 12 weeks to unite. Fractures in the cancellous ends of the long bones and in short bones take from 6–8 weeks.

In children the times are proportionately reduced with age down to 2–3 weeks for a fracture of the shaft of a long bone in a baby.

If fixation has been used simply to relieve pain rather than to hold an unstable position, it will usually be possible to discard it after 2–3 weeks in an adult and less in a child.

REHABILITATION

This begins immediately after the primary treatment. The limb is moved and used as much as the method of fixation allows. This helps to stimulate union and to prevent joint stiffness. Internal fixation, if secure, has great advantages in this respect. It is also an advantage if the patient can return to his or her normal occupation whilst healing is occurring. When splintage is discontinued a further period of exercises or physiotherapy is often necessary before full joint function is restored.

RE-TRAINING

This is occasionally needed after severe injuries.

CHAPTER 9

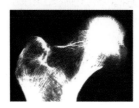

Fractures —
methods of fixation

EXTERNAL FIXATION

Before deciding which method of external fixation to use, it must be decided how accurately the fracture needs to be held. Many fractures can be adequately immobilized with a simple device such as a splint made of wire, metal or polythene, bandaged in place, and a sling or crutches may be used to avoid load-bearing. These devices are often used to relieve pain rather than to secure immobilization.

PLASTER OF PARIS

This material is still widely used for making splints, open or closed casts, jointed casts, etc. (Chapter 50).

On the whole, the advantages outweigh the disadvantages (see below). Other types of moulded splint, e.g. polythene, plastazote etc., are usually less convenient to make and fit, although they may have other advantages.

There is a new generation of cast-making materials on the market. Most of these are made from a fabric base impregnated with a resin which undergoes a setting process when activated by heat or water. They all have slightly different characteristics, but, in general, they have advantages over Plaster of Paris in that they are light in weight, but very strong. This means that the patient may be able to bear weight on an unprotected cast and nursing and moving a patient with a larger cast may be

PLASTER OF PARIS—ADVANTAGES

It is:
- cheap and easily available;
- versatile and readily applied and fashioned;
- reasonably comfortable;
- absorbs secretions to some extent;
- fairly strong; and
- radio-translucent.

PLASTER OF PARIS–DISADVANTAGES

It is:
- rather heavy and warm;
- unyielding, so may cause pressure problems, or uncertain immobilization;
- difficult to inspect the limb, so it may conceal trouble, e.g. wound breakdown or sepsis; and
- not waterproof unless specially treated.

simplified. Most of the newer materials are waterproof, but to make full use of this property, lining and padding materials also need to be waterproof or, at least, quick drying. The main disadvantages of these new materials are that they are less easy to apply, each requiring its own technique, they tend at present to be less comfortable than Plaster of Paris, and they are much more expensive. For these reasons they are at the moment mainly used for special purposes such as making splints and orthoses or for the occasional circumstance where their advantages can justify their cost. Nevertheless, it is likely that in the future they will become much more widely used.

CAST-BRACING

The use of Plaster of Paris and the newer cast materials to make hinged and jointed casts has become popular over the last few years, although internal fixation is tending to displace it. It has been used particularly for fractures of the femur and tibia, although the principle is now being extended to the treatment of other fractures. The cast is accurately moulded around the limb using some of the techniques developed by limb-fitters, and specially designed hinges are used to connect the various segments. The femoral cast-brace has the advantages of allowing the joints to be exercised and the patient to be mobilized whilst avoiding the risks of internal fixation. If a cast-brace is to be used, it is usual to treat a femoral shaft fracture by traction until it is considered to be stable, usually at about 3–6 weeks. The cast is then applied and the patient allowed to mobilize (see Fig. 9.14). Full weight-bearing is usually permitted and, indeed, encouraged.

Traction

This may be used both to secure reduction and then to hold the position. Its use has diminished with the increasing interest in internal fixation.

USE OF THOMAS' SPLINT WITH FIXED TRACTION

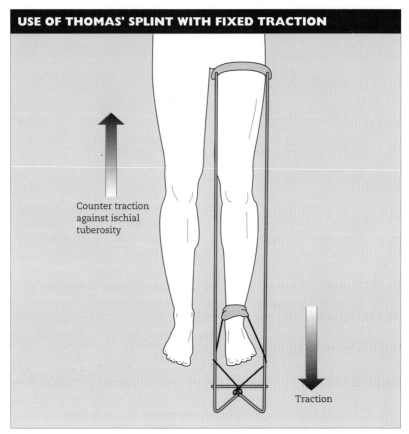

Counter traction
against ischial
tuberosity

Traction

Fig. 9.1

1 FIXED TRACTION

The traction is applied against a counter force applied to the patient's body, e.g. a collar and cuff sling utilizes the weight of the arm to apply traction to the upper arm or shoulder. The counter force is applied to the part of the sling which passes around the patient's neck. The Thomas' splint is the best example of fixed traction using an orthopaedic appliance, the counter force being applied to the ischial tuberosity (and the overlying skin and soft tissues) (Fig. 9.1).

2 SLIDING OR BALANCED TRACTION

The patient's weight is balanced against an applied load, utilizing frictional and gravitational forces to counterbalance the applied traction. Sliding traction can be applied in many ways, but the principle is always the same. It allows the patient to move about the bed or to move the limb whilst the traction continues to act in the desired line (Fig. 9.2).

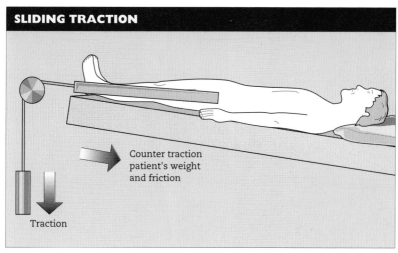

SLIDING TRACTION

Counter traction
patient's weight
and friction

Traction

Fig. 9.2

METHODS OF APPLYING TRACTION

1 Skin traction

The force is exerted tangentially along the skin by using adhesive strapping to attach the cord and weight. This is satisfactory for many purposes, but the force which can be applied is limited by the damage it may cause to the skin. Many people become sensitive to the adhesive.

2 Skeletal traction

This is applied by means of a pin or similar device applied directly through bone. It enables greater force to be used, but may allow infection into the bone. The pins are sometimes incorporated into plaster-casts to give greater stability (Fig. 9.3).

Traction may be applied to the skull by means of tongs inserted into the calvarium (Fig. 9.4).

COMMON TYPES OF SLIDING TRACTION

1 Simple traction

This is applied as in Fig. 9.2, usually to the skin. It is useful for many conditions, but particularly for those affecting the hip and the spine, e.g. a prolapsed intervertebral disc.

2 Longitudinal traction

This is used, for example, for fractures of the femur. It is an alternative

SKELETAL TRACTION

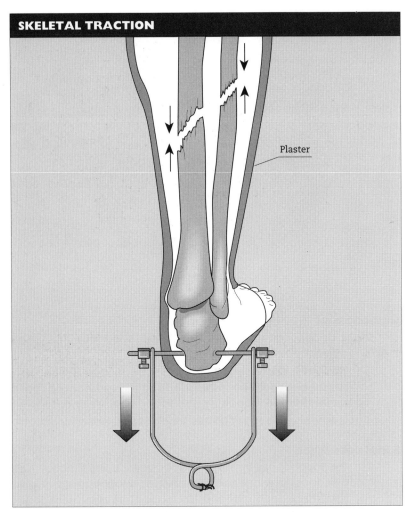

Plaster

Fig. 9.3

to the use of the Thomas' splint as a fixed traction device. The traction is applied through a pin in the upper tibia and the leg is supported on the Thomas' splint with a special knee attachment (Pearson) to allow the knee to be flexed (Fig. 9.5). The splint is usually suspended by cords from an overhead beam. If the tibia is also fractured this may be immobilized in a below knee plaster-cast incorporating the tibial pin.

3 Hamilton–Russell traction

This was designed to apply a traction force in line with the shaft of the

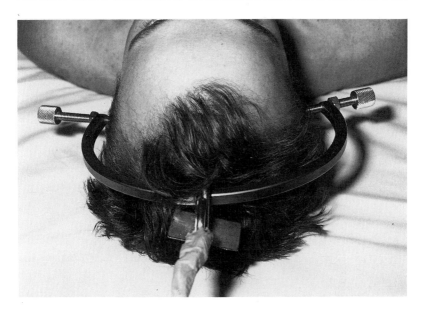

Fig. 9.4 Gardner–Wells skull calipers.

THOMAS' SPLINT WITH KNEE ATTACHMENT AND SKELETAL TRACTION

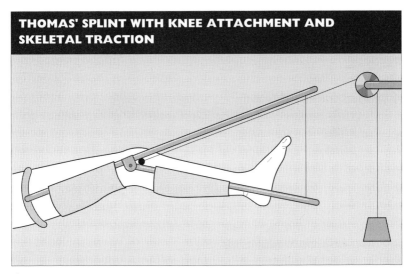

Fig. 9.5

femur whilst allowing movement of hip and knee. This is achieved by applying a pull in two directions, giving a resultant force in the desired line in all positions of the limb. It is usually applied with skin extensions and is mainly used for hip conditions and fractures of the upper femur (Fig. 9.6).

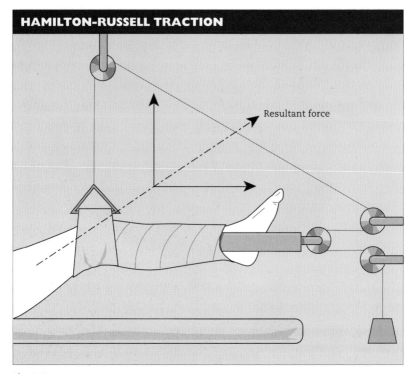

HAMILTON-RUSSELL TRACTION

Resultant force

Fig. 9.6

4 Gallows traction (Bryant)

This is a simple method (Fig. 9.7) of applying longitudinal traction to the femur in a child up to the age of 2 years. In older children vascular complications may occur. The traction is arranged to raise the buttocks just clear of the bed.

5 Sliding traction using the Böhler–Braun frame

This is a useful method for applying traction to a tibial or femoral fracture. The leg is supported in good alignment on slings stretched across the frame (Fig. 9.8).

INTERNAL FIXATION

This has undoubtedly become more popular as techniques have improved. It is usually reserved for those fractures where accurate reduction is necessary and when mobilization of the limb or the patient is particularly important. Accurate reduction is usually desirable for fractures involving joint surfaces. Internal fixation can be used,

'GALLOWS' TRACTION

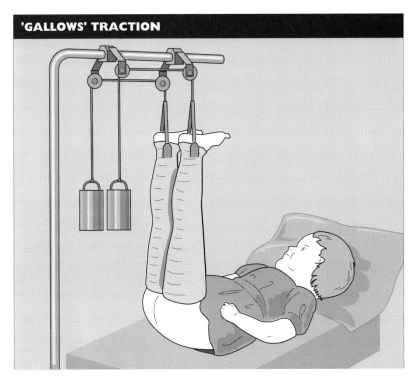

Fig. 9.7

but with more danger, in open fractures. The time from injury to operation then becomes important, and the 6-hour rule is worth remembering.

Many types of internal fixation device are used: screws, plates, compression plates, intramedullary nails, etc. The latest techniques utilize advanced engineering principles, and scientifically designed implants, usually arranged to allow compression and firm fixation of the fragments. These have the disadvantage that they partially replace the load-bearing functions of the bone so that they may need to be removed when the

INTERNAL FIXATION–ADVANTAGES

- It allows accurate reduction and maintenance of position.
- It allows the patient and his joints more mobility, thus encouraging rehabilitation and avoiding joint stiffness.
- It may encourage union, but only if sufficiently strong.
- It may diminish time spent in hospital.

INTERNAL FIXATION–DISADVANTAGES

- It may introduce infection.
- It is often technically exacting and operative complications may occur.
- If it is inadequate or infection occurs, union may be long delayed or may not occur.
- It may not be sufficiently strong to allow the advantages of full mobilization.
- Excessively rigid fixation may delay union.
- Further surgery may be needed to remove the device.

fracture is united. The fracture then requires further protection.

There is currently interest in designing internal fixation devices which allow a degree of flexibility at the fracture site. The idea is that this may restore some of the natural processes of fracture healing which can be inhibited by rigid devices (Chapter 4).

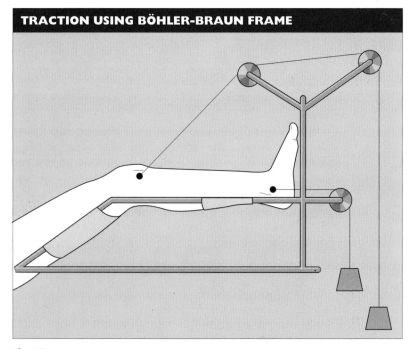

TRACTION USING BÖHLER-BRAUN FRAME

Fig. 9.8

SCREW FIXATION

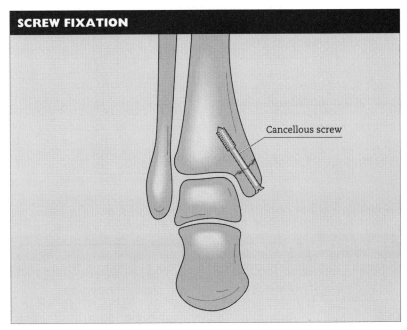

Cancellous screw

Fig. 9.9

Common techniques of internal fixation

1 SCREW FIXATION

Simple screw fixation is usually used to attach small bony fragments, e.g. the malleoli. The screw may have a large self-tapping thread which is wider than the shank to give a good grip on cancellous bone (Fig. 9.9), or it may be designed with a standard thread, in which case it is usually necessary to screw into the opposite cortex. This type of screw may be self-tapping, but in modern designs (e.g. the AO/ASIF technique) the holes are tapped. A single screw placed at right angles to the fracture line can be used to compress the fracture provided the thread is arranged to bite only into the farther fragment (Fig. 9.10). Such a screw is not in itself sufficient to hold the fracture and a plate or some form of external fixation is required in addition.

2 PLATE FIXATION

Many sizes and shapes of plate are used to hold fractures. The plate can be designed to apply compression to the fracture in order to give firmer fixation. The shape of the screw heads and the walls of the slot are designed to ensure this in the AO/ASIF design (Fig. 9.11).

SINGLE SCREW FRACTURE COMPRESSION

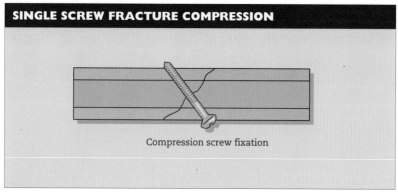

Compression screw fixation

Fig. 9.10

COMPRESSION PLATING

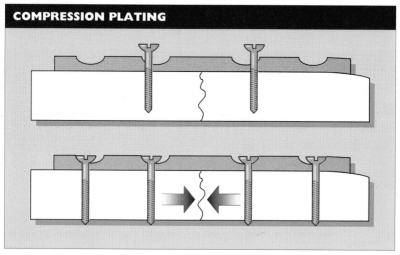

Fig. 9.11

3 INTRAMEDULLARY NAIL

This technique was devised by Kuntscher. In his design a hollow rod, which is trefoil-shaped in cross-section to diminish rotation, is passed along the medullary cavity. It is either introduced retrogradely through the fracture site or from one end (closed nailing). It is slotted to give it a good grip on the medullary cavity and, since most bones have a slight longitudinal curve, it works on the principle of 3-point fixation (Fig. 9.12). If correctly inserted it gives good fixation, enabling the patient to mobilize early. More modern designs are curved to fit the medullary cavity which is reamed to ensure a tight fit. The AO design uses this principle.

THE RUSSEL-TAYLOR INTERLOCKING INTRA-MEDULLARY NAIL

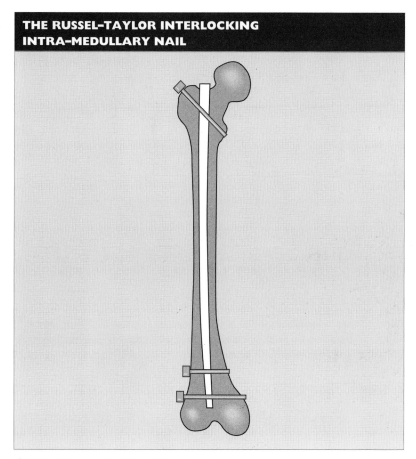

Fig. 9.12 Courtesy of Smith and Nephew Surgical.

4 INTERLOCKING INTRAMEDULLARY NAILS

If an intramedullary nail does not fit tightly in the medullary cavity, rotation at the fracture site is likely to occur and the fragments may slide along the nail, opening a fracture gap or causing the nail to back out. To overcome these problems the so-called 'locking' or 'interlocking' nail has been devised. This allows for the insertion through the nail of cross screws at the upper and lower ends of the shaft (see Fig. 9.12). These nails give very firm fixation and can be used to bridge significant gaps at the fracture site. If desired, the screws can be removed from one end of the bone when the fracture becomes reasonably stable, to allow some degree of 'telescoping' which may help to stimulate union.

Infection following intramedullary nailing is usually more difficult to treat than with other methods of internal fixation. If infection occurs, the

WIRE FIXATION OF OLECRANON FRACTURE

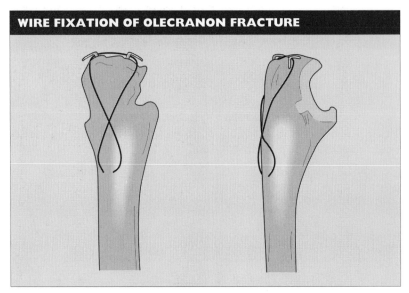

Fig. 9.13

nail is usually left *in situ* until the fracture is healed and then removed. Intramedullary nailing is used mainly in the femur and tibia, less frequently in the humerus.

5 WIRES

These are occasionally used to hold small bone fragments in position, e.g. stiff Kirschner wires or encircling wire bands (Fig. 9.13 AO/ASIF).

Summary

Internal fixation should be used in the situations listed below.

1 When adequate reduction cannot be maintained by external fixation (frequently fractures involving joint surfaces).

2 When it is important to allow early movement of a limb or a joint.

3 When it is important to avoid a long period of immobilization in bed, e.g. the elderly patient with a femoral neck fracture.

4 In cases of multiple trauma, where internal fixation of one or more of the fractures may simplify treatment of other injuries and has been shown to reduce mortality. A fracture associated with a severe vascular injury requiring repair may well come into this category.

5 Certain pathological fractures, particularly those resulting from malignancy, where union may be uncertain and the patient's life expectancy may be short.

With many fractures these criteria do not apply, and closed techniques are perfectly adequate to secure good results.

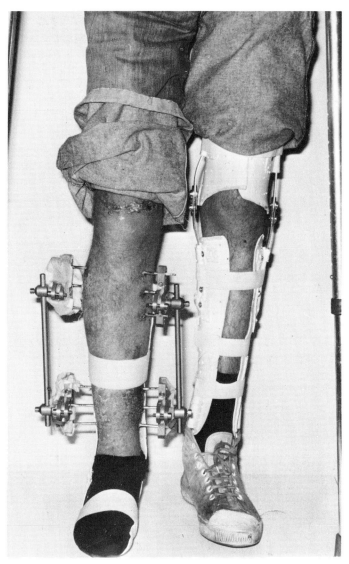

Fig. 9.14 An intero-external fixation frame and one type of femoral cast-brace.

FRAME FIXATION

There are situations where external fixation using Plaster of Paris or traction may not be adequate or may have other disadvantages, but, on the other hand, internal fixation may be hazardous or technically impossible. In these circumstances it may be possible to insert pins into the bones above and below the fracture and connect these together rigidly by means of a frame assembly (Figs. 9.14 and 11.4). There are many designs of such frames, both for general use and for specific purposes such as fractures of the pelvis. They have the advantage of giving good fixation whilst allowing access to the fracture site. This may be important if there is a wound requiring attention. They also avoid the dangers of introducing foreign material into the fracture site. However, they tend to be expensive and rather clumsy for general use. Furthermore, there is some evidence that rigid fixation of this type, if maintained for too long, may inhibit union and the frame is often used until the fracture appears stable and is then replaced by a cast. Frames are available which allow some movement at the fracture site, whilst still maintaining overall stability. There are, however, some theoretical objections to this and the correct technique for such devices has not yet been fully evaluated.

CHAPTER 10

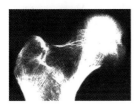

Fractures – complications

IMMEDIATE COMPLICATIONS
(i.e. occurring at the time of injury)

1 Severe haemorrhage.
  (a) External.
  (b) Internal.
2 Injury to important internal organs—brain, lung, liver, etc.
3 Injury to local nerves or vessels.
4 Skin loss or damage.

EARLY OR INTERMEDIATE COMPLICATIONS
(i.e. occurring during the period of treatment)

LOCAL

1 Skin and soft-tissue necrosis.
2 Gangrene from vascular damage or external pressure.
3 Pressure sores and nerve palsies from splintage or traction.
4 Infection and wound breakdown.
5 Loss of alignment. Failure of internal fixation.
6 Tetanus and gas gangrene (p. 239–40).

GENERAL

1 Deep vein thrombosis and pulmonary embolism. The former may occur in the immobilized leg or elsewhere. It is commoner in patients confined to bed. There is no general agreement as to the best form of prophylaxis. *(TEDs + Sc hep)*
2 Hypostatic pneumonia.
3 Renal calculus, acute retention and other urinary tract problems.
4 Fat embolism—usually occurring 3–10 days after fractures of long bones, and particularly after major trauma. The cause is unknown. It was originally thought to be caused by fat released into circulation from the fracture site, but it is now thought to be a metabolic phenomenon

associated with a period of circulatory insufficiency. It manifests itself as confusion and respiratory difficulty (often detected by a lowered arterial oxygen tension), and a petechial rash which varies in severity. It is sometimes fatal, but its severity can be diminished by correct fluid replacement, early immobilization of the fracture and intensive respiratory care.

5 'Crush syndrome' — this is usually associated with extensive soft-tissue damage or ischaemia of a large volume of tissues, for example, following occlusion of the femoral artery. Its cause is complicated, various factors such as fluid loss, release of toxic materials from the site of damage, and possibly diffuse intravascular coagulation, all contributing to an effect on the kidneys resulting in acute tubular necrosis with renal failure. It may be prevented by removal of the damaged tissue before severe renal changes have occurred, e.g. by amputation of the limb. If the renal changes become established, dialysis may be necessary in anticipation of recovery of renal function.

LATE COMPLICATIONS

1 Delayed and non-union. Mal-union, i.e. union in bad position (Chapter 11).

2 Late wound sepsis with skin breakdown.

3 Failure of internal fixation, e.g. breakage or cutting out of plates or nails.

4 Joint stiffness and contracture.

5 Sudek's atrophy (algodystrophy) — a condition in which the limb becomes painful, swollen and discoloured, with obvious circulatory changes and X-rays showing diffuse, patchy porosis of the bones. It is thought to be due to a sympathetic malfunction, but is ill-understood. It appears to be precipitated by trauma, either external or surgical and is usually seen after Colles' fractures and other common injuries. It is a distressing condition, but usually settles after several weeks or months. During this period it is important that the patient be encouraged to exercise the limb despite the pain. There is evidence that treatment with calcitonin may shorten the course of the condition in some patients.

6 Osteoarthritis resulting from joint damage or occasionally from mal-alignment of the limb.

7 Compensation neurosis and other psychological disturbances.

CHAPTER 11

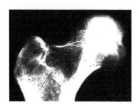

Fractures –
problems of union

The decision as to whether a fracture is united or not is essentially a clinical one: it depends on the disappearance of the original signs of the fracture, i.e. pain, tenderness, abnormal mobility, swelling, etc. There is usually some residual loss of function after a period of immobilization, so this is not a helpful physical sign in diagnosing union.

X-rays are helpful in that they may show callus (Fig. 11.1a). This may be visible as early as three weeks after a shaft fracture, but when rigid internal fixation is used callus may be minimal. Even profuse callus may not mean that the fracture is safe, but it is usually an indication that union is proceeding. It can be difficult to assess whether movement is still occurring at the fracture site and it is sometimes helpful to stress the fracture under the X-ray image intensifier to detect minor degrees of movement.

Absence of callus with mobility at the fracture site are indications of *delayed union*. This means delay beyond the normal time, but still with the possibility of union if immobilization is continued. When the fracture has been fixed internally it is usually difficult to judge when union has occurred on clinical and radiological grounds and the decision to allow unprotected load-bearing may have to be made on the basis of average union times. Occasionally, this leads to load-bearing on an un-united fracture and in these circumstances the fixation device will usually break or cut out of the bone.

Many fractures take longer to unite than the average times suggested (Chapter 8) and protection may still be needed from full load-bearing beyond these times, even though union may apparently have occurred.

Non-union is a clinical and radiological diagnosis. The most useful X-ray sign is that the medullary cavity has become sealed off and there is an obvious gap between the bone ends (Fig. 11.1b). True radiological union, characterized by trabeculae crossing the fracture site, is often not evident until long after clinical union has occurred and remodelling may continue for many months after that (Fig. 11.1c). Non-union is commoner with fractures through cortical bone than with fractures of cancellous bone which are often impacted.

PROBLEMS OF UNION

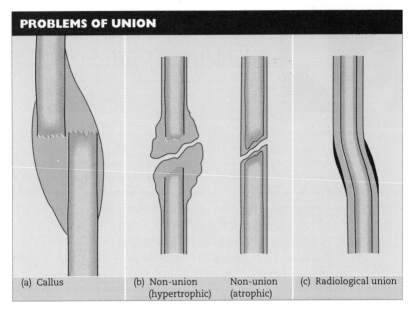

(a) Callus   (b) Non-union   Non-union   (c) Radiological union
(hypertrophic)   (atrophic)

Fig. 11.1

A decision to treat delayed union is usually made before true non-union occurs. It is usually apparent after 4–5 months that union is not occurring, but in most cases the decision can be made long before this.

MAL-UNION

This expression means that the fracture has united in an unsatisfactory position—judged either from a functional or cosmetic point of view. It should not occur if management of the fracture has been adequate, but circumstances are not always favourable and some patients are left with a degree of deformity or shortening of the limb. In children, considerable compensatory remodelling can be expected and even length defects often correct by the end of growth. In adults, much less correction can be expected although when the swelling and thickening associated with the fracture has settled, the appearance may be much more satisfactory than might at first have been expected. In some cases, a corrective osteotomy or even bone lengthening may have to be considered. The latter can be a hazardous procedure and in most cases shortness, which is usually only a problem in the lower limb, can be compensated by modifications to the shoes.

FACTORS INFLUENCING UNION

1 Age. This is a favourable factor in children, especially young children and babies. In adults, age affects union very little, even into old age, unless the patient is severely malnourished.

2 Fracture site. Here the important feature is usually the blood supply, especially when one fragment is rendered avascular by the fracture, e.g. scaphoid and femoral neck fractures.

3 Degree of violence. Comminuted fractures with much soft-tissue damage can be expected to unite slowly.

4 Infection. Severe infection, with osteomyelitis, usually delays union.

5 Immobilization—some fractures need more immobilization than others. Fractures of the clavicle, for example, usually unite rapidly with minimal immobilization. In the early stages following the injury, excessively rigid fixation may delay union, but rigid fixation is often used later as a method of treating delayed union.

6 Bone or generalized disease. Local pathology may prejudice union, e.g. malignant disease or infection. Generalized bone disease may or may not matter, e.g. osteoporosis does not necessarily impair healing. Severe malnutrition, vitamin deficiency or steroid excess may interfere with union.

7 Distraction of the bone ends is harmful and is usually avoidable. Interposition of soft tissue may delay or prevent union, although this is by no means always the case. If there is evidence that the bone ends are being held apart by soft tissues, it is usually advisable to carry out an open reduction (but not necessarily internal fixation).

TREATMENT OF DELAYED OR NON-UNION

To some extent, the management depends on whether the non-union is infected or not. An infected non-union usually fails to heal on antibiotic treatment alone because of the presence of dead bone, either as a separate sequestrum or still attached to the living bone.

THE NON-INFECTED FRACTURE

Non-union is sometimes classified as:
1 hypertrophic, i.e. with much callus at the bone ends (Fig. 11.1b); or
2 atrophic, i.e. with no obvious callus (Fig. 11.1b).

TREATMENT

The hypertrophic type will often unite if the fracture is rigidly immobilized, usually by internal fixation, e.g. by a plate or intramedullary nail. A compression plate gives particularly firm fixation.

CORTICO-CANCELLOUS GRAFTS

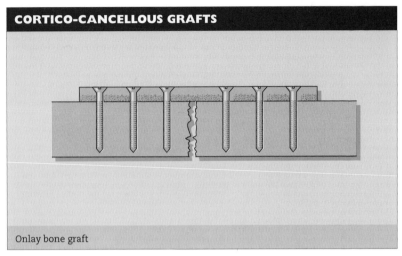

Onlay bone graft

Fig. 11.2

CANCELLOUS STRIPS (PHEMISTER)

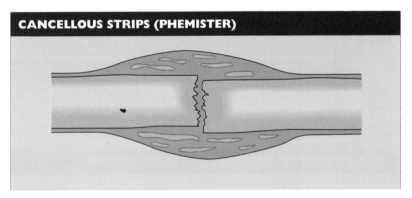

Fig. 11.3

The atrophic type also requires firm fixation, but union tends to proceed more quickly if a bone-graft is used to stimulate bone formation. There are two common techniques of bone-grafting.

1 Cortical grafts—onlay or sliding, may be used to provide both fixation and some osteogenic stimulus (Fig. 11.2). They are now rarely used.

2 Cancellous grafts (Phemister), usually taken from the iliac crest, may be laid as strips around the site of non-union, without breaking it down if realignment is not necessary (Fig. 11.3). This technique is often combined with internal fixation.

Theoretically, the best osteogenic stimulus is provided by live bone-marrow working upon a bony scaffold. The usual graft of cancellous bone

RIGID INTERO-EXTERNAL FIXATION

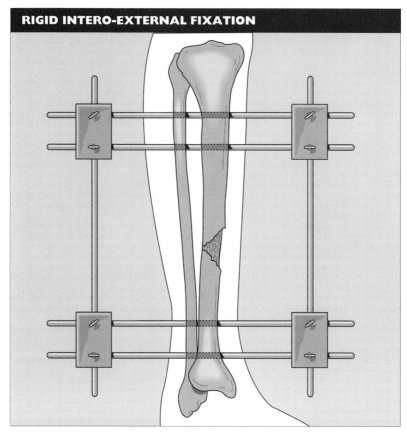

Fig. 11.4

chips provides both of these conditions, the bony scaffold being dead, but the marrow cells surviving the transplant.

THE INFECTED FRACTURE

Union will not usually occur until the infection is overcome. Firm fixation of the fracture and excision of bone which is obviously dead will often eliminate or reduce the infection, enabling a bone-graft to be carried out. If the defect after removal of dead tissue is large, a considerable quantity of bone may be needed to bridge the gap. Cancellous bone chips are usually used rather than large inlay or onlay cortical grafts. Immobilization of the fracture needs to be continued until solid union occurs. In severely infected non-unions, a rigid form of intero-external fixation, using a frame, is safer than implanting metal plates or nails (Fig. 11.4). A less rigid

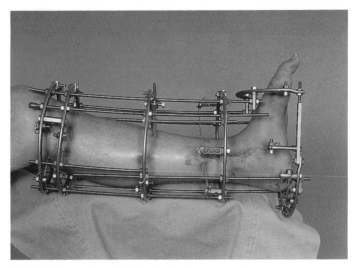

Fig. 11.5 Ilizarov frame fixation for fracture non-union.

but more adaptable type of frame devised by Ilizarov has also been suggested for this situation (Fig. 11.5). Composite grafts of skin, subcutaneous tissue, muscle and bone, with vascular anastomosis may be needed for the difficult case—usually a tibial fracture. Securing union in such cases can take many months or even years and in some patients amputation may be a better option.

ELECTRICAL STIMULATION OF BONE UNION

There is interest in the idea of stimulating fractures to unite by means of an electrical current passed through or induced at the fracture site. In one technique the limb is immobilized in plaster and an electrical coil is arranged to surround the fracture site. An alternating current is passed through the coil and this in turn induces an alternating field in the bone. A second method involves implanting wires in the bone close to the fracture site and stimulating the fracture directly through these. The scientific evidence for these techniques remains equivocal.

CHAPTER 12

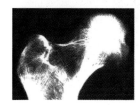

Injuries of the spine and trunk

The spine consists of a complex system of bones and articulations. Its mobility varies at different levels.

A typical intervertebral articulation is shown in Fig. 12.1. The posterior ligament complex is at least as important as the intervertebral disc in maintaining the stability of one vertebra on another. In the cervical region the facet joints are in a horizontal plane (Fig. 12.2); in the lumbar region they are vertical and almost in a para-sagittal plane (Fig. 12.3). In the thoracic spine they are intermediate in alignment, giving this region more stability. The ribs also contribute to this stability. Because of these variations, different types of injury occur at the different levels. Stability is lost when both the intervertebral disc and the posterior ligament complex are disrupted.

In the adult the spinal cord extends from the foramen magnum to the lower border of the 1st lumbar vertebra, and below this level the roots of the cauda equina lie within the theca as far as the lower border of the 2nd sacral vertebra. These nervous structures are vulnerable when the spine is injured and characteristic patterns of neurological loss occur at the different spinal levels.

Any patient suspected of having a spinal injury, particularly if unconscious, must be moved with great care, with a number of helpers lifting the patient 'in one piece', avoiding any flexion or rotation of the spine. The head may be supported on a stretcher with sandbags on either side of the neck.

CERVICAL SPINE

Injuries of the cervical spine are usually the result of road traffic or sporting accidents and represent the commonest injuries of the spinal column. The injury is often caused by a fall on to the head, with the neck being forcibly bent. The patient is often unconscious following the head injury, so the injury to the cervical spine may not be immediately apparent. This possibility should be considered in all patients who are uncon-

INTERVERTEBRAL ARTICULATIONS

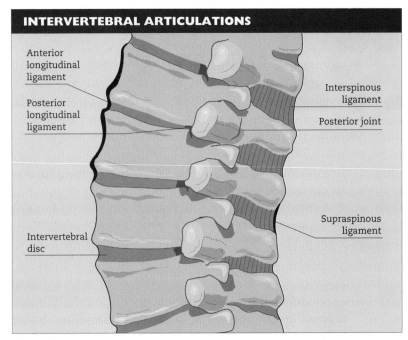

Anterior longitudinal ligament

Posterior longitudinal ligament

Intervertebral disc

Interspinous ligament

Posterior joint

Supraspinous ligament

Fig. 12.1

CERVICAL INTERVERTEBRAL JOINTS

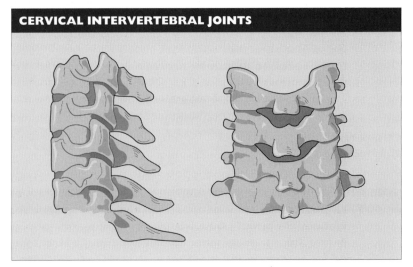

Fig. 12.2

LUMBAR INTERVERTEBRAL JOINTS

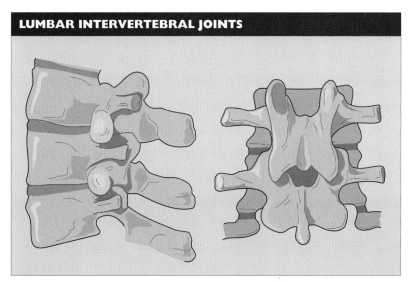

Fig. 12.3

scious following an injury and a lateral X-ray of the cervical spine should be obtained *in all cases.*

The most serious injuries are usually caused by flexion and rotation and these result in subluxation or dislocation of one or both facet joints, together with disruption of the intervertebral disc—an unstable injury (Fig. 12.4).

The cervical spine can also be injured by forced extension, as might occur from a fall on the face or forehead. This usually causes a ligamentous injury and rarely renders the spine unstable.

Radiography

Good X-rays are essential for the diagnosis of suspected cervical spine injuries, and should be obtained routinely for any patient who is unconscious following a head injury and any patient with pain in the neck or radiating down the arm or who has a cervical twist or torticollis following an accident. A patient who has had a severe shoulder injury may also warrant X-rays of the cervical spine.

The X-rays required are: a lateral film of the *whole* cervical spine, including one taken with firm traction on the head and an assistant applying traction to the arms to draw down the shoulders, giving a view of the C7–T1 region; an AP view, including one through the open mouth, and 30 degree oblique views which show the facet joints in detail. If, on

CERVICAL SUBLUXATION

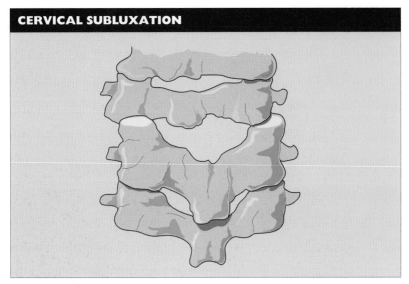

Fig. 12.4

the lateral film, one vertebral body appears to be displaced forwards on the one below by less than half a diameter this usually means subluxation of one facet joint. More displacement than this usually means a subluxation or dislocation of both joints (Fig. 12.5).

If the ordinary X-rays show no abnormality, then either the fracture may be in the region of the atlas or axis, or the injury may be of the hyperextension type which often reduces spontaneously. The only evidence for this may be a small flake of bone which is pulled off by the anterior ligament from the lower anterior margin of the upper vertebral body. Occasionally, a flexion injury may also have reduced fully by the time the film is taken. In this case there may be a small bony flake off the upper anterior margin of the body below the disc involved. If this is suspected, flexion and extension X-rays may be advisable, but these must be carried out with great care.

Computed tomography (CT) scanning has helped to clarify the pathological anatomy of many types of cervical injury.

Clinical features

In the conscious patient, a cervical injury is usually suggested by pain and muscle spasm with localized tenderness. The presence of a retropharyngeal haematoma seen through the open mouth is evidence of a fracture or dislocation at C1 or C2. Occasionally, there may be a twist

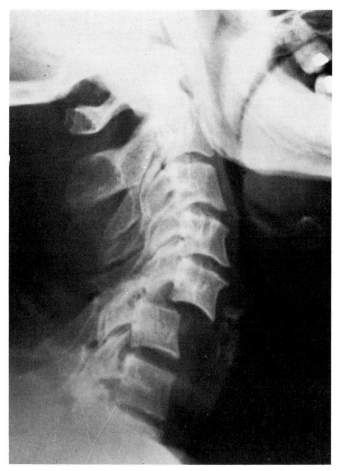

Fig. 12.5 Cervical subluxation–lateral X-ray.

of the neck or torticollis. Neurological loss may be gross, minimal, or absent, but in all cases careful examination of arms and legs is essential.

Treatment

This depends on whether the injury is stable or unstable. As a general rule, any displaced flexion injury will be unstable. Most authorities agree that any dislocation or subluxation should be reduced whether there is neurological loss or not. This may be achieved by either:

1 manipulation under anaesthesia with X-ray control; or

2 continuous traction applied through skull tongs (see Fig. 9.4): if this method of reduction is used, gradually increasing weights are applied to

the traction apparatus and the patient's neurological state is carefully monitored during the period of reduction, which may take a few hours.

Following reduction if there is a fracture as well as a subluxation, traction is usually maintained until signs of bony fusion between vertebrae start to appear on X-ray, normally at about 3–4 weeks. Traction may be by skull tongs or, if the patient is fit to mobilize, a halo-vest may be used. If spontaneous fusion does not occur, a decision is usually then made to fuse the two segments surgically to ensure long-term stability. Pure subluxations without a fracture usually remain unstable and fusion is advisable at an early stage.

Extension injuries are often not unstable and symptomatic immobilization in a collar is usually sufficient.

Fractures of the vertical compression type are not common and may be of the burst type (see Fig. 7.5). These are usually unstable to some extent and, as a minimum, require immobilization in a collar.

Fractures of the atlas

The ring of the atlas is usually fractured in four places as a result of a vertical compression force. This is usually a stable injury and cord damage is uncommon. Treatment in a collar is adequate.

Fractures of the odontoid

These are uncommon and easily missed. The fracture is usually at the base and displacement may be considerable, while still allowing survival. An X-ray taken through the open mouth shows the fracture best. Union usually occurs after treatment on traction, followed by a protective collar for a total of 3 months. If non-union occurs then surgical fusion is necessary for safety and this may be done either anteriorly (through the mouth) or posteriorly.

Hangman's fracture

This is characterized by fractures of the pedicles of C2 with forward displacement of the body. It was typically found after judicial hanging.

Whiplash injuries

This type of injury typically occurs when the car in which the patient is sitting is struck from behind by a second vehicle. The sudden acceleration causes the neck to extend and then, as the car decelerates, to flex violently forwards. The main damage is to the ligaments and other soft tissues of the spine and the symptoms are usually of pain in the neck, sometimes with radiation down the arm and occasionally with paraesthesiae or numbness in the arm or hand. The onset of symptoms is occasionally delayed by a few hours or even days. The neck is usually stiff and there may be objective neurological signs. X-rays are usually normal or show degenerative changes only and treatment is essentially conservative, initially with a collar and then by gradual mobilization with physiotherapy. The prognosis is variable; some patients recover completely, others continue to have troublesome symptoms over a long period and occasionally the disability proves to be permanent.

THORACIC INJURIES

The thoracic spine is essentially a stable structure, but the canal is narrow and paraplegia is common.

Flexion injuries

These may result in crush or wedge fractures which are commonest in this part of the spine. These fractures are stable, often without neurological damage, and heal well. Symptomatic treatment is sufficient, usually rest and analgesics initially, followed by mobilization as the pain settles. In the absence of severe violence, a search should be made for underlying pathology. Many conditions may weaken the vertebral body to the point where a fracture occurs after minimal trauma, or even after bending or lifting. Osteoporosis in the elderly, multiple myeloma, and secondary neoplasms are the commonest causes of pathological wedge fractures (Chapter 13).

Paraplegia may occur with more severe, displaced or unstable fractures (Chapter 13).

Fracture dislocation at the thoraco-lumbar junction

This injury is common and is caused by flexion and rotation violence, e.g. a fall from a height on to the shoulder or a rock fall over the flexed back (Fig. 12.6). Instability of the fracture dislocation rests partly on the disc, which is disrupted, but more importantly on the posterior ligament complex, which may rupture completely, producing a palpable gap or step in the line of the spinous processes. There may be other external evidence of the injury such as bruising or abrasions over the shoulder. If a gap is felt on palpating along the line of the spinous processes, the fracture should be regarded as unstable. Typically, the injury occurs at a level somewhere between T10 and L2 and produces a shearing fracture

'MECHANISM' OF THORACO-LUMBAR INJURY

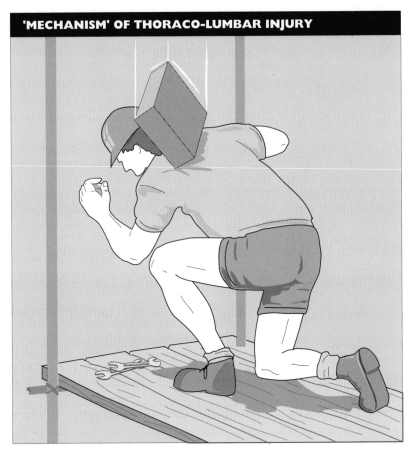

Fig. 12.6

just below the disc. The facet joint is often fractured on one side (Fig. 12.7). Paraplegia is common, and its presence influences treatment (Chapter 13). Computed tomography scanning has demonstrated that the cord damage is often caused by disc material and bone fragments being pushed backwards into the spinal canal. A surprising degree of occlusion of the canal can occur without neurological complications. Removal of this material cannot be guaranteed to improve the neurological prognosis, presumably because the damage to the cord has occurred at the time of injury and is irreversible.

Management of the unstable fracture

If there is paraplegia, good nursing care is essential with regular turning to avoid pressure sores. Some authorities fix the fracture internally to

THORACO-LUMBAR FRACTURE DISLOCATION

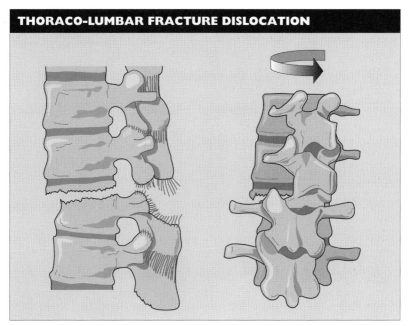

Fig. 12.7

avoid pain during turning and to avoid complications of late spinal deformity. Plates fixed on either side of the spinous processes have been popular and the Harrington instrumentation, designed for the treatment of scoliosis, has been used for selected unstable fractures of the thoraco-lumbar spine. More recently, pedicle screw fixation of the type devised by Cotrel-Dubosset has been recommended for these injuries (Fig. 12.8). It is claimed that internal fixation allows early mobilization of the patient, avoiding some of the problems of a period of bed rest.

Other authorities rely on careful nursing until the fracture unites, usually at 12 weeks. Spinal fusion is not often required for this type of fracture-dislocation.

If there is no paraplegia, the patient can be nursed in bed or on a plaster bed until union occurs because in this case there are no problems of sensory loss. Again, internal fixation allows early mobilization and is becoming more widely used.

FRACTURES IN THE LUMBAR REGION

VERTICAL COMPRESSION FRACTURES

Falls on the head or heels occasionally produce a so-called burst fracture in the mobile areas of the spine, i.e. cervical or lumbar. These may or may

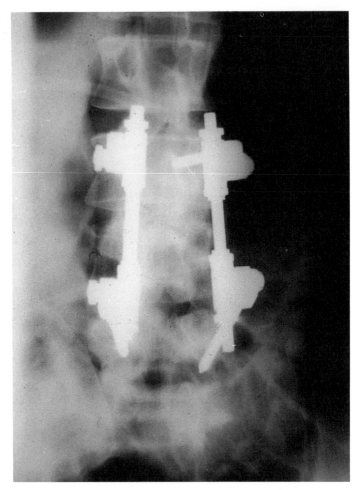

Fig. 12.8 Cotrel-Dubousset fixation. Courtesy of Athrodax Surgical Ltd.

not be associated with paraplegia, and are variably unstable. If there is no paraplegia, external support with a moulded polythene or plaster jacket until union occurs is adequate.

FRACTURES OF TRANSVERSE PROCESSES

These are particularly common in the lumbar region. They are usually caused by severe crushing or forcible lateral flexion of the trunk. They are treated symptomatically, but often take a long time to become painless because of the associated soft-tissue damage. They are commonly associated with injuries to the kidneys.

FRACTURES OF SACRUM AND COCCYX

These occasionally occur from direct impact and can produce neurological problems, particularly affecting the bladder, and may occasionally cause long-term pain.

Coccydinia is a condition in which there is chronic pain in the coccygeal region, often following an injury or after childbirth, but sometimes for no obvious reason. The pain interferes with sitting. It is difficult to cure, but may be helped by injections of local anaesthetic and steroids or by manipulation of the coccyx via the rectum and under anaesthesia. Excision of the coccyx may rarely be necessary, but is not always curative.

CHAPTER 13

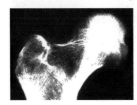

Paraplegia

The importance of spinal injuries is their liability to produce damage to the spinal cord and nerve roots.

CERVICAL INJURIES

If the cord is damaged above the level of C4, survival is unlikely because of paralysis of all respiratory muscles. Below this level, various degrees of quadriplegia occur. The nerve roots emerge horizontally at the disc above the correspondingly numbered vertebra, except for the 8th root which emerges below C7 vertebra. The roots do not run downwards alongside the cord in the cervical spine so that transection of the cord produces a clear-cut level which may be determined by simple neurological examination of the arms, measuring muscle power and sensory loss.

If the injury is to the lower cervical spine, a common site, a good deal of arm function may remain.

Incomplete and complex lesions also occur, e.g. the Brown-Séquard syndrome, in which there is partial neurological loss in one arm and in the opposite leg, and the 'central-cord' syndrome in which there is flaccid weakness of the arms and spastic weakness of the legs. This condition is usually caused by an extension injury of the cervical spine in an older person whose spine shows changes of spondylosis.

THORACIC INJURIES

These are usually complete and with a well-defined neurological level.

Thoraco-lumbar injuries

Paraplegia is common in fracture dislocations at the thoraco-lumbar junction. The neurological picture may be complex because at this level the lumbar and sacral roots run down alongside the cord which terminates at the lower border of L1 (Fig. 13.1). Because of this, various

ANATOMY OF SPINAL CORD AND ROOTS AT THE THORACO-LUMBAR REGION

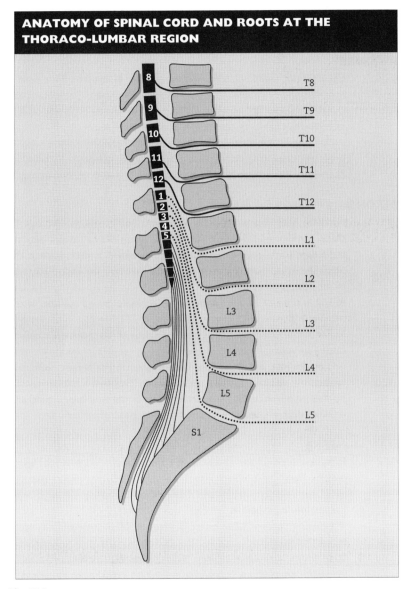

Fig. 13.1

combinations of cord and root transection occur, producing some upper motor neurone, and some lower motor neurone phenomena.

RECOVERY

Considerable neurological recovery may occur at any level if the cord is not completely transected but only traumatized. Complete cord transection does not recover. Damaged roots are theoretically capable of recovery since they behave like peripheral nerves.

Injuries at the thoraco-lumbar junction, therefore, have a variable prognosis depending on whether the cord is completely transected or not and on how much of the neurological loss is due to root damage.

DIAGNOSIS

Accurate neurological diagnosis is essential for prognosis, and this includes motor and sensory testing, especially in the sacral and perineal regions. If some residual sensation or movement is detectable in the paralysed area, then recovery is possible because the lesion must be incomplete.

• The anal reflex is a response of the sphincter to stimulation of the surrounding skin.

• The bulbo-spongiosus reflex is a contraction of the cremasteric muscle caused by squeezing the glans-penis.

Spinal shock is a short-lived phenomenon in the human. Complete motor loss associated with a positive anal reflex and bulbo-spongiosus reflex which have appeared in the first few hours after injury, especially if the tendon jerks also reappear quickly, is a bad prognostic sign.

MANAGEMENT

Paraplegic patients are usually nursed and rehabilitated in special Spinal Injuries units. The problems are those of providing adequate nursing to avoid complications whilst the spinal injury is healing. These complications are listed below.

1 Pressure sores—caused by the patient's inability to move and loss of protective sensation.

2 Urinary tract problems due to bladder paralysis. This is usually treated initially by intermittent catheterization and later by the establishment of adequate drainage either by training in the use of appliances, self-catheterization, or occasionally by surgery. Artificial sphincters are currently under trial.

3 Bowel problems, stasis, incontinence, etc.

4 Chest problems due to immobilization and paralysis of respiratory muscles—usually treated by physiotherapy and antibiotics.

5 Bone demineralization due to inactivity, sometimes with renal stone formation.

6 Psychological problems.

The rehabilitation period is prolonged and requires a skilled team effort. Appliances such as calipers, wheelchairs and modifications in the home, together with extensive retraining, are often necessary, and some supervision is usually needed throughout life.

CHAPTER 14

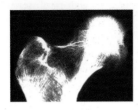

Fractures and dislocations of the shoulder and upper arm

FRACTURE OF THE CLAVICLE

This is one of the commonest fractures in childhood and early adult life and is usually caused by a fall on the outstretched hand, or directly on the shoulder. The fracture is rarely open. In a child the fracture is usually of the greenstick type.

CLINICAL FEATURES

The patient complains of pain in the shoulder region and supports the weight of the arm with his other hand. The bone typically breaks in the middle of the shaft or at the junction of the middle and outer thirds, and the outer fragment is pulled downwards and forwards by the weight of the arm (Fig. 14.1).

COMPLICATIONS

These are rare, but the brachial plexus may be injured, as may the subclavian artery or vein. Occasionally the dome of the pleura may be penetrated by a bony fragment, producing a pneumothorax. Non-union is very rare and is more likely after internal fixation.

TREATMENT

For most clavicular fractures, adequate treatment consists of supporting the weight of the arm in a broad sling. With the more severely displaced fractures, an attempt is sometimes made to secure a partial reduction by means of a figure-of-eight bandage (Fig. 14.2), but this is not an effective device and may be uncomfortable. Very occasionally, displacement may be sufficiently severe to warrant internal fixation, particularly if the fracture is at the lateral end. A small plate or tension band wiring may be used. It should be emphasized that the majority of clavicular fractures heal well, give excellent function and after remodelling are cosmetically satisfactory.

Three weeks of support is normally sufficient and subsequent recovery of function is usually rapid.

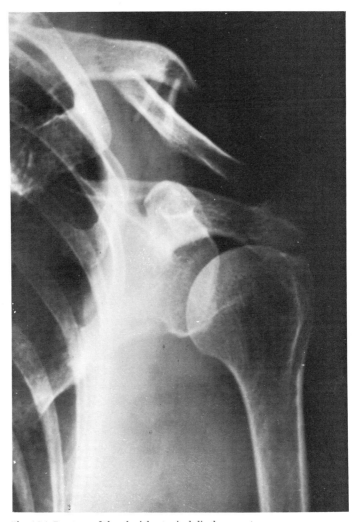

Fig. 14.1 Fracture of the clavicle – typical displacement.

FRACTURES OF ACROMION AND SCAPULA

These are often caused by a direct blow or fall and are rarely displaced. They are usually of little significance. Fractures of the scapula may be associated with rib fractures.

TREATMENT

Simple support in a broad sling is sufficient, with early movement when the pain allows.

SLING AND FIGURE OF EIGHT BANDAGE

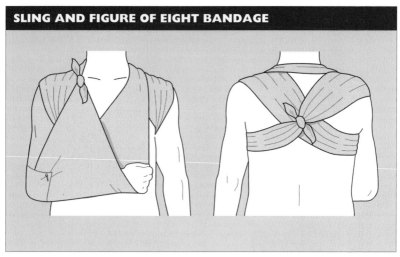

Fig. 14.2

SUBLUXATION AND DISLOCATION OF ACROMIO-CLAVICULAR JOINT

These injuries are not common. They are usually caused by a severe fall on the top of the shoulder, often as a result of sport. Subluxations are associated with tearing of the joint capsule but with the coraco-clavicular ligament remaining intact. A complete dislocation involves rupture of the ligament (Fig. 14.3). In both cases the displacement is difficult to reposition, but function is usually good even without full correction.

CLINICAL FEATURES

The outer end of the clavicle is abnormally prominent and tender, usually with some additional swelling. Shoulder movements are restricted. The injury is frequently missed on X-rays, but the displacement may be more obvious if the patient holds a weight in the hand.

TREATMENT

A broad sling is often sufficient, sometimes supplemented by strapping over the acromio-clavicular joint. The subluxation will usually persist, but function is likely to be normal. Rarely, more likely in athletes, surgical repair or reconstruction of the coraco-clavicular ligament is indicated. The repair may be protected by driving a screw across the clavicle and into the coracoid process or a threaded pin or figure-of-eight wire may be passed across the acromio-clavicular joint. Subluxation may recur

ACROMIO-CLAVICULAR DISLOCATION

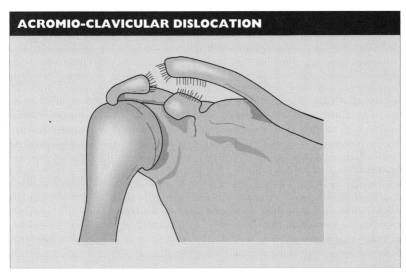

Fig. 14.3

ANTERIOR OR SUB-CORACOID DISLOCATION

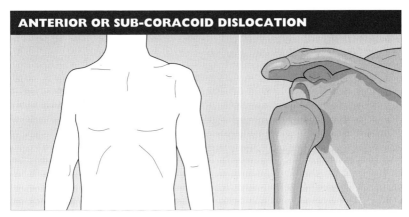

Fig. 14.4

when these devices are removed, but the long-term appearance may be improved.

DISLOCATION OF THE SHOULDER

This is a common injury, usually following a fall on the arm or shoulder. It usually occurs in an anterior direction (sub-coracoid) (Fig. 14.4), or occasionally posteriorly or inferiorly.

CLINICAL FEATURES

Diagnosis is usually easy in the typical *anterior dislocation*, because of the flattening of the deltoid muscle which produces a straight drop in the line of the shoulder from the tip of the acromion (see Fig. 14.4). The injury is a painful one and the patient supports the arm against all movement. The humeral head may be palpable below the coracoid or in the axilla. *Posterior dislocation* is more difficult to diagnose because the abnormality in contour of the shoulder is less obvious and the X-ray appearances may be misleading, the rotation of the upper end of the humerus producing a so-called 'light-bulb' appearance. The dislocation is best seen on an axillary view if this can be obtained. *Inferior dislocation*, sometimes called 'luxatio erecta', is rare and is characterized by the fact that the arm lies in a vertical position alongside the patient's head.

COMPLICATIONS

Occasionally the circumflex (axillary) nerve is damaged, causing paralysis of the deltoid. This may be checked by testing sensation over the insertion of the deltoid. Recovery is usual. The brachial plexus and axillary artery may also be damaged.

TREATMENT

Reduction should be carried out as soon as possible. Many methods are available:

1 The patient lies face down with the arm hanging over the side of a couch, and with an analgesic injection the muscles gradually relax allowing the operator to slip the head back into joint.

2 The Hippocratic method—under general anaesthesia with patient supine the operator pulls downwards on the arm whilst applying countertraction in the axilla with his stockinged foot, and uses his toes to slip the head into position.

3 Kocher's method. The elbow is flexed and traction applied to the arm. The arm is then externally rotated, adducted across the chest and flexed at the shoulder and then internally rotated until the forearm touches the chest. There is a risk of fracturing the humerus, and the other methods are generally to be preferred.

After reduction an X-ray is taken to confirm the position and the arm immobilized for 3 weeks in a broad sling, then exercised. This period is usually shortened in the elderly where stiffness tends to be a problem.

Recurrent dislocation

This occasionally follows one or more traumatic dislocations. It is said to be less likely to occur if the first injury is immobilized long enough for capsular healing to occur. After several dislocations a defect may be

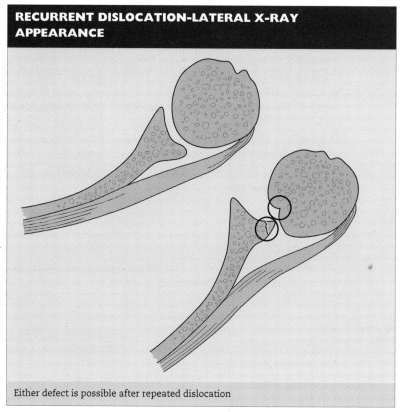

RECURRENT DISLOCATION-LATERAL X-RAY
APPEARANCE

Either defect is possible after repeated dislocation

Fig. 14.5

visible in the head or the edge of the glenoid on a lateral X-ray film (Fig. 14.5), and at operation the cartilaginous glenoid labrum and capsule may be found to be avulsed from the anterior margin of the glenoid (Bankart lesion).

TREATMENT

Several operations are available, e.g. the Putti–Platt and Bankart procedures. These involve tightening and reinforcing the anterior capsular structures and the overlying tendons of the rotator-cuff muscles. They usually restrict external rotation of the shoulder to some extent, but almost always control the instability. It is essential that the direction of dislocation is confirmed before surgery.

FRACTURES OF THE HUMERAL NECK

These fractures are often classified as abduction or adduction types, depending on the relative positions of the proximal and distal fragments. They are often comminuted, with the greater tuberosity forming a separate fragment. This classification is of little value unless manipulative reduction is to be attempted, in which case it may help to decide if the fracture is stable or unstable. The stable fractures are impacted and may be safely mobilized early. Unimpacted fractures may be considerably displaced and may be associated with damage to the brachial plexus or axillary artery. Many of these fractures occur in elderly people from a fall on the arm or shoulder. The degree of displacement varies and is often not severe. Nevertheless, a stiff shoulder is a common outcome and it is rarely worth attempting to produce an anatomical reduction even if there is gross displacement.

TREATMENT

In this group of patients a broad sling is used to support the arm initially, but mobilization is encouraged as soon as possible. The patient begins to swing the arm in the sling within a few days and as the pain settles more vigorous physiotherapy is commenced.

In younger people severe displacement may necessitate manipulation under anaesthesia or even open reduction. The period of immobilization may be much longer without necessarily producing long-term stiffness in young adults. Displacement of the upper humeral epiphysis in a child often requires manipulation.

Fracture dislocation of the shoulder is a complex injury and priority is usually given to reducing the shoulder dislocation. Severely displaced fractures and fracture dislocations are difficult to manage at all ages. Manipulation may fail and an open procedure be necessary. There may be technical difficulties with open reduction and, even if satisfactory alignment of the fragments is achieved, fixation can present problems. The head of the humerus is not easy to fix adequately. The AO technique makes use of special plates with cancellous screws entering the head (Fig. 14.6). As with the femoral head, ischaemic necrosis of the head of the humerus may occur. In this case, or if it proves impossible to achieve primary fixation, it may be appropriate to replace the humeral head with a prosthesis, that designed by Neer being the most widely used. This procedure tends to give disappointing results in terms of movements, but may give a reasonably painfree shoulder.

Fractures of the greater tuberosity may cause a large fragment to be pulled upwards by the rotator-cuff muscles and this may need open reduction and internal fixation to avoid impingement on the acromion.

INTERNAL FIXATION OF FRACTURE-DISLOCATION (AO)

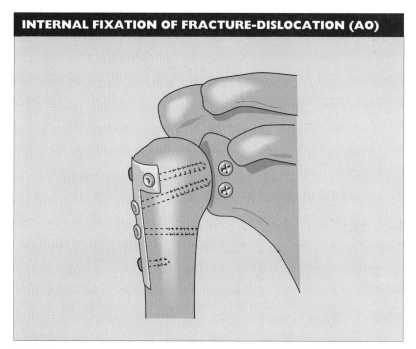

Fig. 14.6

FRACTURE OF THE HUMERAL SHAFT

This is fairly common in all age groups and may be caused by a fall on the outstretched hand or, more usually, by a direct blow.

CLINICAL FEATURES

It is frequently spiral and may be considerably displaced, usually making diagnosis easy.

COMPLICATIONS

The radial nerve is vulnerable as it winds round the shaft of the humerus and is occasionally injured. Rupture of the brachial artery is a rare complication.

TREATMENT

In principle, this consists of using the weight of the arm to realign the fragments (Fig. 14.7). A collar and cuff sling, together with metal gutter-splints surrounding the fracture, extending higher on the lateral side and bandaged in position, is usually adequate. The splints need adjustment

METHODS OF TREATING FRACTURES OF THE HUMERAL SHAFT

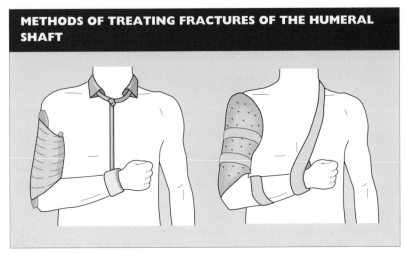

Fig. 14.7

weekly in the early stages. As an alternative, a polythene encircling splint fastened by Velcro strips can be used and the patient can tighten this daily. Immobilization is usually needed for 8–12 weeks. Non-union is relatively uncommon.

Patients who need to be nursed in bed for other injuries may require internal fixation of the fracture with a plate or intramedullary nail. This is usually also necessary if an arterial repair is to be carried out. Severely comminuted fractures may warrant the use of an interlocking intra-medullary nail (p. 69).

For most purposes perfect reduction is not necessary and provided alignment is good, function and appearance will be satisfactory.

CHAPTER 15

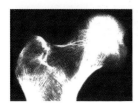

Fractures and dislocations of the elbow and forearm

Injuries around and involving the elbow are very prone to result in stiffness and a long period of mobilization may be necessary to regain full movements, even in children.

DISLOCATION OF THE ELBOW

This is usually produced by a fall on the hand with the elbow partially flexed.

CLINICAL FEATURES

The elbow is swollen and held in a flexed position. The ulna is displaced backwards on the lower end of the humerus (Fig. 15.1). The radial head may be fractured, as may the coronoid process.

COMPLICATIONS

Median nerve palsy occasionally occurs, but the prognosis for recovery is good. Brachial artery damage is rare.

TREATMENT

Reduction is usually easy, sometimes without anaesthesia. The operator, keeping the elbow flexed, puts his fingers around the epicondyles from behind and pushes forwards on the olecranon with his thumbs. The elbow is immobilized for three weeks in a simple sling or collar and cuff, and the patient then mobilizes the joint with or without supervised physiotherapy.

FRACTURE DISLOCATION OF THE ELBOW

This is usually a severe injury, e.g. the 'side-swipe' injury sustained by a blow to the elbow hanging out of a car window. There may be fractures of the condyles of the humerus or the radial head, or, most commonly, of the olecranon. In the worst injuries there may be multiple fractures.

DISLOCATION OF THE ELBOW

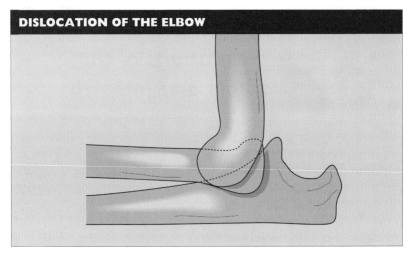

Fig. 15.1

TREATMENT

Manipulative reduction or internal fixation may be necessary, but a stiff elbow is the usual outcome. Attempts are usually made to stabilize the elbow so that early mobilization can be attempted. If it is completely detached or badly shattered, the radial head may need to be removed, but its absence increases the instability. A prosthetic replacement for the head is available.

SUPRACONDYLAR FRACTURE OF THE HUMERUS

This is essentially an injury occurring in childhood, usually arising from a fall on the outstretched hand. The lower fragment is typically displaced and rotated backwards (Fig. 15.2). The elbow usually swells considerably and is held in a semi-flexed position. Crepitus may be felt on attempting to move the joint.

COMPLICATIONS

The sharp anterior margin of the upper fragment may kink the brachial artery which may also be injured if the elbow is flexed before reducing the fracture. The radial pulse is often not palpable, but usually the circulation remains adequate. Nerve injuries are uncommon but both median and ulnar palsies may occur. Late deformity occasionally occurs because of mal-union ('gunstock' deformity).

TREATMENT

This is by manipulation under anaesthesia with X-ray contol. The elbow

SUPRACONDYLAR FRACTURE OF THE HUMERUS

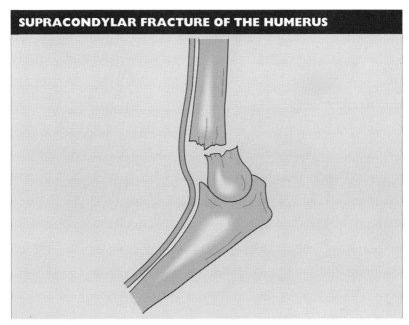

Fig. 15.2

is kept flexed to about 60 degrees and the epicondyles are held between the operator's fingers whilst the fragment is pulled downwards and forwards. The epicondyles must be kept level, otherwise the fracture may unite with a tilt. Having reduced the fracture and checked it by X-rays, the position of the arm in a collar and cuff sling against the chest usually gives reasonably accurate rotation of the lower fragment on the upper. The elbow should not be flexed much above 90 degrees, particularly if swelling is severe.

POST-OPERATIVE MANAGEMENT

The patient is admitted and the circulation in the limb watched over the next 24 hours. The pulse may not return after manipulation, but this in itself is not a cause for alarm, provided the circulation remains adequate.

Pain in the forearm flexor region and particularly on passive extension of the fingers is a warning sign of ischaemia of the forearm muscles. If this is untreated it will result in muscle necrosis and later contracture of the fingers — Volkmann's ischaemic contracture.

If circulation is not restored by extending the elbow, the artery should be explored and if damaged, a segment may need to be resected and grafted.

Occasionally, the fracture is unstable in the flexed position and traction (Fig. 15.3) or even immobilization in extension may be necessary.

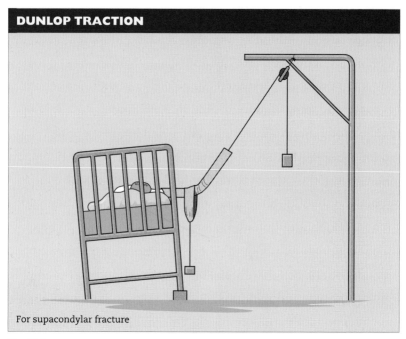

DUNLOP TRACTION

For supacondylar fracture

Fig. 15.3

If instability is difficult to control by an external technique, internal fixation may be the best option. The position can usually be held with two Kirschner wires driven across the fracture line from the lateral side of the distal fragment. They are removed after 3 weeks.

FRACTURES OF THE EPICONDYLES

These injuries usually occur in children from a fall on the arm.

Medial epicondyle

The medial epicondyle may be avulsed by the medial ligament (Fig. 15.4), and when this happens it occasionally becomes trapped in the medial side of the elbow joint and is visible there on a lateral X-ray film (Fig. 15.5).

TREATMENT

Manipulation may be possible by abducting the elbow and attempting to draw out the fragment by extending the wrist and fingers. If this fails, surgery is necessary to extract the fragment from the joint and reposition it. It may be stable in its normal position or may need to be pinned.

FRACTURE OF MEDIAL EPICONDYLE

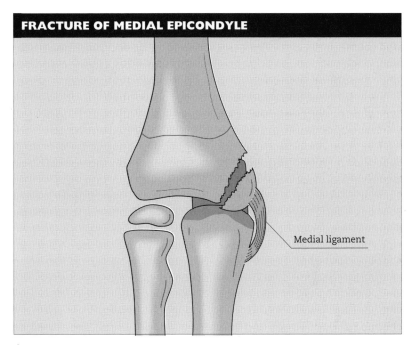

Medial ligament

Fig. 15.4

FRACTURE OF MEDIAL EPICONDYLE

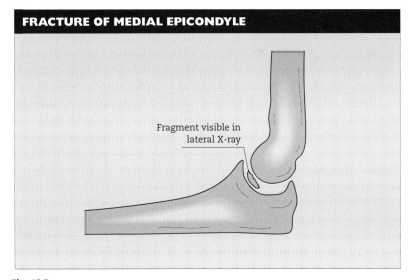

Fragment visible in lateral X-ray

Fig. 15.5

FRACTURE OF LATERAL EPICONDYLE IN A CHILD

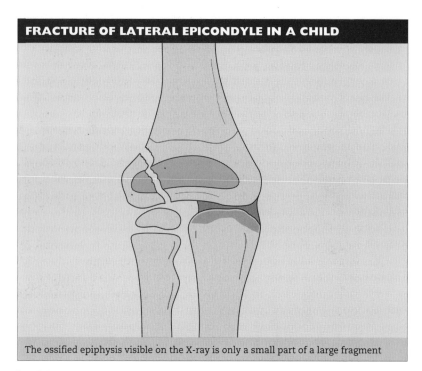

The ossified epiphysis visible on the X-ray is only a small part of a large fragment

Fig. 15.6

Lateral condyle

A fracture of the lateral condyle in a child involves a much larger piece of bone than is obvious on X-ray (Fig. 15.6).

TREATMENT

The fragment usually needs pinning back in position to avoid non-union and later deformity due to interference with the growing epiphysis. In particular, cubitus valgus may occur and this is often associated with ulnar palsy later in life (Chapter 6).

INTERCONDYLAR OR T-SHAPED FRACTURE OF THE HUMERUS

This usually occurs in adults, as a combination of a supracondylar fracture and a vertical break between the two condyles.

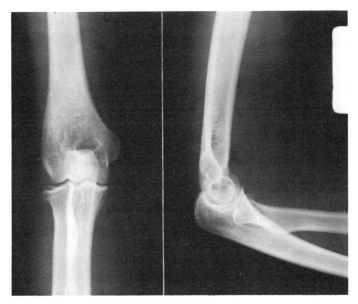

Fig. 15.7 Fracture of the radial head.

TREATMENT

It may be possible to manipulate the fracture, but more usually, the two fragments may need to be internally fixed together and the combined piece fixed to the shaft. Stiffness of the elbow is common, whatever method of treatment is used.

FRACTURES OF THE RADIAL HEAD (Fig. 15.7)

These are essentially produced by abduction injuries in which the head is driven against the capitulum, and the medial ligament is strained.

CLINICAL FEATURES

The elbow is swollen and painful and there is localized tenderness over the radial head and also usually on the medial side. All movements are restricted, particularly, in the severe injuries, pronation and supination.

TREATMENT

Minor cracks and undisplaced fractures may be supported in a sling and mobilized early. Comminuted fractures usually restrict rotation severely and are best treated by excision of the radial head at the earliest opportunity. It is helpful, in deciding whether to excise the head, to check the range of pronation and supination. If this range is good, it is reasonable to leave the head *in situ* and concentrate on mobilizing the elbow.

Single fragments off the head may, if large enough, be suitable for replacement and fixation with a tiny screw or pin. With severe comminution, the radius may move upwards causing subluxation of the inferior radio-ulnar joint. In these circumstances a radial head prosthesis may be useful in restoring joint alignment.

In the child, the radial head represents the epiphysis and may be displaced and tilted. It is often possible to correct this by manipulation and it is then reasonably stable. Open reduction is occasionally needed, but again the fracture is usually stable after reduction. The head should not be excised.

PULLED ELBOW

This is an injury of young children who have been pulled forcibly by the arm. It is caused by the radial head slipping out of the annular ligament, and is usually easily treated by simply rotating the elbow and allowing the head to click into position—a click may be felt once only as the head reduces.

FRACTURE OF THE OLECRANON

This may occur as part of a fracture-dislocation of the elbow, or as an isolated injury. The proximal fragment is usually pulled away from the distal fragment by the triceps muscle (Fig. 15.8).

TREATMENT

In an elderly patient, the position may be accepted and the elbow mobilized in the hope of avoiding stiffness. There will usually be some residual weakness of extension, for example, when reaching up to a shelf above shoulder height.

In all other patients, open reduction and internal fixation using a long screw or the tension-band technique gives the best results and almost full movements may be achieved (Fig. 9.13).

FRACTURE OF THE SHAFTS OF THE RADIUS AND ULNA

These are common and usually caused by direct violence. They are often open. A displaced fracture of the mid-shaft of either bone alone can only

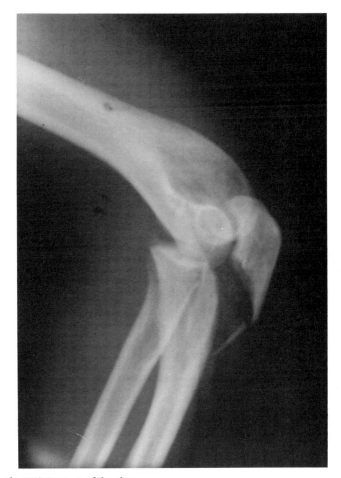

Fig. 15.8 Fracture of the olecranon.

occur if either the radial head subluxates with an ulnar fracture (Monteggia fracture, Fig. 15.9) or the lower end of the ulna subluxates with a fracture of the radius (Galeazzi fracture, Fig. 15.9). Fractures of both bones are more usual.

TREATMENT

Accurate alignment is essential for all these shaft fractures to allow pronation and supination. They are usually treated by open reduction and plating at the earliest opportunity. Following plating, a period of 4–6 weeks in plaster is usual, followed by mobilization of the elbow, wrist and forearm, but avoiding heavy pressure until the fracture is soundly united,

FRACTURES OF THE RADIUS AND ULNA

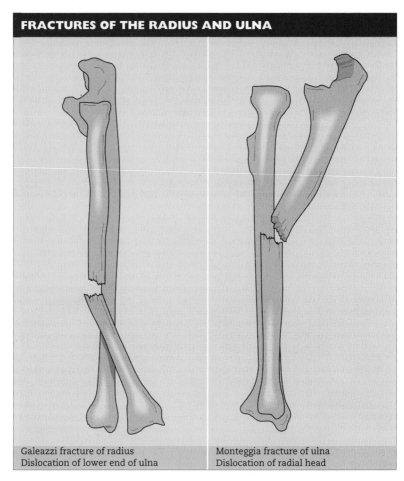

Galeazzi fracture of radius
Dislocation of lower end of ulna

Monteggia fracture of ulna
Dislocation of radial head

Fig. 15.9

e.g. at 12 weeks. Greenstick fractures in children may be manipulated and held in a plaster-cast which must include the wrist and the elbow, bent to 90 degrees, to control rotation of the forearm. Even minor degrees of mal-union may severely restrict pronation and supination. Corrective osteotomies rarely restore normal rotation. Non-union, particularly of ulnar fractures, is fairly common. The risks are lessened by secure internal fixation.

CHAPTER 16

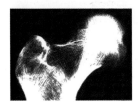

Fractures and dislocations of the wrist and hand

FRACTURE OF THE LOWER END OF THE RADIUS

1 Colles' fracture

The term has come to mean a fracture within 2.3 cm of the lower end of the radius with backward tilt, backward displacement and, often, impaction of the distal fragment producing shortening of the radius and radial deviation of the wrist (Fig. 16.1). The fracture may be comminuted. The styloid process of the ulna is often avulsed by the triangular articular disc so that the inferior radio-ulnar joint is disrupted. It is one of the commonest fractures of middle-age, but is much less common in young adults. The bone is usually porotic and the injury commonly occurs in post-menopausal women. In these circumstances the fracture may be regarded as being pathological.

A Colles' fracture is almost always produced by a fall on the outstretched hand. It produces a characteristic 'dinner fork' deformity of the forearm and wrist (Fig. 16.2).

TREATMENT

If the fracture is only minimally displaced, reduction is not necessary. A useful way of assessing the need for reduction is to draw a line between the two lips of the articular surface of the radius on the lateral film. If this line is at right angles or slightly tilted forwards relative to the line of the radial shaft, then reduction is not necessary. Any backward tilt of this line suggests the need for reduction (Fig. 16.3). Significant backward and proximal shift of the distal fragment with shortening of the radius is also an indication for manipulation, since it is this which is largely responsible for the ugly 'dinner fork' deformity and for the malalignment of the inferior radio-ulnar joint. This is an important joint and there is a risk, if alignment is not restored, of the patient being left with restriction of pronation and supination.

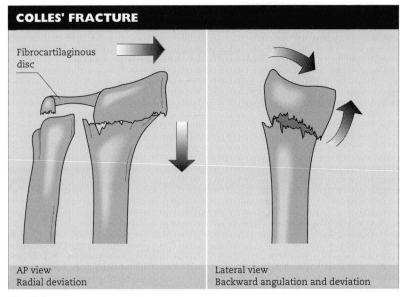

COLLES' FRACTURE

Fibrocartilaginous
disc

AP view
Radial deviation

Lateral view
Backward angulation and deviation

Fig. 16.1

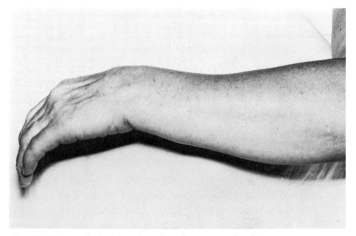

Fig. 16.2 Dinner fork deformity of the forearm and wrist.

The usual method of reducing the fracture is by manipulation under anaesthesia.

A dorsal plaster slab is prepared, of a size sufficient to cover the forearm and wrist to the level of the knuckles and to extend around the sides of the forearm, but not meet at the front. The elbow is held by an

COLLES' FRACTURE–DEGREE OF DISPLACEMENT

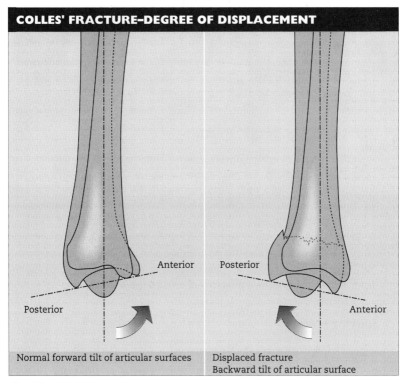

Anterior

Posterior

Posterior

Anterior

Normal forward tilt of articular surfaces

Displaced fracture
Backward tilt of articular surface

Fig. 16.3

assistant and traction is applied to disimpact the distal fragment which is then flexed, pushed forwards and towards the ulnar side. Keeping traction on the thumb in line with the forearm, the slab is applied directly to the skin or over a layer of stockinette, but with no padding and the wrist is held in slight flexion and in ulnar deviation. The slab is held in place with a *wet* gauze bandage and whilst the plaster is setting, the fracture is moulded using the ball of the thumb. A check X-ray is then taken and, if all is well, the arm is supported in a sling. If the fracture is severely comminuted, the cast should be extended above the elbow with the latter flexed to a right angle in order to control forearm rotation and with the forearm in pronation. Swelling is usual, but subsides with use of the hand. It is important to instruct the patient to exercise her fingers by pressing the fingertips into the palm of her hand, and her shoulder by frequently placing her hand behind her neck and behind her back. It is usual to see the patient next day to check the cast and again one week later when an X-ray is taken to check that the position has not been lost.

The plaster may then be completed. The cast is removed at 5 to 6 weeks and exercises started if the tenderness has almost disappeared, as is usual.

In the child, the fracture is usually of the greenstick type and reduction is rarely necessary. Two or three weeks in a plaster slab is sufficient to allow healing to occur.

Complications of Colles' fracture

Median nerve symptoms are not uncommon, but usually subside after reduction. Median nerve compression also occurs occasionally as a late complication of a badly reduced fracture. Malunion may be associated with pain from the subluxated inferior radio-ulnar joint, the pain tending to occur on rotation of the forearm. Occasionally, excision of the lower end of the ulna may be worth considering, but this weakens the wrist and is not always successful in relieving the pain. A residual deformity at the fracture site may also be complicated by rupture of a tendon crossing the fracture line. Sudek's atrophy is a rare complication (p. 74).

2 Smith's fracture

This is a fracture of the lower end of the radius with forward angulation.

TREATMENT

Smith's fracture is usually treated by manipulation under anaesthesia. It is essentially caused by pronation and is, therefore, best held after manipulation in a full-arm cast to control rotation, with the forearm fully supinated. Rarely, the fracture may need a small plate on the front of the radius to control forward displacement.

3 Slipped lower radial epiphysis

This injury is similar to a Colles' fracture, but occurring through the epiphyseal line in a child. It is usually Type II in the Salter and Harris classification (p. 51). It is easy to manipulate if this is done within the first 3 days and 3 weeks' immobilization in a plaster back slab is sufficient.

4 Fractures of the scaphoid

A distinction is made between fractures of the waist and fractures of the tubercle. The injury usually occurs in working men as a result of a blow to the palm of the hand or a fall on the hand.

DIAGNOSIS

This is partly clinical and partly radiological, the main physical signs being swelling and tenderness in the 'anatomical snuff box' with pain on wrist movements and on longitudinal compression of the thumb. In addition to the usual AP and lateral views, oblique or 'scaphoid views' of the wrist are necessary because the fracture may be hairline. It is usually suggested that if the clinical signs suggest a fracture, but the X-ray is negative, the wrist should be immobilized for 1 or 2 weeks, then re-X-rayed, when the fracture will be revealed if present. In practice, if there is a fracture it will almost always be visible on the original films.

COMPLICATIONS

Fractures through the waist may deprive the proximal half of the bone of its blood supply which enters through the distal half. When this occurs, union becomes uncertain and avascular necrosis of the proximal fragment may occur, causing subsequent degeneration of the wrist (Fig. 16.4).

Treatment of scaphoid fractures

The wrist is immobilized in a scaphoid plaster in the neutral position, the plaster extending from elbow to knuckles, including the thumb to the base of the nail (Fig. 16.5). Immobilization must be continued until the clinical signs disappear and there is radiological evidence of union. This takes at least 6 weeks and may take several months. Non-union of a scaphoid fracture may be treated with a bone-graft or screw placed across the fracture line. A useful screw for this purpose has been devised by Herbert. It has threads on each end which are of different pitches, so that when tightened it compresses the fragments together. Internal fixation is occasionally useful for the severely displaced fresh fracture or when the fracture is associated with a dislocation of the wrist.

An established non-union or painful ischaemic necrosis may also necessitate surgery, either excision of the necrotic fragment or the radial styloid or, more effectively, arthrodesis of the wrist. It is worth remembering, however, that many non-unions remain completely symptom-free, and indeed may only be discovered accidentally when the wrist is X-rayed for some other reason.

DISLOCATIONS OF THE CARPUS

These are uncommon injuries but are often missed because of a failure to compare a lateral X-ray with the normal. The whole carpus may be dislocated forwards or backwards and one or more bones of the proximal row may be left *in situ*, usually the lunate (Fig. 16.6). Occasionally, the

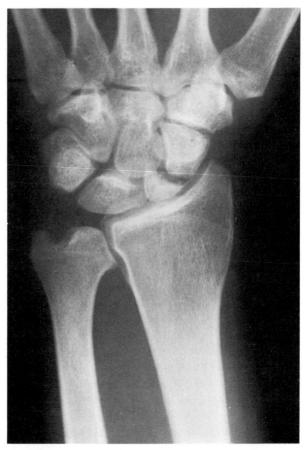

Fig. 16.4 Fracture of the scaphoid–avascular necrosis.

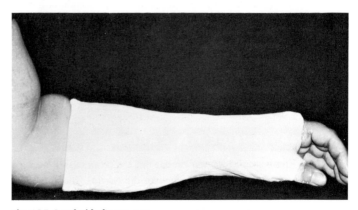

Fig. 16.5 Scaphoid plaster-cast.

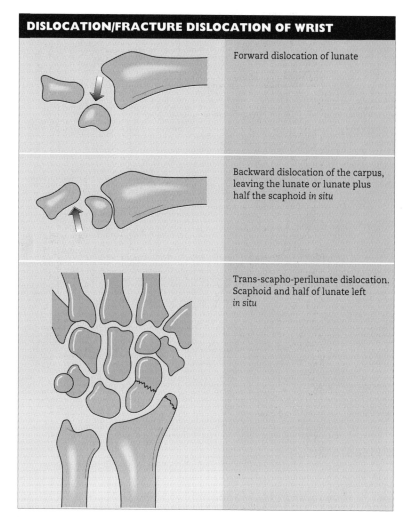

DISLOCATION/FRACTURE DISLOCATION OF WRIST

Forward dislocation of lunate

Backward dislocation of the carpus, leaving the lunate or lunate plus half the scaphoid *in situ*

Trans-scapho-perilunate dislocation. Scaphoid and half of lunate left *in situ*

Fig. 16.6

scaphoid fractures through the waist and, when displacement occurs, the proximal pole of the scaphoid and the whole of the lunate are left behind—trans-scaphoid-perilunate dislocation.

TREATMENT

This is by manipulation or open reduction, followed by immobilization in plaster for approximately 6 weeks. In a trans-scaphoid-perilunate disloca-tion, the scaphoid fracture frequently fails to unite and primary internal fixation of the scaphoid is usually advisable.

BENNETT'S FRACTURE

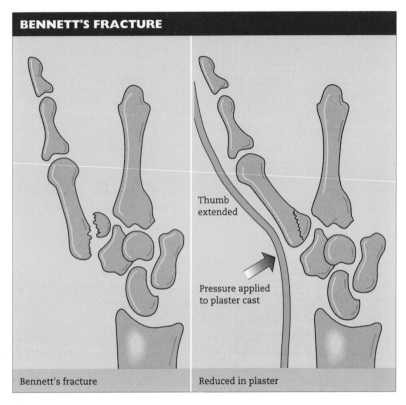

Thumb
extended

Pressure applied
to plaster cast

Bennett's fracture   Reduced in plaster

Fig. 16.7

COMPLICATIONS

Median nerve compression commonly accompanies these injuries.

BENNETT'S FRACTURE

This is a fracture dislocation of the carpo-metacarpal joint of the thumb. It can usually be treated by extending the thumb, applying a plaster-cast and exerting pressure on the base of the thumb whilst the plaster sets (Fig. 16.7). There is a move towards the use of a percutaneous Kirschner wire to stabilize the fragment. Four to six weeks in plaster is usually sufficient for union. Rarely, open reduction may be necessary, in which case the fragment is pinned in position.

FRACTURES OF THE METACARPALS

These are common and frequently stable unless grossly displaced. They usually need little or no manipulation, and may be supported in a plaster slab for 3–4 weeks, allowing the hand to be used whilst union is progressing. It is important that the fracture does not unite with mal-rotation because this affects the plane of finger flexion. Spiral fractures, particularly, may require plating to avoid this complication. A fracture of the neck of the 5th metacarpal often follows a blow with the fist. An attempt is usually made to reduce it by manipulation and it is then held by extending the dorsal slab to include the little finger with the metacarpophalangeal joint in extension. Three weeks in plaster is sufficient.

FRACTURES OF THE PHALANGES

These are serious injuries and are difficult to treat. They are often compound and associated with tendon and nerve damage.

TREATMENT

Fractures of intermediate phalanges can often be manipulated and held by flexing the fingers over a malleable metal splint. Strapping the finger to the adjacent one helps to control rotation, which if it is allowed to occur can severely affect finger flexion and function.

The more difficult fractures, especially at the ends of the bones, may need open reduction and fixation with crossed Kirschner wires. Small plates are available for phalangeal shaft fractures.

Fractures of the terminal phalanges are caused by crush injuries. They are often compound and associated with much damage to the pulp and may result in the nail and bed being lifted off the phalanx. Closed injuries may be treated symptomatically or, if very tense, by removing the nail or boring a hole through it with a hot wire. This usually gives instant relief.

Partial amputation of the tip may be treated by primary split skin-grafts, occasionally by flap grafting, using the thenar eminence as a donor site (Fig. 16.8). It is often simpler to carry out a partial amputation of the phalanx to allow flaps to be fashioned to cover the finger end.

Mallet finger

This is an avulsion injury of the extensor tendon from the base of the terminal phalanx – usually caused by stubbing the finger (Fig. 16.9).

TREATMENT

It is sometimes possible to secure union by using a malleable splint to hyperextend the terminal interphalangeal joint and allow flexion of the proximal interphalangeal joint (Fig. 16.10). Union is more likely to occur if the tendon has avulsed a fragment of bone from the base of the

FLAP GRAFT

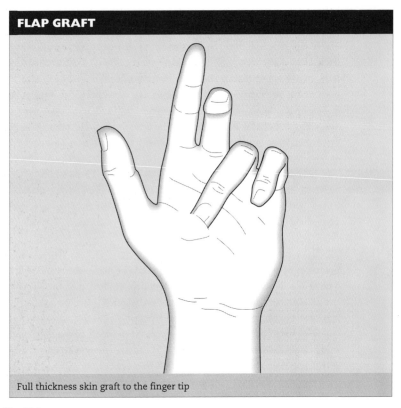

Full thickness skin graft to the finger tip

Fig. 16.8

MALLET FINGER

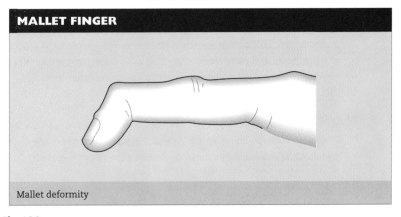

Mallet deformity

Fig. 16.9

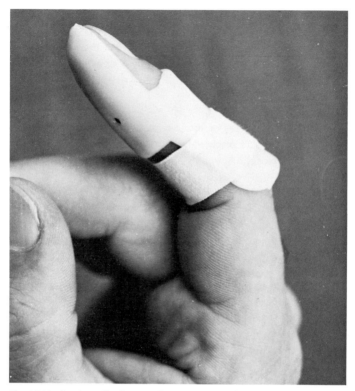

Fig. 16.10 Plastic mallet finger splint.

phalanx. At least six weeks' splintage is usually necessary. Treatment is not always successful and the patient may be left with an extension lag, i.e. the inability to extend the terminal joint actively, even though passive extension is full. This is not usually troublesome, however, if the finger tip tends to 'get in the way', the interphalangeal joint may need fusion later.

Dislocations of the finger joints

These can usually be reduced easily and are reasonably stable. They are supported by strapping adjacent fingers together and movement is allowed immediately.

Rupture of the ulnar collateral ligament of the thumb

Sometimes known as 'gamekeeper's thumb', the injury is a partial or complete rupture of the ulnar collateral ligament of the meta-carpophalangeal joint of the thumb and is caused by forced abduction. If it is unrecognized and allowed to heal with lengthening, it results in instability which interferes with the 'pinch' grip of the thumb against the index finger. It should be suspected if there is tenderness over the ligament and the instability may be demonstrable by comparing with the opposite side.

TREATMENT

Minor degrees of instability, suggesting a strain or partial tear, may be treated in a scaphoid-type plaster-cast. If the instability is obvious, surgical repair, followed by plaster immobilization is advisable.

MANAGEMENT OF HAND INJURIES

All these injuries, especially serious open ones, are prone to stiffness and treatment should aim at early movement and use of the hand as soon as possible.

HAND INJURIES

There are several principles worth remembering:
- severely damaged fingers may be better amputated rather than trying to preserve a finger which may prove to be useless and may interfere with rehabilitation of the hand;
- the index and little fingers contribute most to the power grip;
- as much of the thumb as possible should always be preserved;
- a digit deprived of sensation is almost useless; and
- severe crush injuries of the hand are complex to treat and are best managed in a specialized hand service where decisions as to conservation, internal fixation, reconstruction, rehabilitation, etc., can be based on wide experience.

CHAPTER 17

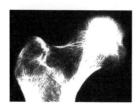

Fractures
of the pelvis

Pelvic fractures are common, particularly following road and industrial accidents. The associated soft-tissue injuries are usually more serious than the fractures themselves.

STABLE FRACTURES

The true pelvis forms a ring structure which is intrinsically stable. Fractures which do not enter the ring or which break it in one place only are stable, e.g. fractures of the iliac wing, or pubic bones (Fig. 17.1a, b, c). They may be associated with bleeding, but other complications are rare.

TREATMENT

This consists of rest until the patient can walk, usually after 2–3 weeks.

UNSTABLE FRACTURES

These are fractures in which the pelvic ring is disrupted in two or more places, one of which is above the level of the hip, e.g. through the waist of the ilium, the sacro-iliac joint or sacrum. Various combinations are possible (Fig. 17.1e, f, g). Many of these injuries are produced by compression forces, either from front to back or from side to side, as may occur if the patient is crushed by machinery or run over by a vehicle. A double fracture below the level of the hip joints is technically unstable, but may be treated as stable (Fig. 17.1d).

DISPLACEMENT

The pelvis may open like an oyster or one side may be displaced upwards—hindquarter dislocation. Either of these is likely to be associated with bladder or urethral damage. Occasionally, if the fracture is produced by side-to-side compression, the fragments of the pelvic ring may overlap, narrowing the ring. In addition to standard AP X-ray films, inlet and outlet views of the pelvis may be necessary to make an accurate diagnosis.

FRACTURES OF THE PELVIS

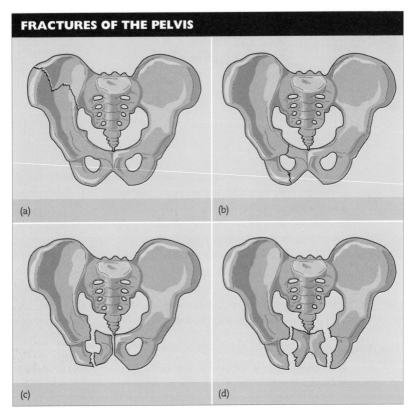

Fig. 17.1

TREATMENT

The management of the fractures themselves is usually relatively simple, but that of the complications is much more difficult. The unstable oyster-type fracture will often close if the patient is turned on one side and the hindquarter dislocation can usually be manipulated under anaesthesia by applying traction to the leg. Some form of fixation is required and the current trend is to use a specially designed external frame with bone screws introduced at various points around the iliac crest (Fig. 17.2). This technique, if properly applied, gives firm fixation. It may then be possible to mobilize the patient, although standing and walking is not usually advised for the first few weeks.

If a suitable frame or the necessary expertise is not available, the fracture can be held reduced by nursing the patient on pelvic slings (Fig. 17.3) with traction on the legs. These are so arranged that the weight of the patient with the sling underneath the buttocks causes the sides of the sling to compress the pelvis and close the fracture. Sufficient weight is

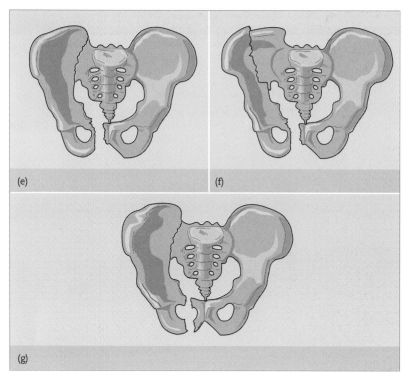

(e)

(f)

(g)

Fig. 17.1 (*Continued*)

used just to support the patient off the bed. The legs are flexed to prevent their tendency to roll outwards. Pelvic slings are not appropriate for side-to-side compression injuries since they may cause the pelvis to unite in a distorted position.

The unstable fracture usually requires 12 weeks of fixation before stability is achieved. If the sacro-iliac joint has been damaged by the fracture, the patient may later complain of chronic pain in this area and fusion of the joint may become necessary. Distortion of the true pelvis does not usually cause symptoms, but may interfere with childbirth.

COMPLICATIONS

Haemorrhage

All pelvic fractures produce some bleeding, but this can be catastrophic from the large plexus of vessels which line the inside of the pelvis.

FIXATION WITH EXTERNAL FRAME (ORTHOFIX)

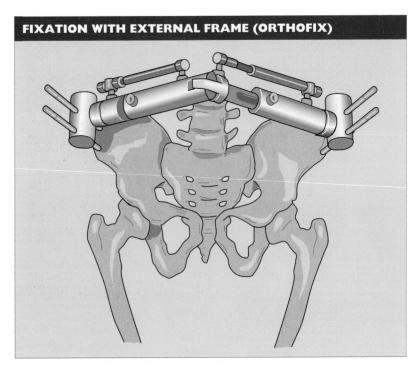

Fig. 17.2 Courtesy of EBI Medical Systems Ltd.

Internal bleeding can be recognized by the usual signs of impending shock and by the palpation of a mass in the supra-public region and particularly on rectal examination. Pelvic bleeding is one of the causes of shock which should be considered in the patient with multiple injuries and an X-ray of the pelvis is usually regarded as routine in such patients. If there is a palpable supra-public mass this should be marked on the abdomen to assess whether it is increasing in size.

TREATMENT

This involves blood transfusion, sometimes massive, and often, for this reason, requiring fresh blood. Stabilizing the fracture helps to control the bleeding and should be done as soon as possible. If frame fixation is not readily available, pelvic slings may be used as a temporary measure or for definitive treatment. If control of the bleeding is not achieved, surgical exploration is likely to be necessary. It may be possible to ligate a major bleeding vessel or, alternatively, the wound may have to be packed. Control may still not be possible and death can occur from exsanguination.

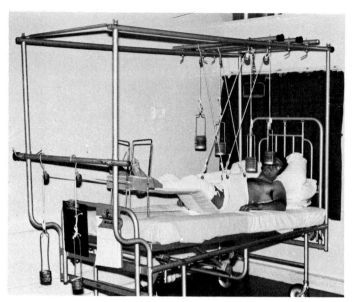

Fig. 17.3 The method of using pelvic slings.

Injuries to bladder and urethra

These are common and diagnosis may be difficult. The badly injured patient may not be able to pass urine for many reasons, such as fear, shock or pain, as well as damage to the bladder or urethra.

TYPES OF INJURY

The bladder may be ruptured either intra- or extra-peritoneally. The urethra may be ruptured anywhere along its length in the male, but particularly at the junction of the prostatic and membranous parts.

DIAGNOSIS

The patient may be asked to pass urine, but not to persist if the attempt fails. Percussion of the bladder is helpful in that a distended bladder cannot have been ruptured, but urethral injury is still a possibility. Rectal examination may reveal a pelvic swelling representing blood in the Pouch of Douglas. With a rupture of the membranous urethra, the prostate may be displaced upwards and be impalpable. There may be bleeding from the urethra.

Investigations and treatment

There are at least two schools of thought.

1 A soft catheter is passed gently down the urethra. If this passes easily into the bladder and a moderate quantity of clear or slightly bloodstained urine is obtained, the system is usually intact and the catheter is left *in situ*. If the catheter fails to pass, this may be because the urethra is damaged. In this case there is often bleeding *per urethram* and bruising in the perineum. Urethroscopy may be helpful in making the diagnosis. If the catheter passes into the bladder and blood or a very small quantity of urine is obtained, the bladder may be ruptured and a cystogram is advisable. In either of these cases surgical exploration will be necessary.

2 Catheterization is considered dangerous and supra-pubic drainage is established if the patient fails to pass urine. The bladder or urethral rupture is then investigated at leisure and repaired as appropriate.

Injuries to the rectum

These are less common. They may be suspected by the presence of bleeding *per rectum* and diagnosed by rectal examination and sigmoidoscopy. They are usually treated by suture and a temporary colostomy.

Vaginal injuries

These are also uncommon. They are treated by suture.

Sciatic nerve injuries

These are relatively uncommon. Recovery may occur, but occasionally the nerve is trapped in the fracture and persistent pain may result. Exploration may be necessary to free it.

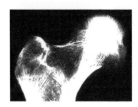

CHAPTER 18

Fractures and dislocations of the hip and femur

The hip joint is anatomically strong, but dislocation can occur, usually as a result of considerable violence.

Fractures occur both in the pelvic and femoral components of the hip joint.

These injuries are often caused by car accidents in which a front seat traveller is involved in a head-on collision and strikes his knee under the dashboard. Depending on the degree of flexion of the hip, a simple dislocation may occur or there may be a fracture dislocation involving the head or acetabulum. The acetabular fracture may be through the back, the floor or, less commonly, the front of the acetabulum.

DISLOCATION OF THE HIP

Simple dislocation of the hip is usually posterior. It is very rare in children. The patient presents with the leg flexed, adducted and short-ened and the femoral head may be palpable in the buttock (Fig. 18.1). The sciatic nerve, particularly the lateral popliteal division, may be damaged.

TREATMENT

Reduction is usually easy. It is carried out under general anaesthesia with the patient lying supine, preferably on the floor or a low couch, and by flexing the hip and simply lifting the head of the femur into the joint. Once reduced, it is usually stable and the leg is then held on longitudinal skin traction for 3 weeks to allow the capsule to heal, followed by a further 3 weeks of protected weight-bearing. Stiffness of the joint is rarely a problem.

FRACTURE DISLOCATION OF THE HIP

The acetabulum can be regarded as being formed from a strong roof, an anterior or ilio-pubic column and a posterior or ilio-ischial column (Fig. 18.2a). On this basis, fractures of the acetabulum can be classified into four simple groups (Judet, p. 134).

POSTERIOR DISLOCATION OF THE HIP

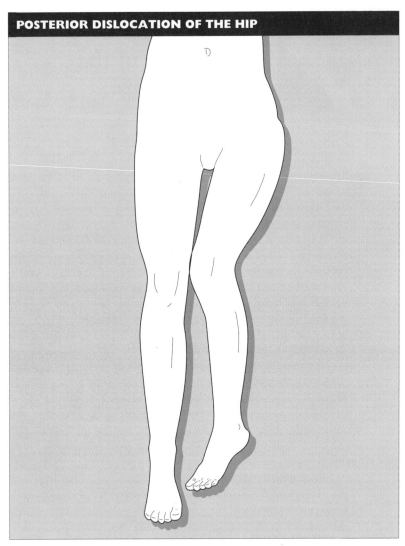

Fig. 18.1

JUDET FRACTURE GROUPS

1 fracture of the posterior rim (Fig. 18.2b);
2 fracture of the ilio-ischial column (Fig. 18.2c);
3 transverse fracture (Fig. 18.2d); and
4 fracture of the ilio-pubic column (Fig. 18.2e).

In each case the femoral head tends to subluxate or dislocate from its normal relationship with the pelvis considered as a whole.

Fracture of the posterior rim (Fig. 18.2b)

Stability after reduction depends on the size of the posterior fragment. If the hip is easily re-dislocated, the posterior fragment will need internal fixation with a screw.

Other fracture dislocations of the hip

Fractures in Judet groups 2, 3 and 4 above are often, sometimes rather inaccurately, called 'central' dislocations of the hip.

The fracture should be assessed fully by taking standard antero-posterior, lateral, and several oblique X-rays, the latter taken with the patient rotated in a vertical axis through 45 degrees. These will give an indication of the procedures which will be necessary to restore the continuity of the acetabulum. Computed tomography (CT) scanning may also be helpful.

Rarely, a dislocation of the hip is complicated by a fracture of the femoral head. A large fragment may need to be fixed in position and a small fragment excised.

TREATMENT

Some of these fractures may be treated adequately by applying traction to the leg. This may reduce the head and cause the fragments to realign themselves. If the reduction is reasonably good, the traction will need to be maintained for 12 weeks until union of the fragments occurs. In some cases, on applying traction to the leg, the femoral head may reduce, leaving the fragments displaced. The head is then prone to re-dislocate. In this case, open reduction and internal fixation of the fragments may be necessary, but the technique is exacting and perfect reduction may not be achieved. Even severe degrees of residual displacement of acetabular fractures can allow surprisingly good hip function. There is an increasing tendency to refer patients with severely displaced acetabular fractures to centres specializing in these injuries. This can be done after the patient's condition has been stabilized.

FRACTURES OF THE FEMORAL NECK

These are essentially injuries of the elderly and the bones are frequently osteoporotic. They are, therefore, pathological fractures. Femoral neck fractures occasionally occur through normal bone in younger patients and, very rarely, in children.

The mental and social condition of the patient at the time of injury is all-important in determining the ultimate outcome of all femoral neck fractures. Relatively few patients return to full mobility following these

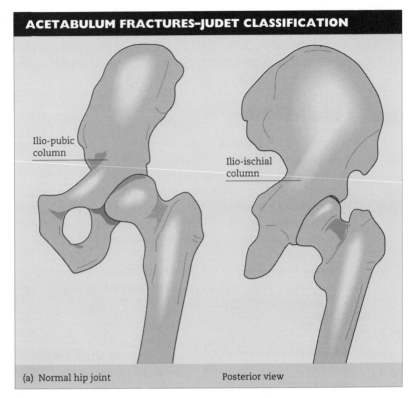

ACETABULUM FRACTURES–JUDET CLASSIFICATION

Ilio-pubic column

Ilio-ischial column

(a) Normal hip joint   Posterior view

Fig. 18.2

injuries. Fractures of the femoral neck in children and young adults carry a much worse prognosis from the point of view of vascularity of the head.

Intracapsular fracture

This type of fracture occurs through the femoral neck usually just below the head. Good quality X-rays, especially a lateral film, are necessary for accurate diagnosis, particularly if the fracture is undisplaced or impacted. The typical displacement is for the leg to slip into external rotation and adduction which makes it easily distinguishable from a dislocation.

CLINICAL FEATURES

The injury is often relatively minor, such as a stumble and it is probable that at least some of these fractures actually occur before the fall, causing it, rather than being produced by it. Occasionally, the patient may still be able to walk on the limb, but restriction of movement at the hip is usual.

ACETABULUM FRACTURES (CONTINUED)

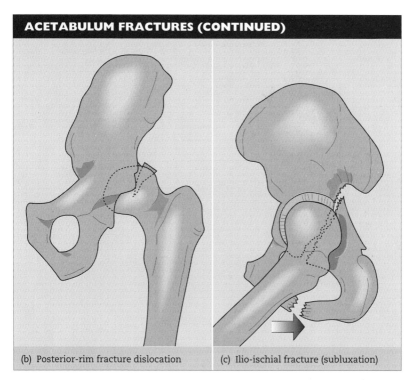

(b) Posterior-rim fracture dislocation   (c) Ilio-ischial fracture (subluxation)

Fig. 18.2 (*Continued*)

COMPLICATIONS

Because the fracture is intracapsular, the blood supply to the head, which reaches it via the neck, may be interrupted (Fig. 18.3). This makes healing less certain and may result in ischaemic necrosis of the head, even if union is successful. There is no reliable method of assessing the vascularity of the head, but grossly displaced or long-standing, unreduced fractures may be presumed to have a poor prognosis.

TREATMENT

The survival of the patient is the first consideration with this fracture which carries a poor prognosis for life, 30–40% of patients dying within the following 6 months.

Virtually all authorities believe that early mobilization is essential to avoid the complications of long periods in bed.

Essentially, two methods of treatment are available.

I Manipulation of the fracture and internal fixation. Many methods are available. The simple Smith–Peterson trifin nail which used to be widely used has been superseded by various kinds of screws, sliding nails, etc. With all these devices it is difficult to get a good grip on the proximal

ACETABULUM FRACTURES (CONTINUED)

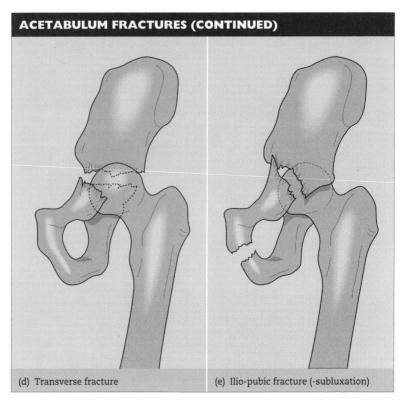

(d) Transverse fracture | (e) Ilio-pubic fracture (-subluxation)

Fig. 18.2 (*Continued*)

fragment. The Garden Screw technique can give good fixation if correctly used and fixation with three cannulated screws is also satisfactory (Fig. 18.4).

2 The femoral head may be excised and replaced by a prosthesis of the Moore or Thompson type (Fig. 18.5). This technique may also be used following failed internal fixation.

The mortality of immediate surgery is high and it is usual to spend 2–3 days assessing the patient's general condition and correcting any medical problems. During this time, if the fracture is to be fixed it can be reduced gradually and simply by applying traction and internal rotation (Wainwright). The decision can then be made, on the basis of check X-rays, to fix the fracture or to replace the head.

Some surgeons nail the less displaced fractures and replace the more severely displaced ones. Others make the decision mainly on age, tending to replace the head in patients over seventy. Any fracture which has been left displaced for more than 24 hours can be presumed to have a bad prognosis and replacement is advisable. In the best hands, internal fixation can give up to 90% union, but a proportion of the united heads

INTRACAPSULAR FRACTURE

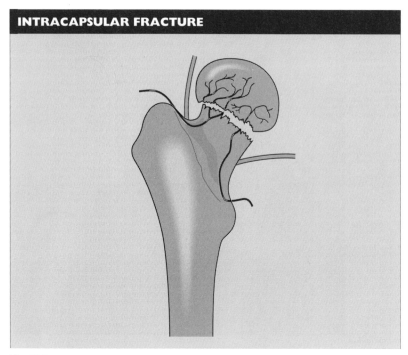

Fig. 18.3

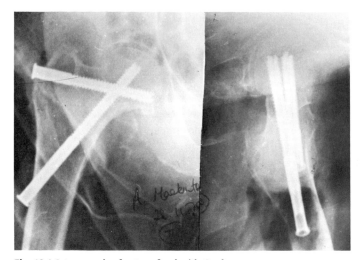

Fig. 18.4 Intracapsular fracture fixed with Garden screws.

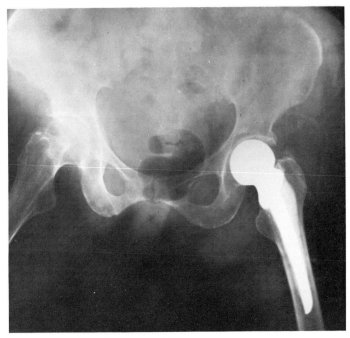

Fig. 18.5 Thomson hip prothesis.

will disintegrate from ischaemia and some of these will require later replacement because of pain.

Following the nailing or replacement procedure the patient can walk with support, but mobilization is usually very slow.

INTER-TROCHANTERIC FRACTURES

These fractures occur through the base of the neck in the inter-trochanteric region (Fig. 18.6). They usually affect the somewhat younger patient. Because the blood supply is adequate, they tend to unite without difficulty. The physical signs are similar to the intracapsular fracture and X-ray diagnosis usually presents no problems.

TREATMENT

For the younger patient, traction for 3 months in bed may be satisfactory, although it is rarely the preferred option these days. For the older patient, bed rest is inadvisable and internal fixation is usually employed. Many devices are available. The simple nail plate (Fig. 18.7), which used to be widely used, does not give adequate fixation for all types of inter-trochanteric fracture and inadequate fixation allows the fracture to drop

INTER-TROCHANTERIC FRACTURE

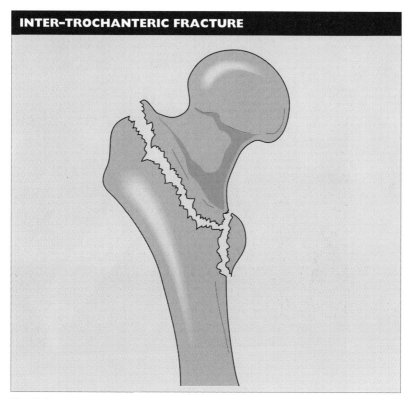

Fig. 18.6

into varus on weight-bearing. Modern devices allow the nail to slide along a holder which is part of the plate. This allows the fracture to compact during weight-bearing. The Richard's screw works on this principle (Fig. 18.8).

FRACTURES OF THE FEMORAL SHAFT

This fracture is common in all age groups. The fracture occurs at various levels in the shaft and is frequently compound and associated with other injuries. The diagnosis is usually obvious.

COMPLICATIONS

Gross swelling should arouse suspicion of a rupture of the femoral artery. Shock is rare with an isolated fracture, but blood replacement may be necessary. Sciatic nerve injury occasionally occurs.

TREATMENT

The aim of treatment is to restore length and alignment and to encourage

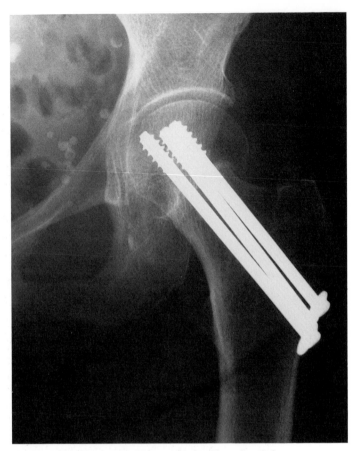

Fig. 18.7 AO screw fixation of intracapsular femoral neck fracture.

union and early rehabilitation. Few fractures can be treated in more diverse ways. Anatomical reduction is not essential, provided alignment is good. Slight overlap of less than 1 cm is not detrimental. In a child, if anatomical reduction is obtained, slight overgrowth may occur but this usually corrects before maturity, as does a moderate length deficiency. Manipulation under anaesthesia is usually followed by one of the following methods of fixation.

1 Fixed traction, in a Thomas knee splint (pp. 60, 63) with countertraction, against the ischial tuberosity. If skeletal traction is needed, the splint is modified with a Pearson knee attachment. The Thomas splint requires attention to detail and careful nursing if complications are to be avoided and good position maintained.

2 Sliding traction, usually with the thigh supported on a frame or on pillows (p. 66). Gallows traction is appropriate for infants (Fig. 9.7).

3 A plaster hip spica extending from toes to the level of the chest. This

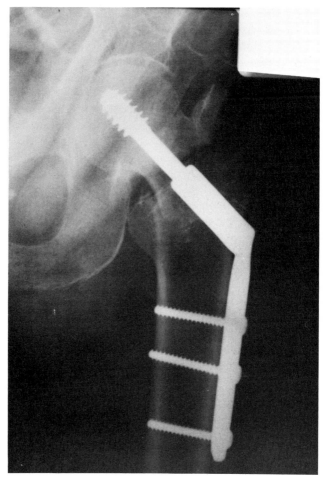

Fig. 18.8 Richard's screw and plate fixation of an inter-trochanteric fracture.

is uncomfortable and gives relatively poor fixation. It is now rarely used except in children.

4 The cast-brace. This is a technique which employs a closely fitting full-leg plaster moulded around the thigh and including a hinge at the knee. It permits weight bearing after 2–3 weeks. It has its advocates, but appears to be giving way to internal fixation.

5 Internal fixation. The Kuntscher intramedullary nail is of historical interest (p. 68). It was designed to allow accurate reduction and to enable mobilization of the joints and the patient. It relied on the principle of three-point fixtion and was usually introduced through the fracture site, which involved opening the fracture, thereby increasing the risk of infection and subsequent osteomyelitis. This is a serious complication which may interfere with union and cause long-term drainage even when the nail is removed.

Modern techniques, requiring X-ray control, introduce the nail by a closed method through the upper end of the femur. Their proponents claim the highest percentage of successful results of all methods. Simple intramedullary nailing, which depends on a close fit within the medullary canal, is not suitable for all fractures because of the widening of the canal below the middle of the bone allowing rotation of the distal fragment to occur around the nail. To overcome this problem, the so-called 'interlocking' nail has been introduced and has extended the scope of nailing to more difficult fractures, sometimes with extensive bone loss. There are various designs, but in principle the nail is provided with transverse screws passing through the femoral cortices and the upper and lower end of the nail. This gives very firm fixation and, if required, the upper screws can be left out or removed to allow a little telescoping movement at the fracture site to stimulate union (Fig. 9.12).

Internal fixation is usually indicated for multiple fractures, pathological fractures and vascular injuries, but is now being used for simpler fractures and is proving to be safe provided theatre facilities are good and technique is meticulous.

Twelve to sixteen weeks is the normal time for union of a femoral shaft fracture to occur. If external fixation has been used, it is often wise to protect the fracture for a further period in a cast-brace. Internal fixation normally allows full weight-bearing from about 3–4 weeks.

Knee stiffness is common with most methods of treatment, but usually disappears with exercise.

FRACTURES OF THE LOWER SHAFT AND SUPRACONDYLAR FRACTURES

These are difficult fractures to manage. The lower the fracture, the more the fragment tends to be pulled out of alignment by the gastrocnemius attachments. They are common in elderly patients and are often comminuted or T-shaped.

TREATMENT

These fractures can sometimes be held in fixed traction by a Thomas splint. If traction is used, it will usually be needed for 12 weeks, although a cast-brace may be used in the later stages. Internal fixation is often a better option, although difficult with the porotic bone of elderly patients. It usually involves introducing a nail into the distal fragment, if necessary fixing several fragments together with screws, connected to a plate applied to the side of the femur.

CHAPTER 19

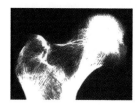

Fractures and dislocations of the knee and tibia

This is a rare injury. It is inevitably associated with rupture of ligaments and the direction of dislocation is variable. It may be associated with damage to the popliteal artery and careful assessment of the vascularity of the limb should be carried out, if necessary by arteriography.

TREATMENT

Reduction by manipulation is usually easy, although occasionally, open reduction and ligament repair may be necessary. After reduction, immobilization on traction for 1–2 weeks, followed by controlled mobilization in a cast-brace for up to 6 weeks is usually adequate. Persistent instability may be a problem, necessitating an attempt at ligament reconstruction.

DISLOCATION OF THE PATELLA

This is an injury of children and young adults, usually from a fall or blow to the side of the knee. The patella dislocates laterally and the knee remains flexed until the patella is reduced. The injury involves a tear of the medial capsule and quadriceps expansion. Some knees seem to be prone to recurrent dislocation and patients with this tendency exhibit the so-called 'apprehension sign' if an attempt is made to dislocate the patella laterally (Chapter 28).

TREATMENT

Reduction can usually be achieved by straightening the knee. A short period in a cast or firm bandage to allow the capsule to heal can be followed by active mobilization.

LIGAMENTOUS INJURIES AROUND THE KNEE

The cruciate ligaments and the collateral ligaments are frequently strained or torn, especially in sportsmen. Incomplete healing may lead to long-term instability of the joint, with a feeling of 'giving way'.

1 Strains of the collateral ligaments

These are common following sporting injuries. They are usually associated with an acute effusion in the knee and tenderness over the damaged ligament. Stressing the ligament causes pain, but the joint remains stable.

TREATMENT

These injuries usually settle with a short period of rest, followed by support and exercises.

2 Complete ruptures of the collateral ligaments

These are diagnosed by demonstrating clinical instability and by stress X-rays, carried out best under anaesthesia. When tested by varus or valgus stressing, an isolated collateral ligament rupture will not result in significant instability if the test is performed with the knee fully extended, but at 10 degrees of flexion there will be significant opening of the joint on the damaged side. If, in addition, one of the cruciates is torn then the joint will open widely on the affected side, even in full extension.

3 Anterior cruciate tears

A tear of the anterior cruciate frequently accompanies a tear of the medial meniscus and may also accompany a tear of the medial ligament. The diagnosis is made by the presence of an effusion or haemarthrosis and by a positive 'draw sign' (Fig. 19.1). The 'Lachman test' may be a more sensitive indicator in some cases (p. 367). An isolated anterior cruciate rupture may not produce sufficient instability to give a positive draw sign.

4 Posterior cruciate tears

Posterior cruciate tears are unusual except when associated with a collateral tear and a tear of the posterior capsule. Posterior instability is diagnosed by the posterior 'set back' when testing for the draw sign (p. 367).

DIAGNOSIS AND TREATMENT OF LIGAMENTOUS RUPTURES

All these injuries can be difficult to diagnose accurately and the current trend is to classify them in terms of the direction of instability e.g., lateral,

DIAGNOSIS OF AN ANTERIOR CRUCIATE TEAR

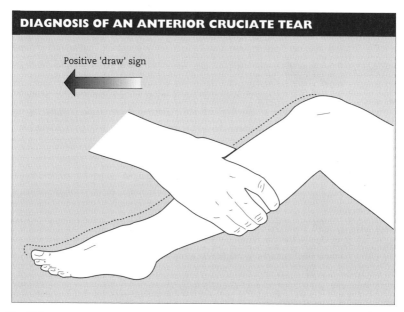

Positive 'draw' sign

Fig. 19.1

postero-medial, etc. It is usually advisable to carry out a full examination under anaesthesia to assess what type or combination of instability is present.

There is no general agreement as to the best way to deal with the various injuries. Repair of isolated cruciate ruptures by simple suture is often unsuccessful unless the ligament has avulsed a fragment of the tibial tuberosity (usually in young people), in which case this may be fixed back surgically with a reasonable chance of union. An isolated anterior cruciate rupture with no significant collateral instability is usually treated conservatively, either in a plaster cylinder or by using a brace designed to allow some movement while protecting against excessive stress on the ligament. Isolated collateral ligament ruptures may also be treated in the same way, but an attempt is often made to suture the ligament. Complex multiple ligament injuries are usually treated by surgical repair, but the results are unpredictable at best, and there is often persistent instability when knee movements are regained. There is general agreement that a long period of protection is necessary following ligament repair, usually in a cast-brace or similar orthosis.

The treatment of chronic ligamentous instability of the knee has become a specialized field involving accurate diagnosis and multiple reconstructive procedures. Attempts have been made to stimulate the regeneration of new ligaments using such materials as carbon and plastic fibres and there are a number of ligament substitutes on the market. These can give good early function, particularly valued by the professional sportsman, but their long-term effects have not been evaluated. At the moment, the trend appears to be to use autogenous materials for grafting, a strip of patellar tendon being the favoured material for replacing the damaged cruciates. Anchoring the graft to bone sufficiently to allow early stressing presents some problems, but the long-term aim is for the graft to be re-vascularized and, in effect, to form a new ligament. In order to do this some controlled longitudinal stress appears to be important. In skilled hands, the repair can be carried out arthroscopically which makes early mobilization much easier.

Many patients can, to some extent, overcome instability and the tendency for the knee to give way by developing the quadriceps and hamstring muscles by vigorous exercise, making surgery unnecessary.

FRACTURES OF THE PATELLA

These are of two types.

1 The comminuted fracture

This type of fracture is caused by a direct blow, often against the parcel shelf of a car. There is likely to be damage to the underlying femoral condyles (Fig. 19.2).

TREATMENT

If the fragments are severely displaced, the patella is best excised and the quadriceps tendon reconstituted. After 3 weeks in a plaster cylinder, physiotherapy is needed to mobilize the knee and regain quadriceps power.

2 The avulsion or transverse fracture

This is caused by violent contraction of the quadriceps against resistance (Fig. 19.3). The patella is frequently torn in two horizontally, and the split extends laterally into the quadriceps expansion.

TREATMENT

Open reduction is carried out and the position held with a circumferential wire suture or a longitudinal screw. Mobilization is possible after 3 weeks in a plaster cylinder.

STAR-SHAPED FRACTURE OF THE PATELLA

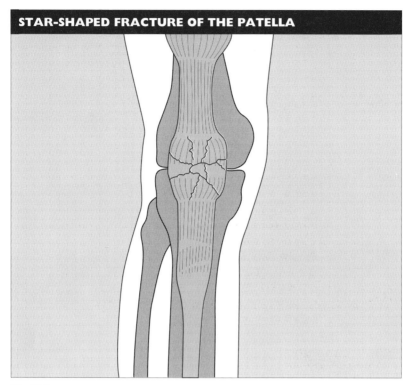

Fig. 19.2

A late complication following any patellar fracture may be osteoarthritis of the patello-femoral compartment, usually leading to generalized osteoarthritis of the knee.

Rupture of the quadriceps or patellar tendon

The same mechanism which causes a transverse fracture of the patella may also result in a transverse rupture of the quadriceps tendon just above the patella, or alternatively, of the patellar tendon. Occasionally, the tibial tubercle is avulsed by the patellar tendon. These injuries tend to occur in middle age. Diagnosis rests on the inability of the patient to extend the knee actively and on the palpation of a gap in the tendon.

TREATMENT

Surgical suture is required for these injuries with protection in a plaster cylinder for 3 weeks, then mobilization with physiotherapy.

TRANSVERSE FRACTURE OF THE PATELLA

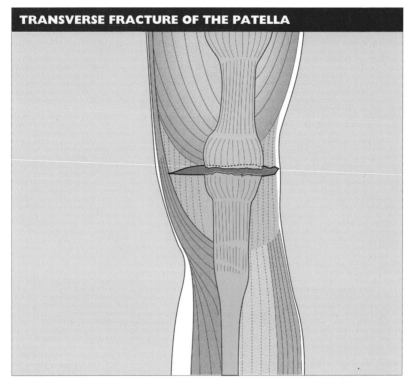

Fig. 19.3

FRACTURES OF THE UPPER TIBIA

Fractures of the intercondylar region are essentially avulsion injuries and have been mentioned in connection with the anterior cruciate ligament.

Fractures of one or other condyle are usually caused by a forcible valgus or varus strain, e.g. by being struck by a car bumper (Fig. 19.4). The knee fills with blood and may feel unstable on lateral and medial stressing.

TREATMENT

If the fractured condyle is not depressed more than 2 mm, the knee may be mobilized using a CPM device (p. 414) or, if this is not available, a sliding traction system. More severe depression is treated by open elevation of the joint surface and a bone-graft to fill the underlying defect. A transverse screw may be used to maintain the elevated position. In some cases the procedure can be carried out arthroscopically. Mobilization should be encouraged as early as possible to avoid stiffness, and a cast-brace is useful to provide protection when the patient leaves hospital.

FRACTURE OF THE MEDIAL TIBIAL CONDYLE

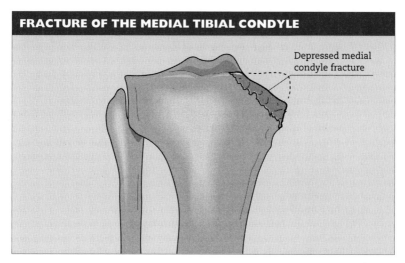

Depressed medial
condyle fracture

Fig. 19.4

A late complication is osteoarthritis of the damaged half of the joint.

FRACTURES OF THE TIBIAL SHAFT AND FIBULA

These are extremely common injuries in all age groups and are frequently open, sometimes with a very extensive and contaminated wound. They often follow road traffic and sporting accidents. Diagnosis is easy. The X-ray gives some indication of the mechanism of injury and of the likely stability of the fracture after reduction. Oblique and spiral fractures of the tibia are usually unstable after reduction. If the fibula is not fractured, closed reduction of the fracture of the tibia may be difficult and if conservative treatment is adopted there is always a tendency for the tibial fracture to displace into a varus position. In these circumstances internal fixation may be preferred.

TREATMENT OF FRACTURES OF THE TIBIA AND FIBULA

Wound management is all-important in securing early union of open fractures. The wound is treated in the usual manner and closed as quickly as possible. Grossly contaminated wounds are usually best left open after removal of all necrotic and foreign material. Plastic surgical techniques, using rotated or free full thickness grafts with vascular anastomosis, often incorporating muscle, have become important in achieving early soft-tissue healing.

Transverse tibial shaft fractures are reasonably stable when reduced, with little tendency to shorten. They can usually be held in a well-fitting full leg plaster-cast with the knee flexed to 20–30 degrees to prevent rotation at the fracture site.

If the tibial fracture is spiral or comminuted, some means must be found to prevent shortening. A full leg plaster-cast alone is rarely sufficient. There are many possibilities and the choice will often depend on available resources and facilities.

1 Internal fixation is becoming the most popular choice for most unstable tibial fractures, its proponents claiming earlier mobilization, more certain union and better alignment. Plating, usually with a compression plate, has been widely used, but has now largely given way to intramedullary nailing, particularly with locking nails (p. 49). The complication rate, however, can be high with any form of internal fixation and infection is a constant risk, particularly if the fracture is compound. Considerable expertise is needed to obtain consistently good results from internal fixation and if this is lacking or theatre facilities are poor, conservative management is often the safer option.

2 Internal fixation carries particular risks if the fracture is associated with an extensive or badly contaminated wound. In these circumstances frame fixation, with pins placed above and below the fracture (p. 71) gives good fixation and allows access to the wound for dressing, grafting etc. This type of fracture is often slow to unite and union may be further inhibited by rigid fixation (p. 75). Frames which allow controlled mobility of the fracture in the early stages may prove better in this respect.

3 Conservative treatment usually relies on some kind of plaster-cast fixation. One technique involves the application of a below-knee cast with a Steinmann pin through the os calcis or lower tibia to apply traction with the leg supported on a Braun frame. After 3 weeks, the fracture is usually stable, traction can be discontinued and the cast can be completed above the knee (see Fig. 9.3) or a cast-brace may be used (see below). An alternative is to insert transverse Steinmann pins through the bone above and below the fracture, often with the lower pin through the os calcis, and to embed these in the plaster-cast (Fig. 19.5).

4 A close-fitting cast-brace which allows knee movement (Sarmiento) can give good results, but needs considerable expertise. Weight-bearing is permitted after 3 weeks.

Methods 1, 2 and 4 allow early mobilization of the ankle and knee and enable to patient to walk, initially non-weight-bearing.

LENGTH OF TREATMENT

Opinions vary as to when weight-bearing should be started. Most tibial

TRANSVERSE STEINMANN PINS EMBEDDED IN PLASTER CAST

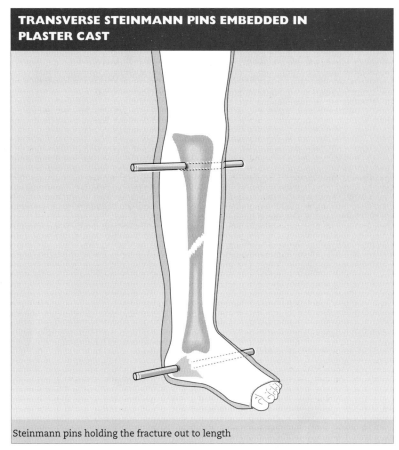

Steinmann pins holding the fracture out to length

Fig. 19.5

fractures require at least 3 months' immobilization and may take 5 or more months to unite. If the fracture is stable, particularly after intramedullary nailing, weight-bearing can be started almost immediately. In other cases it is usually delayed for at least 6 weeks. There is evidence

COMPLICATIONS

- Non-union of tibial fractures is common, especially when complicated by infection.
- Some degree of ischaemia of the deep muscles of the calf is common and may result in the patient developing flexion contractures of the toes.
- Stiffness of knee, ankle and foot may delay full rehabilitation.

that full weight-bearing will tend to be resisted until the fracture is safely united.

ISOLATED FRACTURES OF THE FIBULAR SHAFT

These are of little significance, and can be treated with a supportive dressing or plaster-cast until painless.

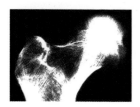

CHAPTER 20

Fractures
of the ankle
and foot

The ankle joint is a stable system, with the body of the talus fitting closely within the mortice of the tibia and fibula. The collateral ligaments are strong and the anterior and posterior ligaments weak, as is usual with hinge joints (Fig. 20.1).

LIGAMENT STRAINS

These are the commonest ankle injuries by far. The anterior talo-fibular part of the lateral ligament is usually strained or the whole ligament is occasionally ruptured by the patient 'going over' on the outside of the foot, i.e. an inversion stress with a twisting component.

CLINICAL FEATURES

The ankle is swollen and painful with restriction of movements and tenderness localized over the lateral ligament. When an attempt is made to invert the foot there is pain and muscle spasm in the peronei. Differentiation from a fracture of the lateral malleolus is difficult and X-rays are essential.

TREATMENT

1 A simple strain can be protected by strapping or, if the ankle is very swollen, by a below-knee walking cast for 2–3 weeks.

2 If the signs are severe, and particularly if the ankle is swollen on both sides, complete rupture should be suspected and stress X-rays should be taken, either with local anaesthetic injected into the ligament or a general anaesthetic. The normal side should also be stressed for comparison. A complete rupture may be repaired surgically or treated conservatively. In either case, a weight-bearing below-knee cast is necessary for 6 weeks. Alternatively, early mobilization may be allowed provided the ligament is protected by a suitable brace. An inadequately treated rupture may result in persistent instability, with the joint tending to 'give way' during normal use.

LIGAMENTS AROUND THE ANKLE JOINT

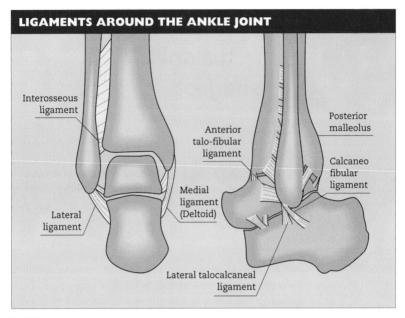

Interosseous ligament

Anterior talo-fibular ligament

Posterior malleolus

Calcaneo fibular ligament

Medial ligament (Deltoid)

Lateral ligament

Lateral talocalcaneal ligament

Fig. 20.1

3 Long-term instability, with opening of the joint on stressing, may require surgical reconstruction of the lateral ligament, usually using the peroneus brevis tendon.

4 Medial ligament strains are uncommon and may be treated conservatively.

FRACTURES AND DISLOCATIONS OF THE ANKLE

Many fractures of the ankle are associated with subluxation or dislocation of the joint surfaces. It is this combination which is known as the 'Potts' fracture' although this term is not now often used.

The variety of such injuries is wide and many classifications have been attempted. Most of these are based on speculation as to the precise mechanism by which the injury has been caused, and none can be regarded as entirely satisfactory in covering all the possibilities.

A frequently-used modern classification (based on that devised by Lauge-Hansen in 1950) divides the injuries as follows:

1 inversion (or adduction) injuries;
2 inversion and external rotation injuries;
3 eversion (or abduction) injuries;
4 eversion and external rotation injuries; and
5 vertical compression injuries.

It should be emphasized that this classification is based on the static X-ray appearances. There is considerable inter-observer error in classifying the injuries and there is much to be said for simply analysing each fracture in terms of the degree and direction of instability.

The subject can be simplified by understanding that the joint can be injured on one side only or on both sides. In the most severe rotational injuries, both sides may be injured together with the posterior lip of the lower end of the tibia which is knocked off by the talus as it rotates out of the ankle. This structure is often called the 'third' malleolus (posterior malleolus).

Most ankle injuries are caused by the weight of the falling patient applying a force to the ankle with the foot in a fixed position.

The degree of instability depends on how much of the ankle complex is damaged i.e.:

• one side only, i.e. one malleolus or one collateral ligament−unimalleolar;

• both sides, i.e. both malleoli or both ligaments or any combination of one malleolus and the opposite ligament−bimalleolar; and

• both sides and the posterior lip of the tibial articular surface−usually called trimalleolar.

On the lateral side, the damage may in some cases extend as high as the upper end of the fibula, in which case the interosseous ligament and membrane may be ruptured.

INVERSION (ADDUCTION) INJURIES

• Rupture of the lateral ligament (Fig. 20.2a). This is produced by an adduction force, in most cases with a twisting component.

• Avulsion of the tip of the lateral malleolus2the equivalent of a lateral ligament rupture (Fig. 20.2b), i.e. unimalleolar.

• Rupture of the lateral ligament combined with a fracture of the medial malleolus, of typical oblique shape (Figs. 20.2c, d), i.e. bimalleolar.

EVERSION (ABDUCTION) INJURIES

These are produced by a pure abduction force without rotation.

• Simple rupture of the medial ligament. This rarely, if ever, occurs i.e. unimalleolar.

• Rupture of the medial ligament or avulsion of the tip of the medial malleolus and a transverse fracture of the fibula (Fig. 20.3a, b), i.e. bimalleolar.

• As above, but the fibular fracture is above the interosseous tibio-fibular ligament which ruptures and there is lateral shift of the talus. This is called a diastasis of the inferior tibio-fibular joint (Fig. 20.3c),

INVERSION (ADDUCTION) INJURIES

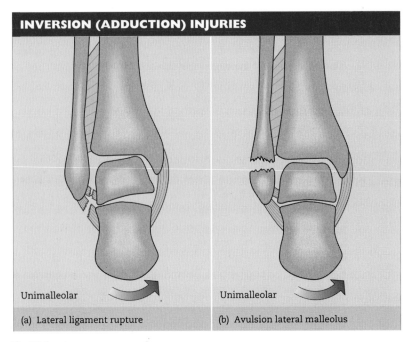

Unimalleolar

Unimalleolar

(a) Lateral ligament rupture

(b) Avulsion lateral malleolus

Fig. 20.2

i.e. bimalleolar. It is doubtful if this ever occurs without an element of rotation.

Rotational injuries

It has been convincingly demonstrated that when a patient 'goes over' forcibly with his/her full weight on the ankle, the violent inversion of the foot is converted by the oblique direction of the subtalar joint into a force causing the talus to rotate outwards in the ankle mortice ('torque convertor' mechanism). It is the talus attempting to rotate externally within the fixed ankle mortice which causes this type of fracture. A rotational force appears to cause various types of injury with combinations of fractures and ligament damage. The Lauge-Hansen classification attempts to explain the different types in terms of the position of the foot at the time the rotational force occurred. In practice, although there is some experimental evidence for these mechanisms, for any given patient the precise mechanism of injury is rarely known and from the point of view of management it is convenient to consider all rotational fracture-dislocations together. An important structure in maintaining ankle stability is the strong interosseous ligament between the lower ends of the

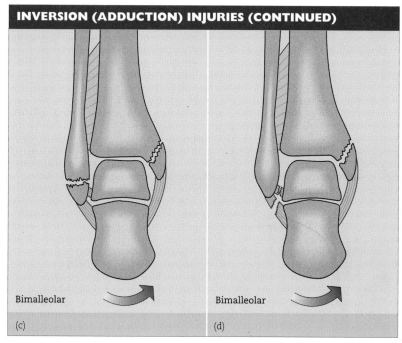

INVERSION (ADDUCTION) INJURIES (CONTINUED)

Bimalleolar

(c)

Bimalleolar

(d)

Fig. 20.2 (*Continued*)

tibia and fibula, and fractures can be subdivided into those where this ligament is intact and those in which it is completely ruptured.

1 ROTATIONAL FRACTURES WITH THE INTEROSSEOUS LIGAMENT INTACT (Fig. 20.4)

1 A spiral fracture of the lateral malleolus is a very common injury (Fig. 20.4a). It is difficult to differentiate from a lateral ligament strain, but maximum tenderness is usually over the bone. It may only be visible on a lateral X-ray and is usually little displaced (unimalleolar).

2 Less common is a spiral fracture of the lower fibula, leaving the upper fibular fragment attached to the tibia by the interosseous ligament, but coupled with an avulsion fracture of the medial malleolus or rupture of the medial ligament (Fig. 20.4b) (bimalleolar). If the medial malleolus is avulsed the fragment is always small. With the higher fibular fractures, part of the interosseous ligament may be ruptured but the upper fibres may bind the tibia and fibula together.

3 As in **2** above, but with the posterior lip of the tibial articular surface fractured (Fig. 20.4c).

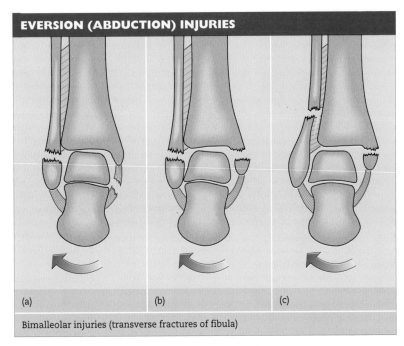

EVERSION (ABDUCTION) INJURIES

(a)   (b)   (c)

Bimalleolar injuries (transverse fractures of fibula)

Fig. 20.3

2 ROTATIONAL FRACTURES WITH THE INTEROSSEOUS LIGAMENT RUPTURED: DIASTASIS OF THE INFERIOR TIBIO-FIBULAR JOINT (DUPUYTREN'S FRACTURE)

1 Spiral fracture of the fibula with rupture of the interosseous ligament and with the medial structures remaining intact is rare (unimalleolar).

2 Spiral fracture of the fibula with disruption of the medial structures – the medial ligament may be ruptured or the tip of the medial malleolus may be avulsed, again usually a relatively small fragment (Fig. 20.5b, c). The fibular fracture may be as high as the upper end of the bone (Fig. 20.5a). With the higher fractures there may be extensive damage to the interosseous membrane which increases the instability. An X-ray of the whole fibula is essential since there may be no fracture at ankle level.

3 As in **2** but with a fracture of the back of the lower end of the tibia. This is usually only the lateral part of the posterior margin, sometimes called the posterior tubercle (trimalleolar).

Vertical compression fractures

These are caused by a fall on the foot from a height. The talus is driven into and shatters the lower end of the tibia (Fig. 20.6). This is a

ROTATIONAL FRACTURES

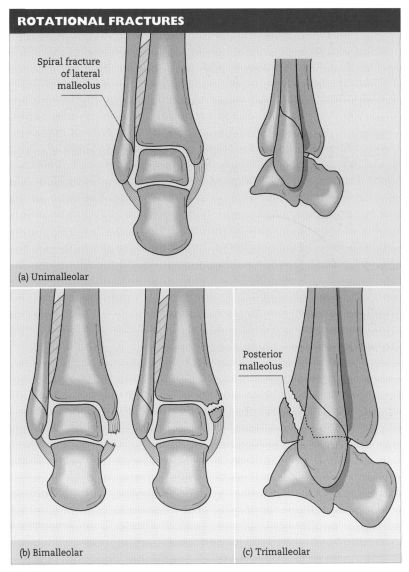

Spiral fracture of lateral malleolus

(a) Unimalleolar

(b) Bimalleolar

(c) Trimalleolar

Posterior malleolus

Fig. 20.4

severe injury usually leading to stiffness and pain and to late arthritic changes.

TREATMENT OF ANKLE FRACTURE DISLOCATIONS

The evidence suggests that anatomical reduction of the fractures, with

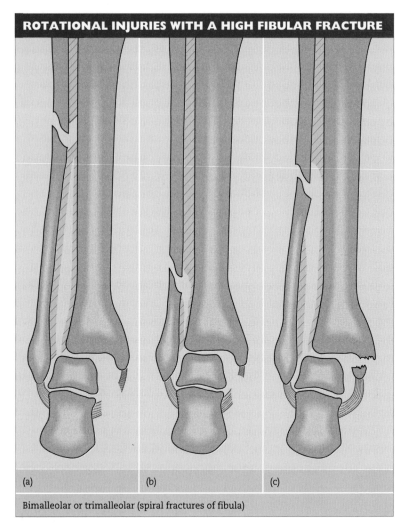

ROTATIONAL INJURIES WITH A HIGH FIBULAR FRACTURE

(a)   (b)   (c)

Bimalleolar or trimalleolar (spiral fractures of fibula)

Fig. 20.5

accurate location of the talus within the ankle mortice, gives the best results and that the technique of maintaining reduction is less important. In practice, internal fixation is often the easiest way of maintaining the position, but it is by no means always necessary. Most surgeons follow a middle course, believing that the risks of internal fixation may sometimes outweigh the advantages.

I Single-sided injuries—unimalleolar

These have some intrinsic stability and can usually be controlled in a

VERTICAL COMPRESSION FRACTURE

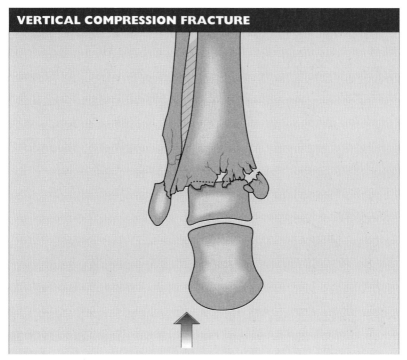

Fig. 20.6

plaster-cast. For the rotational injuries the cast may need to be extended above the knee with the knee slightly flexed. Six weeks' weight-bearing immobilization is usually sufficient.

2 Bimalleolar injuries

These are unstable in several planes. They can sometimes be adequately held in a plaster-cast, particularly if the medial malleolus is partly intact (Fig. 20.7). They need an above-knee plaster with the knee flexed in control rotation. In most cases, internal fixation will be needed and most bimalleolar fractures can be stabilized by fixing the fibula alone, either with screws placed across the fracture line or a plate (Fig. 20.8). A longitudinal screw driven along the medullary cavity from the tip of the malleolus is less satisfactory in controlling rotation. Even higher fibular fractures can be fixed in the same way, with good control of ankle stability. The deltoid ligament need not be repaired, but a large medial fragment, if displaced, may be re-attached with a single screw or tension-band wire. It has been the practice in the past to drive a screw horizon-tally across the inferior tibio-fibular joint if the interosseous ligament is completely ruptured. If the fibula is firmly fixed this is probably unnecess-

BIMALLEOLAR FRACTURE

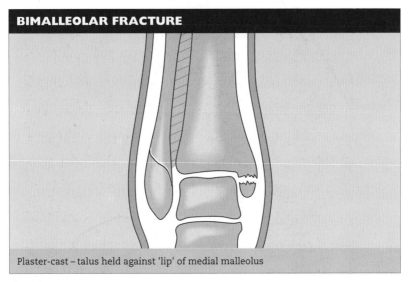

Plaster-cast – talus held against 'lip' of medial malleolus

Fig. 20.7

ary unless there is gross disruption of the interosseous membrane. If such a screw is used, it will need to be removed before the patient bears weight because of the risk of breaking the screw.

3 Trimalleolar fractures

These are always unstable. The posterior malleolar fragment is usually displaced upwards and if on the lateral X-ray it accounts for one-third or more of the articular surface, it needs open reduction and a screw to avoid backward subluxation of the talus. It is usually advisable to fix the fibular fracture and, if necessary, the medial malleolus.

REHABILITATION

With all these fractures, if the ankle is adequately stabilized by internal fixation a plaster-cast is not necessary, although after preliminary mobilization, a cast may be used for protection from full weight-bearing—which is usually avoided for 6–8 weeks.

FRACTURES OF THE FOOT

FRACTURES AND DISLOCATIONS OF THE TALUS

Fractures of the body of the talus are rare but have a poor prognosis for

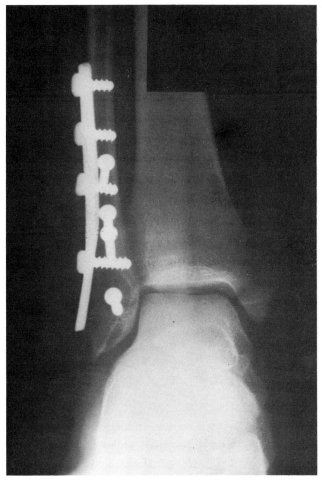

Fig. 20.8 A bimalleolar fracture stabilized by internal fixation of the fibula alone.

ultimate function because of the associated damage to the ankle articular surface. Treatment is usually conservative, allowing movement as soon as possible but avoiding weight-bearing for up to 3 months.

A fracture of the neck is a serious injury and may occur alone or in combination with a subtalar subluxation (Fig. 20.9). It is usually caused by forced dorsiflexion of the ankle. Accurate reduction by manipulation is essential. If the subtalar joint is subluxated, the fracture is best aligned with the foot in plantar-flexion (see Fig. 20.9) in a plaster-cast. A screw may be used to improve stability. Immobilization for 8–12 weeks is usually necessary for union. This injury may be complicated by avascular

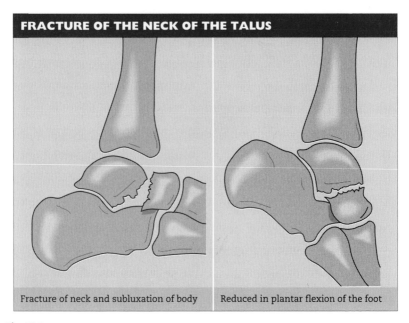

FRACTURE OF THE NECK OF THE TALUS

| Fracture of neck and subluxation of body | Reduced in plantar flexion of the foot |

Fig. 20.9

necrosis of the body of the talus due to interruption of the blood supply by the fracture and by disruption of vessels in the sinus tarsi. This may lead to late arthritis of the ankle.

Occasionally, the talar neck is fractured and the body completely dislocated from the ankle and subtalar joint. The body is displaced medially and may damage the posterior tibial artery. This injury is frequently compound and the risk of avascular necrosis is particularly high. Open reduction is often necessary and wires may be used to stabilize the fracture. A plaster-cast is needed for 12 weeks, initially non-weight-bearing.

COMPLETE DISRUPTION OF THE SUBTALAR AND MIDTARSAL JOINTS

This is a severe injury, usually reducible by manipulation and controllable by plaster fixation, but wire stabilization may be necessary.

FRACTURES OF THE OS CALCIS

These are usually caused by falls from a height onto the heel and are often bilateral. Severity depends on whether the fracture enters the subtalar joint. Because of the way in which the injury occurs, os calcis fractures are sometimes associated with a spinal fracture, usually of the wedge type.

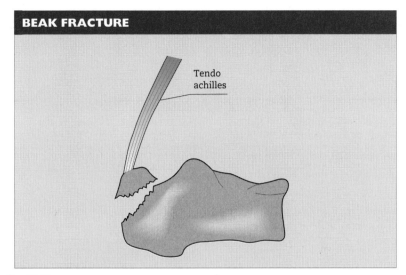

BEAK FRACTURE

Tendo achilles

Fig. 20.10

Clinical features

The heel is usually grossly swollen and bruised and the patient is unable to bear weight. Ankle movements may be moderately reduced, but subtalar movements are often completely absent.

Fractures of the posterior-superior lip of the calcaneus may still be attached to the tendo-achilles and if lifted up may need to be reduced and immobilized with the ankle in equinus, or alternatively by internal fixation ('beak' fracture) (Fig. 20.10).

Fractures involving the subtalar joint usually occur obliquely through the body. Occasionally, the talus acts as a wedge, driving a fragment of the posterior articular surface of the subtalar joint into the body of the calcaneum, causing comminution. Lateral X-rays may show flattening of the normal shape of the subtalar joint (Fig. 20.11) and diminution of 'Bohler's angle'. An axial projection may be helpful in diagnosing fractures of the sustentaculum and disruption of the subtalar joint. Computed tomography scanning can be of value in assessing these injuries.

Treatment

Conservative treatment is usual—elevation in bed until the swelling subsides, then gradual mobilization in a pressure dressing of wool and crepe bandage or a light plaster-cast. Weight-bearing is permitted as the pain allows. Recovery may take many months and improvement can continue for up to 2 years.

Fractures with a large posterior fragment and an elevated heel can

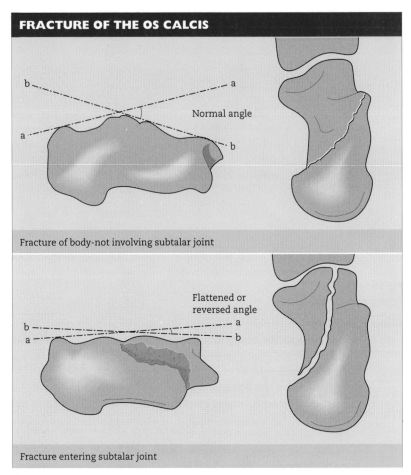

FRACTURE OF THE OS CALCIS

Normal angle

Fracture of body-not involving subtalar joint

Flattened or reversed angle

Fracture entering subtalar joint

Fig. 20.11

sometimes be improved by driving a Steinmann pin or Gissane spike into the os calcis from behind, and using this to lever down the fragment. The pin can be incorporated into a plaster-cast and removed after 3–6 weeks. A depressed central fragment may be elevated surgically and the space below grafted with iliac bone. There is no general agreement as to the merits of attempting to reduce most os calcis fractures by open procedures.

Complications

Occasionally, because of spreading of the heel, the peroneal tendons may become trapped between the os calcis and the lateral malleolus and may require surgical release. Many patients with subtalar damage fail to become painfree and may eventually need a subtalar arthrodesis to restore their ability to walk comfortably. This is usually combined with a midtarsal fusion as the three joints normally move as one round the talus.

Dislocation of the 1st tarso-metatarsal joint

This is a rare injury (Lisfranc dislocation). It is dangerous because the blood supply to the medial ray of the foot may be lost, necessitating partial amputation.

Fractures of metatarsals

BASAL FRACTURES

Fracture of the base of the 5th metatarsal is common and is caused by an inversion strain of the foot so that the base becomes avulsed by the peroneus brevis tendon.

Treatment

A walking plaster-cast for 3–6 weeks.

SHAFT FRACTURES

Metatarsal shaft fractures are common, they are usually caused by crushing and are associated with much soft-tissue damage or swelling.

Treatment

Elevation of the foot, if swollen, is followed by a walking below-knee cast for 6 weeks. If displacement is gross, manipulation and a plaster-cast or open reduction and internal fixation may be necessary.

MARCH FRACTURES

These are common fractures, usually of the neck of the 2nd metatarsal, caused by the stress of long periods of walking. They are usually diagnosed when healing, with callus being visible on the X-ray.

Treatment

A plaster-cast for 3–6 weeks is usually sufficient.

Fractures of toes

These are common injuries and usually of little significance, however, the fracture may interfere with the circulation, necessitating amputation of the toe.

Treatment

They are usually treated by protective dressings and allowing the patient to continue walking.

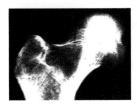

CHAPTER 21

The management of major trauma

Serious, life-threatening injury is relatively uncommon and there is currently debate about the best way of organizing its management. Most patients have major orthopaedic injuries but, apart from pelvic fractures, these do not threaten life. The key to successful management is to have an effective system for resuscitating and assessing the patient, coupled with a service allowing rapid and efficient transfer to a centre with special expertise.

Arrangements for *pre-hospital care* vary in different countries. In the UK this is provided by the ambulance service and advanced training is now provided for ambulance personnel.

In the *Accident and Emergency Department* the trend is towards highly trained teams of surgeons, anaesthetists and nursing staff. The Advanced Trauma Life Support (ATLS) system of training was developed in the USA and has become popular in the UK. In this system, the patient is managed by a team with each member carrying out his/her own tasks and with an experienced team leader providing overall supervision. It is suggested that the ideal team should consist of four doctors and four nurses or operating department assistants. The leader is responsible for pre-planning the activities of each team member and each doctor is in turn required to proceed according to four steps:

1 primary survey;
2 resuscitation;
3 secondary survey; and
4 review, documentation and initial treatment plan.

Doctor 1 is reponsible for looking after the 'head end' of the patient and secures the airway, controls and stabilizes the cervical spine and assesses and assists breathing and oxygenation.

Doctor 2 is responsible for the circulation and should secure at least two good intravenous lines, assess for the presence of shock, commence fluid resuscitation, take blood for cross-matching, obtain blood gases and ensure external haemorrhage has been controlled.

Doctor 3 is responsible for carrying out any urgent surgical procedures, such as cricothyroidotomy, chest drainage, intravenous cut-

GLASGOW COMA SCALE

Verbal response	Orientated	5
	Confused conversation	4
	Inappropriate words	3
	Incomprehensible sounds	2
	Nil	1
Motor function	Obeys	5
	Localizes	4
	Withdraws	3
	Abnormal flexion	3
	Extends	2
	Nil	1
Eye opening	Spontaneous	4
	To speech	3
	To pain	2
	Nil	1
GSC Total score		

down etc., which may be needed as judged by the other team members, and for identifying and controlling life-threatening bleeding.

While these procedures are being carried out, Doctor 4, the team leader, is responsible, helped by information from the other doctors, for the *Secondary Survey* which involves a complete and systematic examination of the patient from head to toe and from front to back, the patient being log-rolled as necessary. At this stage, the level of consciousness is assessed according to the Glasgow Coma Scale and a CT scan may be required. X-rays of the cervical spine, chest and pelvis are performed routinely.

The team leader is also responsible for the *Final Review, Documentation and Initial Treatment Plan*. This involves checking that all resuscitation procedures have been carried out, deciding whether the patient needs to go to theatre immediately for the control of haemorrhage, or alternatively whether urgent investigation is necessary to confirm or rule out life-threatening haemorrhage. A plan is prepared for the further management of the patient and transfer is arranged as necessary. Detailed documentation of the history, physical condition of the patient and all steps taken is carried out before the patient leaves the department.

Many patients require the attention of more than one surgeon for their definitive treatment and it is the duty of the team leader to coordinate the activities of the various experts. There are often multiple fractures and joint injuries and experience has demonstrated that for this type of patient early internal fixation, where appropriate, gives the best prognosis both for survival and for the injuries themselves.

General orthopaedics

CHAPTER 22

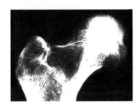

Congenital malformations – principles

Many congenital malformations occur for no obvious reason, but certain factors are known to cause mal-development of the fetus if they act at a time when development is at a critical stage.

1 Genetic disturbances. These may be:
  (a) inherited; or
  (b) due to mutations.

They may arise spontaneously or as a result of external influences such as radiation.

2 Drugs. Thalidomide is the best known example of this, but many others are known, including alcohol.

3 Infections. Syphilis is an example of a bacterial, and rubella an example of a viral infection which may affect the fetus.

4 Trauma. Injury to the mother, particularly during late pregnancy, may damage the fetus. Injury to the baby during labour may produce abnormalities such as brachial plexus damage or cerebral palsy.

5 Anoxia. This may operate during intrauterine life, e.g. as a result of placental separation, or in the immediate postnatal period.

6 Compression *in utero*. There has long been debate about compression as a factor in producing malformations of the limbs such as club foot. Pressure may well be responsible for the more severe resistant deformities. A baby with an intrauterine paralytic condition, such as spina bifida, may fail to make the normal intrauterine movements, so that pressure effects may contribute to the eventual deformities.

MISCELLANEOUS CONGENITAL DEFORMITIES

REDUCTION DEFORMITIES

Part of a limb or a whole limb may be missing. This type of deformity was typically seen following treatment of the mother by thalidomide during early pregnancy (Fig. 22.1). These deformities present complex problems to the limb-fitting specialist, but function may be surprisingly good.

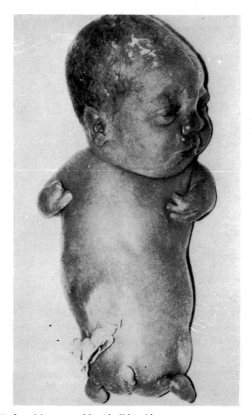

Fig. 22.1 Deformities caused by Thalidomide.

HEMIMELIAS

These are characterized by the absence of one or other component of the limb, e.g. absence or hypoplasia of the radius (radial club hand) or absence of one or more rays of the hand or foot. Absence of individual bones, parts of bones or muscles, occurs occasionally, e.g. the upper end of femur, the clavicles or pectoralis major.

FUSION OF DIGITS

These abnormalities are relatively common and usually minor. They are often of little importance in the foot, but may be disfiguring in the hand, e.g. lobster claw hand.

TRIGGER THUMB

This is a relatively common condition affecting the thumb of babies. The thumb is held flexed at the interphalangeal joint and the condition is due to constriction of the flexor sheath opposite the head of the metacarpal where a nodule can be felt. True 'triggering' of the tendon past the obstruction is rarely seen. The condition is treated by longitudinal division of the tendon sheath.

CONGENITAL DISLOCATION OF THE KNEE

This is a very rare condition. The child is born with the knee hyperextended and with the tibia dislocated anteriorly. Operative reduction may be necessary if manipulation and plaster-cast immobilization fails.

ARTHROGRYPOSIS MULTIPLEX CONGENITA

This is a rare condition in which the child is born with multiple joint deformities, with tight skin and soft tissues. There appear to be at least two main types, one with a myopathic basis, characterized by multiple flexion contractures and deformities of the spine and chest, and the second with an underlying neurological abnormality. There is evidence that in this second group, the deficiency lies in the anterior horn cells. Children in this group usually have flexion deformities of hips, wrists and ankles and fixed extension of knees and elbows. Orthopaedic treatment consists mainly of correcting deformities, muscle re-balancing procedures and appropriate physiotherapy, with splintage as necessary.

DISCOID MENISCUS (p. 369)

In this condition the lateral meniscus fails to develop properly, remaining as a complete disc. It may block movement to some extent and often causes a loud clunk. It is more prone to damage than the normal meniscus and is treated by excision if symptoms are severe.

SPRENGEL'S SHOULDER

A condition in which the scapula is higher and smaller than usual and also rotated into adduction. There may be a ligamentous and bony bar connecting the upper medial border to the cervical spine—the omovertebral bar. This is occasionally worth resecting to give some improvement in appearance: the condition is often associated with Klippel–Feil syndrome (p. 200).

MADELUNG'S DEFORMITY

In this condition the inner part of the lower radial epiphysis fails to grow normally, so that the radius becomes bowed, with an oblique lower end. The ulna, which continues to grow normally, subluxates backwards and can be felt as a prominence. The condition usually occurs in girls, and may be associated with Turner's syndrome. It may be painful and excision of the lower end of the ulna may then be necessary.

CHAPTER 23

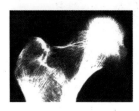

Congenital malformations – congenital dislocation of the hip

True congenital dislocation of the hip (CDH), i.e. a hip which is dislocated at birth, is rare, but the term has come to be used in a wider sense and an attempt has been made to encompass this by renaming the condition Developmental Dysplasia of the Hip (DDH). All babies can be categorized at birth into five groups on the basis of a test devised by Barlow (see p. 182). This classification results from the initial observations of Von Rosen in Sweden that the condition can be diagnosed at birth and that this is the best time to start treatment. It is currently recommended that all newborn babies be examined as soon as possible after birth for evidence of hip instability.

BARLOW'S TEST

The baby is examined when warm and comfortable, preferably after a feed. The child lies supine and the examiner holds the legs with hips and knees flexed and the fingertips behind the hip joint and thumb in front so that the femoral head is between the fingers and thumb (Fig. 23.1). The legs are gradually abducted from the 'together' position and the range of abduction noted. The normal hip in a neonate will abduct until the outside of the thigh lies flat on the couch (Fig. 23.2). An attempt is then made to displace the head of the femur into and out of joint posteriorly by pressure with thumb and fingers. Every child falls into one of five categories.

Pathology

Capsular laxity is the dominant feature in the unstable hip. If treatment is not initiated and if instability persists, acetabular development is affected and the cup becomes shallow and open superiorly. Femoral head and neck development are also abnormal and there may be excessive anteversion of the neck relative to the acetabular alignment. There is some dispute as to which of these changes are primary and which are secondary to the persistent instability.

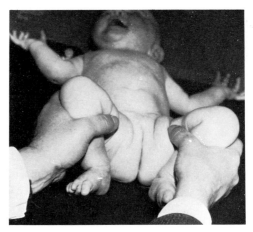

Fig. 23.1 Barlow's test for hip instability.

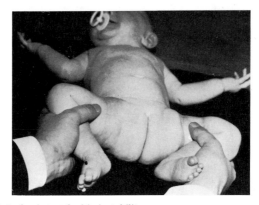

Fig. 23.2 Barlow's test for hip instability.

The so-called 'unstable' hip, i.e. Group 2, undoubtedly stabilizes spontaneously in many cases, but sometimes appears to progress to full dislocation. A possible hypothesis to explain this is that the hip will not develop normally unless the head of the femur rotates about a point axis within the acetabulum. If rotation occurs about an eccentric or movable axis acetabular development will not proceed normally.

Causes

The basic cause of the condition is unknown. Girls are affected more than boys (8:1).

BARLOW'S CATEGORIES

1 The legs abduct fully and the head cannot be displaced, i.e. a normal child.

2 Abduction is full but the head can be displaced backwards—when released it will relocate spontaneously.

3 There may be slight limitation of abduction and as the hip is abducted the head slips over the edge of the acetabulum into joint with a 'clunk'. This is the basis of a test devised by Ortolani. In other words, the head is out of joint in adduction but slips in easily in abduction.

4 Abduction is limited and the head may be palpable in the buttock, the thigh is short and there may be additional skin creases. The head does not relocate on abduction and cannot be manipulated in a true congenital dislocation.

5 Abduction is limited but the head is in joint, i.e. simple limitation of adduction. This may be idiopathic but a neurological condition such as cerebral palsy should be suspected.

Groups 2, 3 and 4 come under the usual definition of CDH.

1 Hereditary factors—the risk is increased to 36% if one parent has a CDH (Wynne-Davies). Familial joint laxity may also be a factor in some cases.

2 Environment—the usual incidence is quoted as 1.5 per 1000 live births, but this varies around the world. This may be due to genetic differences or to differences in the way the newborn child is nursed. In those societies where it is usual to nurse the child with the legs bound together in adduction, the incidence of established CDH is much higher than in those societies where the child is carried on the mother's back with the legs widely abducted. It may be that the birth incidence is the same in both groups but that in the second group, the position of carrying the child actually treats the lax hips.

3 Position *in utero*—breech delivery is more commonly associated with CDH. It is likely here that joint laxity is the primary factor and that the vulnerable hip is dislocated by mal-position either before or after birth.

Diagnosis

AT BIRTH

Barlow's test is described above. Over the last few years there has been increasing concern about the failure of clinical screening to reduce the incidence of late-diagnosed CDH. Barlow's test needs experience to obtain consistent results and there is also a suspicion that in some cases which have been diagnosed late, the hip was either normal to clinical testing at birth or the standard tests are not sensitive enough. This has led to a search for more objective tests and particularly to the use of ultrasound.

X-rays are not always helpful at birth. On an AP film taken with the legs in neutral, the hip may appear to 'stand off', but because the head is not ossified this may be difficult to judge. On a film taken in 45 degrees of abduction, a line drawn along the centre line of the femur may be abnormally high, i.e. may point towards the corresponding anterior superior iliac spine rather than towards the superior lip of the acetabulum (Ortolani). Some hips, however, reduce spontaneously in this position so that the X-ray may appear normal.

Ultrasonic scanning has the advantage that it can demonstrate the soft tissues, including articular cartilage, and it can also be used in 'real time' to see the head moving in relation to the acetabulum. At the moment, there is no general agreement as to the significance of the various ultrasound findings and the test cannot be considered suitable for routine scanning of all neonates.

LATER IN LIFE

The leg may be short and abduction of the hip limited. The femoral head may be felt to move in and out of joint in abduction, or may fail to reduce and be palpable in the buttock, or rarely, deep to the inguinal ligament. Most late cases are spotted when the child walks. Walking is usually delayed and the child usually walks with a characteristic waddle (Trendelenburg gait) due to inefficiency of the abductors. Trendelenburg's test is valuable in assessing hip instability (p. 354).

X-rays usually make the diagnosis obvious (Fig. 23.3). An arthrogram, in which radioopaque dye is injected into the joint, will show the exact position and shape of the head and may show the inverted capsule (limbus) (Fig. 23.4). It is likely, however, that MRI scanning will replace arthrography as the investigation of choice.

Management

IF DIAGNOSED AT BIRTH

These children make up Barlow Groups 2, 3 and 4. Splintage in abduction usually allows stabilization of the hip in 3 months or less. There are many types of splint. Popular ones are the Von Rosen or a modification of this (Fig. 23.5) and the Pavlik sling (Fig. 23.6). All these devices hold the hip in the so-called 'frog' position. With children in Group 2, it is usual to wait for a few days from birth before splinting because many hips become stable within this time. The hips should be X-rayed on the splint. A few

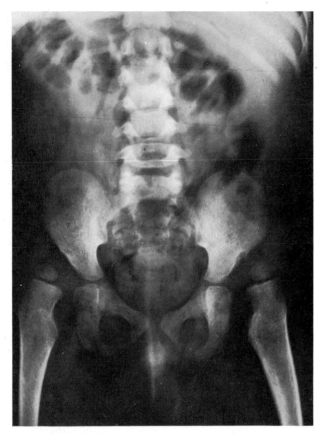

Fig. 23.3 Radiograph of late CDH.

hips fail to stabilize by the end of 3 months and a further period of splintage may be necessary, usually in a plaster hip spica.

DIAGNOSED IN THE FIRST 18 MONTHS

The principle of management is to reduce the hip and maintain reduction until the acetabulum and soft tissues develop sufficiently to contain the femoral head. The head can often be reduced by traction or manipulation but open reduction may be necessary.

Traction

Many methods are available. Longitudinal sliding skin traction is often adequate but alternatively, traction may be carried out on an abduction frame. Over a period of 1–2 weeks the hip may reduce spontaneously,

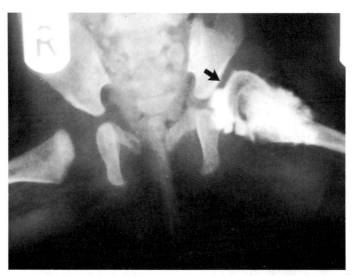

Fig. 23.4 Arthrogram of a late CDH–arrow points to the limbus.

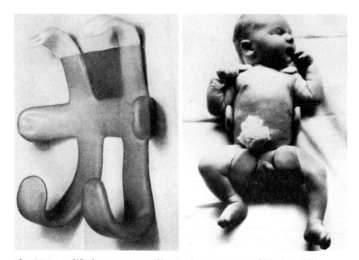

Fig. 23.5 Modified Von Rosen splint in the treatment of hip instability.

but if this fails, gentle manipulation under anaesthesia may produce a satisfactory reduction.

Open reduction

If the above methods fail, open reduction becomes necessary, this usually being carried out through an anterior approach, although an approach

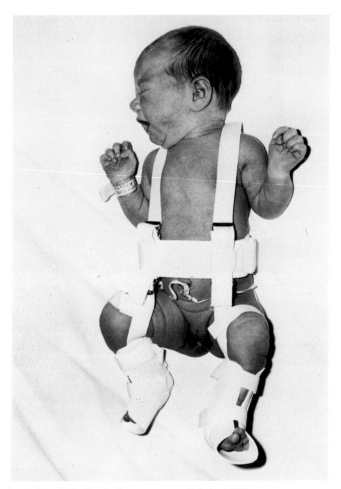

Fig. 23.6 Pavlik's sling in the treatment of hip instability.

through the adductor region has certain advantages. There are usually several obstacles to reduction (Fig. 23.7).

1 The glenoid labrum and superior capsule may be folded inwards to form a crescentric flap in the upper part of the joint. This is usually called a limbus.

2 The psoas tendon may constrict the inferior capsule like an hourglass and any attempt to internally rotate the hip increases this constriction.

3 The inferior capsule may be infolded and adherent to the floor of the true acetabulum.

4 The ligamentum teres may be hypertrophied.

OBSTACLES TO REDUCTION OF LATE CDH

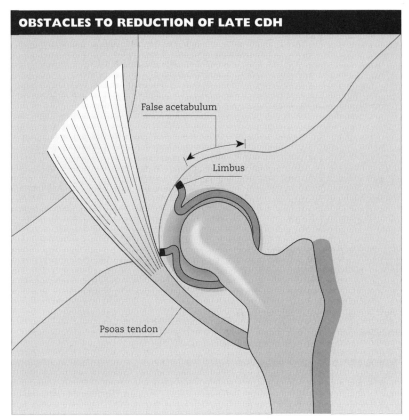

False acetabulum

Limbus

Psoas tendon

Fig. 23.7

5 The acetabulum is usually abnormally shallow and may be orientated so that it looks too far forward relative to the position of the femoral neck, which in turn is almost always anteverted.

The operation consists of opening the capsule, dividing the psoas and inferior capsule and, if possible, reducing the head under the limbus into the true acetabulum. The redundant capsule may need to be tightened. In order to prevent the inferior capsule and psoas from re-forming and tightening up again, the hip should be reduced in the internally rotated position which is also appropriate for the anteverted femoral neck.

Following either closed or open reduction, the hip is held in a plaster hip spica in internal rotation and abduction (Fig. 23.8). The period depends on the age at which treatment is started. It is rarely less than 6 months. In the later stages, some movement may be allowed by keeping the hips in abduction plasters (Fig. 23.9).

INTERNAL ROTATION HIP SPICA

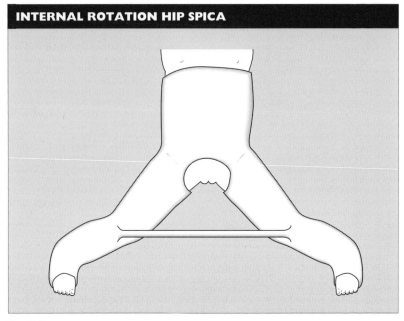

Fig. 23.8

ABDUCTION CYLINDERS

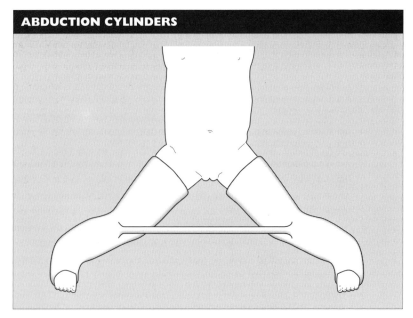

Fig. 23.9

Operative reconstruction

In the older child, hip development may take so long that some form of operative reconstruction may be needed.

1 A shelf may be built out from the margin of the acetabulum (Pemberton).

2 The innominate bone may be divided at the greater sciatic notch, then the lower half rotated over the femoral head (Salter).

3 The femoral neck may be rotated inwards by dividing the upper shaft (Somerville).

These procedures give more rapid stabilization and may avoid long periods of splintage. Their long-term effects are not yet known.

Avascular necrosis of the head is an occasional complication of treatment, especially if forcible manipulation is used.

DIAGNOSED ABOVE THE AGE OF 4 YEARS

If the condition is first diagnosed at this age, the child must be assessed very carefully before any treatment is decided upon. The older the child, the less the chances of obtaining good hip development. Conversely, by this age the fully dislocated hip will usually have formed an adequate false acetabulum and may continue to function reasonably well for an indefinite period, although usually producing a limp.

CONGENITAL SUBLUXATION OF THE HIP

This expression has been widely used without clear definition. In later childhood, it sometimes becomes apparent that certain children have a poorly developed hip, with a shallow and sloping acetabulum (acetabular dysplasia) and a femoral head 'standing wide' and poorly covered by the acetabulum. This is usually nothing more than an X-ray finding, although some children develop pain in early adult life and many appear to progress to osteoarthritis at a relatively young age. It is not known whether some of those hips found to be lax at birth progress to this state or whether it represents a completely separate condition; nor is it known whether preventive treatment has any influence on the condition or whether surgical treatment of the established case is likely to prevent degeneration later in life. Some workers believe it to be a minor degree of true congenital dislocation, perhaps inadequately treated.

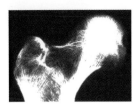

CHAPTER 24

Congenital malformations — club foot

The word 'talipes' means 'club foot'. The name is derived from the resemblance of the common type of equino-varus deformity to a golf putter. The cause is virtually unknown, but there is certainly a paralytic element in some cases, and in others intrauterine moulding may play a part.

Terms used in describing the foot are listed below (also see p. 382).

FOOT TERMINOLOGY

- *Equinus* — means that the hindfoot is plantar-flexed at the ankle.
- *Calcaneus* — the hindfoot is dorsiflexed at the ankle.
- *Varus* — the hindfoot is adducted or inverted when looked at from behind.
- *Valgus* — the hindfoot is abducted or everted when looked at from behind.
- *Cavus* — means that the longitudinal arch is higher than usual.
- *Planus* — the arch is flattened (and the foot is usually valgus).
- *Forefoot adduction*, sometimes called metatarsus adductus. The foot is flat to the ground, but the forefoot is directed medially producing an 'intoeing' appearance.

The forefoot tends to follow the alignment of the hindfoot. When the latter is varus, the sole tends to face medially, i.e. supination, and when the hindfoot is valgus the sole tends to face more laterally than normal, producing a flat foot — pronation. The situation is complicated by the fact that the forefoot may point in a different direction from the hindfoot, e.g. hindfoot neutral or calcaneus, forefoot plantar-flexed. Similarly, the forefoot may be adducted or abducted relative to the hindfoot. In these circumstances it is better to use the full descriptive terms for each part of the foot.

TALIPES CALCANEO-VALGUS

The baby is born with the foot dorsiflexed and everted. This is usually caused by intrauterine moulding and almost always corrects

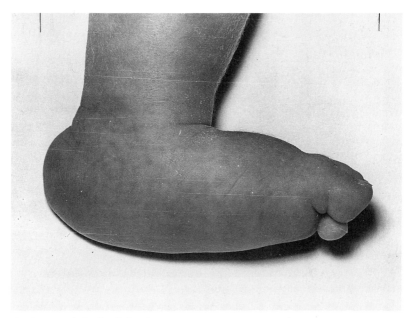

Fig. 24.1 Vertical talus deformity.

spontaneously. No treatment other than stretching by the parent is necessary.

TALIPES EQUINO-VALGUS OR VERTICAL TALUS

This is a rare deformity. The hindfoot is in equinus, the forefoot is dorsiflexed and everted and the talus is abnormally vertical. The condition is difficult to treat and may require surgical correction (Fig. 24.1).

TALIPES EQUINO-VARUS

CLINICAL FEATURES

This is the typical club foot. The condition may be bilateral. The os calcis is small, indeed the whole foot and leg are shortened. The hindfoot is in equinus and inverted and the forefoot is supinated and 'hooked' so that the sole points medially or even upwards (Fig. 24.2). When dorsiflexion and eversion are attempted the dorsum of the foot cannot be made to touch the outer side of the shin as it can be in a normal newborn baby. The talus is directed laterally and its shape is distorted. The navicular is subluxated off the talar head in a medial direction so that it may articulate

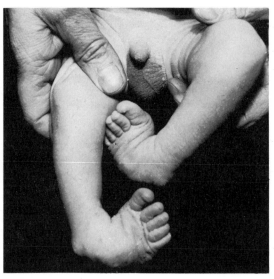

Fig. 24.2 Talipes equino-varus.

CORRECTION OF TALIPES EQUINO–VARUS

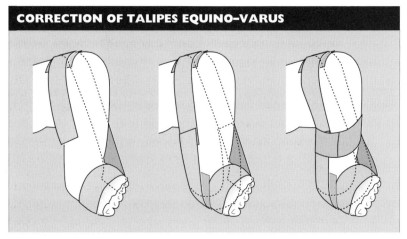

Fig. 24.3 The use of elastic strapping to correct talipes equino-varus (From Fripp and Shaw, 1967).

with the medial malleolus. A search should always be made for a paralytic cause, but the typical case is idiopathic.

TREATMENT

This should begin at birth. The foot is manipulated into slight over-correction and held with a plaster-cast, adhesive strapping or a malleable splint (Fig. 24.3). This is initially changed every 2–3 days with a further

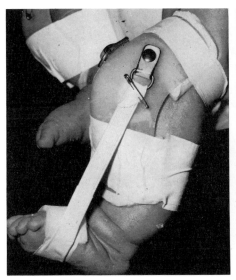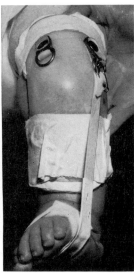

Fig. 24.4 Fitton's elastic splint for talipes equino-varus.

manipulation. When the foot is over-corrected it is splinted continuously, either with elastic strapping or a device such as that shown in Fig. 24.4 which allows some movement but continues the moulding process. Some authorities use plaster-casts continuously but the technique is demanding (Kite). The modern trend is to perform surgery if the foot is not corrected adequately by 2–3 months, or if the midfoot begins to 'break' i.e. the forefoot dorsiflexes and the hindfoot remains in equinus (rocker-bottom foot).

The usual operation is a postero-medial soft-tissue release in which the tendo-achilles and posterior capsule of the ankle are released, the subtalar joint opened and the varus corrected. The talo-navicular joint is then opened and the navicular reduced by swinging the forefoot laterally. The tibialis posterior tendon may need to be elongated. More elaborate procedures are currently being tried, including a technique which employs a transverse posterior incision giving good access to both aspects of the hindfoot.

Following surgery, splintage is continued as before. When the foot is large enough, splints of the type designed by Denis Browne may be used, initially all the time, and later at night only (Fig. 24.5). When the child starts to walk, modified shoes may help to maintain correction. Splintage usually continues until at least the age of one and further follow-up is necessary for many years because relapse is not uncommon.

Late recurrence may occur up to the age of four or even later, and it may then become necessary to correct the residual deformity by bone operations, such as that designed by Evans, in which the calcaneo-cuboid

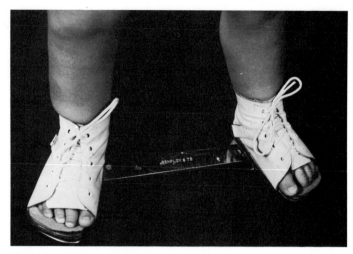

Fig. 24.5 Denis Browne splints.

DILWYN EVANS' OPERATION

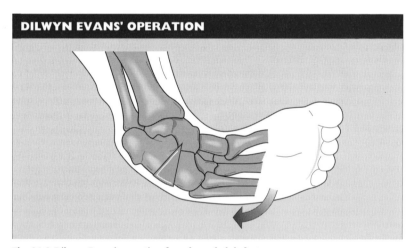

Fig. 24.6 Dilwyn Evans' operation for relapsed club foot.

joint is excised to produce a lateral fusion (Fig. 24.6). This partly corrects the deformity and relies on further growth on the inner side to complete the correction. The operation devised by Dwyer concentrates on taking a wedge from the outer side of the os calcis to correct the inversion of the heel. He also believes that growth corrects the remaining deformity (Fig. 24.7).

Most children born with a club foot should have a well-corrected plantigrade foot by the time they start to walk, although some residual deformity may persist indefinitely. The foot is usually smaller than the normal one.

DWYER OPERATION FOR RELAPSED CLUB FOOT

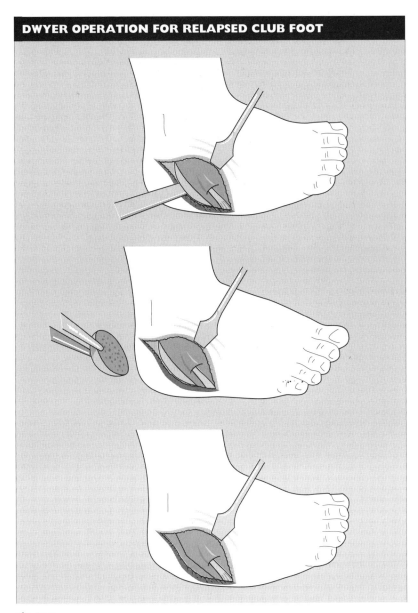

Fig. 24.7

METATARSUS ADDUCTUS

Sometimes called metatarsus varus, although this term is confusing, the foot is essentially plantigrade, but the forefoot points inwards. It may occur as a result of inadequate correction of a talipes equino-varus or as an isolated deformity. If severe at birth it may respond to serial plaster correction and later to the wearing of 'straight last' shoes, i.e. shoes with a straight or flat inner border. The severe, uncorrected case may require midfoot surgery.

CHAPTER 25

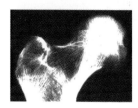

Congenital malformations – spinal malformations

Congenital malformations of the spine are commonest in the lower thoracic, lumbar and sacral regions. Minor malformations of the lumbo-sacral junction are very common, and usually of little significance. Of the more serious deformities, the commonest and most important is spina bifida.

SPINAL DYSRAPHISM

This is a condition in which the neural arches fail to form or close posteriorly. It is often associated with abnormal development of the spinal cord and meninges. Various degrees of the condition occur.

1 Spina bifida occulta is common and usually of no importance (Fig. 25.1a).

2 Meningocele is not necessarily associated with cord abnormality but the sac is continuous with the skin and may need excision and closure of the defect (Fig. 25.1b).

3 Spina bifida with myelomeningocele is one of the commonest congenital malformations (Fig. 25.1c). It has important clinical consequences:

(a) the vertebrae themselves, as well as being defective posteriorly, are often malformed, causing serious spinal deformity, such as scoliosis and kyphosis, the latter usually being localized to the thoraco-lumbar region;

(b) the cord is opened out on the surface and is functionally abnormal, resulting in lower limb and possibly trunk paralysis with paralysis of the bladder and anal sphincter; and

(c) there is frequently an associated malformation of the brain stem resulting in hydrocephalus and often mental defect (Arnold–Chiari malformation).

MANAGEMENT

The condition has received much attention since it became apparent that babies with myelomeningocele could be kept alive by closing the spinal defect surgically and that the hydrocephalus could also be controlled. It

197

VARIETIES OF SPINA BIFIDA

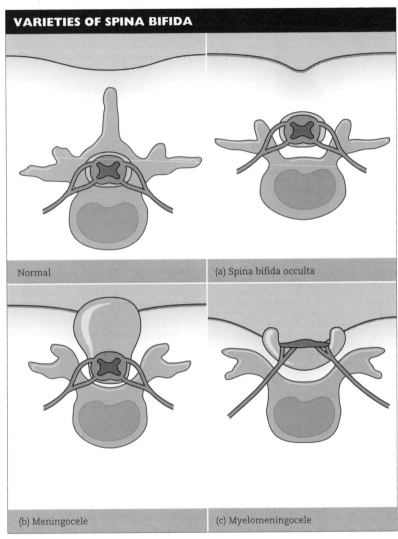

Normal

(a) Spina bifida occulta

(b) Meningocele

(c) Myelomeningocele

Fig. 25.1

has become usual for affected babies to be managed in special centres by a paediatric team.

❙ A detailed assessment at birth by orthopaedic and neurological surgeons, paediatricians, social workers, etc. is essential if an accurate prognosis is to be made. This includes:

(a) accurate assessment of deformities, neurological state of the limbs, both motor and sensory;

(b) assessment of the hydrocephalus; and

(c) assessment of the genito-urinary tract.

2 A decision is then made as to whether the spinal defect should be closed surgically. If this is not done, death is usual. Some babies survive for many years, but, if necessary, the defect can then be closed at a later stage. Those babies who have good innervation of the legs are regarded as suitable for urgent closure, i.e. within the first 24 hours, because of the risk of neurological deterioration if closure is delayed.

3 If the hydrocephalus is progressing, a valve may be used to shunt cerebrospinal fluid from the ventricles back to the circulation, usually into a neck vein.

4 Orthopaedic problems. Several consequences stem from paralysis of the legs:

(a) Deformities may develop due to muscle imbalance. These may affect any of the joints, but particularly the hips and feet.

(b) Activities may be restricted by the motor loss. The joints may lack stability because of muscle weakness.

(c) The limbs may be liable to pressure sores and fractures from lack of normal sensation.

Orthopaedic treatment aims:

1 to avoid or correct deformity by splintage or appropriate corrective surgery;

2 to try to secure muscle balance by partial denervation or tendon transfer; and

3 to improve mobility by the use of appliances.

Neurosurgical treatment is required for the hydrocephalus and treatment is necessary for the urinary tract and bowel problems. This may involve the control of recurrent infection, diversion of the ureters, sphincter surgery, etc.

The majority of children with spina bifida have severe and multiple disabilities and follow-up is likely to continue indefinitely. The tendency at the moment is to concentrate treatment on those most likely to benefit from it. The problem has diminished recently because of the falling birthrate, the reduction in the prevalence of the condition and improved techniques for prenatal diagnosis, offering the possibility of abortion.

CONGENITAL SCOLIOSIS

A scoliosis is a lateral curvature of the spine. It is almost always associated with a rotation of the spine. It is uncommon in the neonate, and in babies most minor curves improve with growth (James). The more severe curves and those with structural abnormalities such as hemivertebrae usually progress and become very severe in later childhood. An attempt is usually made to hold the curve by an external support such as a Milwaukee brace (see Fig. 29.5), but this is of limited value.

CONGENITAL MALFORMATIONS OF THE CERVICAL SPINE

These occur infrequently; they include the *Klippel–Feil syndrome* in which the cervical vertebrae are deformed and often fused so that the neck is shortened and webbed. This is often associated with elevation of one or both scapulae–Sprengel's shoulder (p. 179).

CONGENITAL TORTICOLLIS

This is a condition in which the child develops a fixed, fusiform swelling in one sterno-mastoid muscle, usually during the first 2 weeks after birth. The sterno-mastoid 'tumour' subsides, but the subsequent fibrosis causes a tilt and rotation of the neck to the opposite side. When the condition is well established, the face is usually asymmetrical with the eyes on a different level.

TREATMENT

Passive stretching in the early stages often prevents deformity. Late uncorrected cases may require surgical release of the sterno-mastoid. The operation may correct the torticollis, but the asymmetry of the face remains.

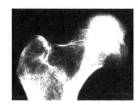

CHAPTER 26

Cerebral palsy

This may be defined as a disorder of movement and posture due to a defect or lesion of the immature brain. It is often present at birth and may be caused by intrauterine developmental defects, by birth trauma and asphyxia, but also by diseases or injuries in early life.

The condition is essentially a *motor* disorder but the child frequently has additional disabilities, such as mental defect, blindness, sensory abnormalities, speech defects, etc. It should be remembered that the condition is a true paralysis in that *voluntary* movements may be weak or absent even though the muscles may be capable of contracting strongly. The motor defects may take several forms and combinations of the following are usual.

SPASTICITY

The defect is essentially of upper motor neurone type and causes variable weakness and spasticity in all four limbs and trunk. Reflexes are exaggerated and the stretch reflex is abnormally sensitive.

LOSS OF COORDINATION

Muscles frequently contract together or out of phase, and the child may have to learn control by laborious exercises. *Athetosis* is a condition in which the limbs move at random, with jerking and incoordinated movements.

RIGIDITY

The limbs are rigid but not spastic in the true sense.

HYPOTONICITY

Occasionally the muscles are *hypotonic* – 'floppy infant'.

MANAGEMENT

The disabilities are variable and complex. The child is usually assessed and managed by a team consisting of paediatricians, orthopaedic surgeons, physiotherapists and various other specialists as necessary.

The orthopaedic problems are best dealt with if the child can be managed in a special centre, from as young an age as possible. The mainstay of treatment is physiotherapy. Many regimes have been worked out, of which the Bobath method may be mentioned as having been particularly influential. Physiotherapy aims to:

- assist in assessment;
- prevent or attempt to correct musculo-skeletal deformity;
- train the child in posture and movements;
- provide suitable sensory stimulation; and
- supervise progress and assist parents.

Surgery has much to offer in cerebral palsy, but it is usually a minor element in a long continued programme of therapy.

ORTHOPAEDIC PROBLEMS

PARALYSIS

This varies in extent:

- arm and leg on one side—hemiparesis;
- one limb—monoparesis;
- both legs—di- or paraparesis; and
- all four limbs—quadriparesis.

On careful testing it is usual to find all four limbs affected to some extent. Depending on the site of the brain lesion, several patterns are seen, but the link between pathology and clinical features is not yet clear. Common examples are the typical hemiplegia with most joints held flexed on one side (Fig. 26.1), and the scissoring pattern with a tendency towards extension of joints (Fig. 26.2).

SPASTICITY

This makes an assessment of muscle power difficult because a muscle may appear weak due to spasticity of the opposing group. Usually, flexors are more spastic than extensors which appear correspondingly weak.

DEFORMITY

This usually develops early as a result of muscle imbalance. Common deformities are flexion of elbow, wrist and fingers with 'clasped thumb', and flexion and adduction deformities of the hip, knee and ankle.

INCOORDINATION AND SENSORY ABNORMALITIES

These cause difficulties with gait and hand function.

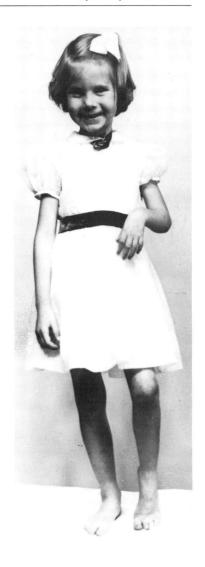

Fig. 26.1 Posture of typical
hemiparetic child with cerebral
palsy.

Surgery

The aims of surgery are listed below.

I To correct any established deformity:

(a) soft-tissue surgery involves dividing tendons, capsules, skin, etc.,
common procedures are elongation of the tendo-achilles, hamstrings
and adductors of the hip; and

(b) bony correction—only needed when deformities are severe,
usually simple osteotomies, e.g. through the lower femur to correct
a flexion deformity of the knee.

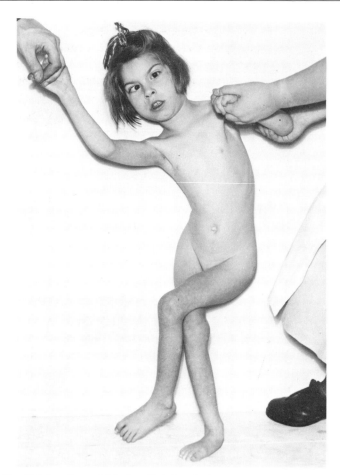

Fig. 26.2 Spastic quadriplegia with 'scissoring'.

2 To restore muscle balance and diminish spasticity:

(a) tendon lengthening achieves this to some extent;

(b) partial denervation, e.g. the anterior branch of the obturator nerve may be divided if the adductors are over-active;

(c) occasionally, tendons may be transplanted, usually in the upper limb;

(d) splintage with calipers, etc., may be needed but can often be avoided.

Surgery is most valuable in the lower limb and may need to be repeated as the child grows. Surgery to the hand should only be used after a comprehensive assessment of potential hand function, including sensation, manipulative ability, etc. The child with one normal hand will usually fail to use the affected one.

Surgery may occasionally be carried out for cosmetic reasons, e.g. tendon transplantation at the wrist, or wrist fusion.

Physiotherapy is essential after surgery as even minor procedures may interfere severely with function, especially in the older child.

Considerable social and psychological support for the child and family is usually necessary and occasionally institutional care.

CHAPTER 27

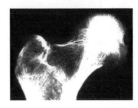

Developmental conditions – general abnormalities of skeletal development

CARTILAGINOUS DYSPLASIAS

DYSPLASIA EPIPHYSIALIS MULTIPLEX

A rare abnormality, which is strongly hereditary in some families. The number of joints affected varies. The child is usually stunted and may have difficulty in walking, with impaired upper limb function. Affected joints are stiff and occasionally painful. The epiphyses ossify late, e.g. the femoral head may ossify at 1–2 years and fragmentation is often extreme. The epiphysis becomes distorted and coxa vara may occur. The metacarpals and phalanges may be shortened. Vertebrae are not usually affected. There are no known biochemical changes.

DYSCHONDROPLASIA (MULTIPLE ENCHONDROMATOSIS – OLLIER'S DISEASE)

A non-hereditary disorder of the growth plate resulting in areas of unossified hyaline cartilage arising around the growth plate area. These tend to increase in size and expand the bone, producing multiple swellings. The condition affects the long bones only and they are often shortened. The hands are particularly affected, and as the lesions grow throughout childhood and into adult life function may be grossly impaired (Fig. 27.1).

Treatment

Usually consists of excising those lesions which are causing trouble, and correcting deformities by osteotomy, so that multiple surgery may be necessary. Sarcomatous change in the lesions is a rare complication.

OSTEOCHONDROMATOSIS (DIAPHYSEAL ACLASIA, MULTIPLE EXOSTOSES)

A strongly hereditary condition affecting the epiphyseal plates of cartilaginous bones. The bones develop exostoses of cancellous bone capped with cartilage and arising from the region of the epiphysis. The

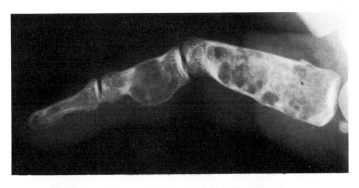

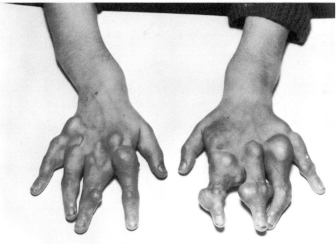

Fig. 27.1 Dyschondroplasia.

exostosis typically points away from the end of the bone (Fig. 27.2). The bones themselves may be deformed. Multiple swellings can be palpated and these increase in size during the growth period. The long bones, iliac crests and scapulae are most usually affected. The swellings may be excised as necessary. The risk of malignancy occuring in adult life is said to be proportional to the number of lesions.

ACHONDROPLASIA

A hereditary condition, occasionally occurring sporadically. It is the commonest of the conditions caused by abnormal maturation of growth plate chondroblasts. It is present at birth and particularly affects the long bones, resulting in dwarfism of characteristic type so that the individual has a long trunk but short, stumpy limbs—the typical circus dwarf. The

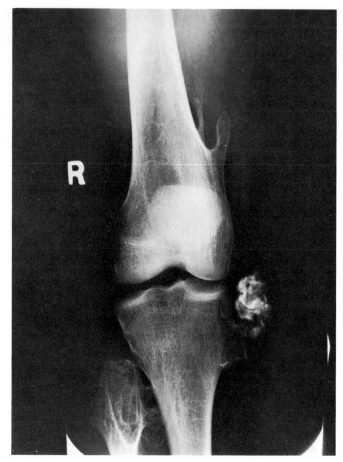

Fig. 27.2 Osteochondromatosis.

head is large and the nose flattened. The hands are short and broad with a short middle finger. X-rays show the bones to be short and dense with flared ends. The acetabulum is broad and flat and the ilium is quadrilateral. The vertebrae are relatively normal, although often wedged and with concave posterior borders and thick pedicles. Mentality is usually normal.

MUCOPOLYSACCHARIDOSES

A series of congenital disorders of growth associated with dwarfism, deformities of bones and joints, and in some cases mental deficiency. They are caused by a defect of mucopolysaccharide metabolism affecting cartilage matrix formation and resulting in deposition of abnormal mucopolysaccharides in the bones and their excretion in the urine (kerato-sulphate).

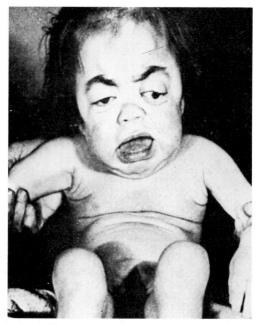

Fig. 27.3 Hurler's disease.

Hurler's disease (Gargoylism)

This was the first to be described—a familial condition with skeletal abnormalities, corneal opacities and mental defect. The facial appearance is characteristic (Fig. 27.3). There are typically deformities of the epiphyses and vertebral bodies.

Morquio's disease—osteochondrodystrophy

A similar condition to Hurler's disease but without mental defect, cranial deformities or corneal opacities. Joints may be more severely affected. Kyphosis is usually present; the joints are deformed and may become stiff. The vertebral bodies are flattened with an anterior tongue. The epiphyses are irregular, particularly at the hips where there may be coxa vara and a fragmented head. Two types are described with slight clinical differences—Morquio–Brailsford and Morquio–Ullrich disease, the latter excreting kerato-sulphate in the urine.

BONE DYSPLASIAS

OSTEOGENESIS IMPERFECTA (FRAGILITAS OSSEUM)

A hereditary disease in which the bones are abnormally thin and delicate, the teeth are poor and the sclerae thin and blue. Sporadic cases also

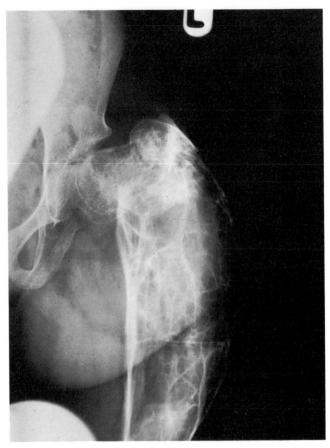

Fig. 27.4 Fibrosis dysplasia.

occur and tend to be more severely affected and dwarfed and have less-blue sclerae. The condition may be present at birth and severe, in which case survival is unusual, or it may appear in early childhood and be less severe—osteogenesis tarda. The characteristic feature is a tendency for the bones to fracture with minimal trauma. The bone is immature and the architecture abnormal. The severity varies, but patients often have multiple fractures over many years. The fractures heal well but may cause multiple deformities and dwarfism. The condition is caused by an abnormality of collagen and it is the defiiciency of collagen in the sclera which allows the blue colour of the retina to show through. Vision is not affected. No treatment is known, but severe cases require protection from everyday injuries. It is possible to strengthen the bones with expanding intramedullary rods which increase in length as the child grows. The tendency to fracture often becomes less in adult life.

FIBROUS DYSPLASIA

A condition in which single or multiple cystic lesions occur in the bones. The proximal ends of long bones are usually affected and the condition is recognized in early adult life, often by the bone fracturing or occasionally because of swelling or deformity. The defects may be localized or may extend to involve the whole bone. When the lesions are multiple they are often associated with endocrine disturbance and pigmented skin patches. The lesions are usually radio-lucent with scalloped edges and occasionally expand the bone (Fig. 27.4), but always leave a layer of cortex. Microscopically, they consist of loose cellular tissue with spicules of bone.

NEUROFIBROMATOSIS (VON RECKLINGHAUSEN'S DISEASE)

In this condition pigmented skin lesions and multiple fibromata in skin and on peripheral nerves are often associated with multiple areas of fibrous dysplasia. Scoliosis occurs in almost half the cases and, occasionally, localized gigantism of part or the whole of a limb.

HYPERPARATHYROIDISM

A defect of parathyroid secretion which is often associated with multiple cystic lesions in bone characteristic of fibrous dysplasia and having similar histology (p. 303).

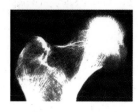

CHAPTER 28

Developmental conditions – localized abnormalities of skeletal development

INFANTILE (OR CONGENITAL) COXA VARA

This is distinct from other causes of a varus femoral neck. The characteristic radiological feature is a separate triangle of bone close to the epiphysis (Fig. 28.1). There is an association with developmental defects or absence of the upper end of the femur. Symptoms usually occur when the child starts to walk or slightly later. The gait is waddling and Trendelenberg's sign is positive. On X-ray, the femoral neck is very horizontal and may even point downwards. The greater trochanter is usually elongated and curves inwards. Surgical correction may be necessary and osteotomy may have to be repeated several times during growth.

SLIPPED UPPER FEMORAL EPIPHYSIS

The upper femoral epiphysis is prone to displacement in certain individuals. Conditions such as rickets, achondroplasia, sepsis etc., may cause it, but in adolescents it may occur spontaneously. The adolescent type is commoner in boys and bilateral in 24% of patients. The child is frequently overweight and may have delayed sexual development. Abnormalities of oestrogen metabolism have been demonstrated in some patients.

CLINICAL PICTURE

Pain is the usual symptom, lasting several days or weeks, and often associated with a limp. The slip occurs through the growth plate and may be acute or may occur gradually over a period of days or weeks. The epiphysis slips backwards, leaving the front of the upper end of the neck exposed and new bone develops in this area, filling the gap. This makes reduction impossible in the later case. The limb may be slightly short, is usually externally rotated and passive internal rotation is diminished.

The condition may not be apparent in the early stages on an AP X-ray, but is detectable on a lateral film. A line drawn through the centre of the femoral neck in any X-ray projection should pass through the

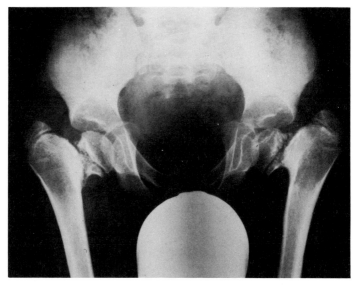

Fig. 28.1 Infantile coxa vara.

centre of the head. If it does not then some displacement has occurred (Fig. 28.2).

TREATMENT

If the symptoms are acute, the head may reduce on traction in internal rotation or by manipulation under general anesthesia. If this occurs, pins are driven up the neck into the head to prevent further slipping (Fig. 28.3). There is some evidence that manipulation may increase the risks of avascular necrosis (see below).

The more usual chronic slip is treated by pinning if the degree of slip is such that this is technically possible. If not, an osteotomy through the neck or in the inter-trochanteric region to correct the deformity should be considered. Following pinning, the epiphysis often fuses early and the external rotation deformity may lessen or disappear spontaneously. Some surgeons pin the opposite hip prophylactically, but in the absence of endocrine abnormality this is probably not justified, although the child should be followed up carefully.

COMPLICATIONS

1 Avascular necrosis of the femoral head occurs in a proportion of cases. The changes are similar to those of Perthes' disease (p. 232) and the head may become distorted or fragmented. Healing eventually occurs and protection from weight-bearing is usually advised during the period when the head is at risk.

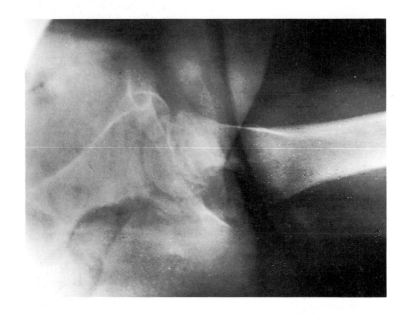

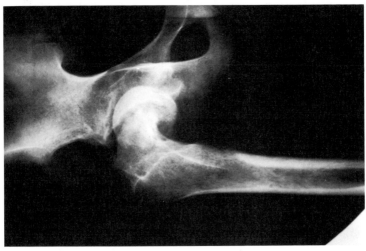

Fig. 28.2 Slipped upper femoral epiphysis.

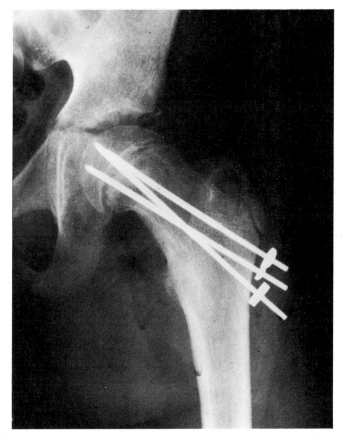

Fig. 28.3 Internal fixation of slipped epiphysis.

2 Chondrolysis is a much rarer condition in which the articular cartilage over the head deteriorates and the joint space appears severely narrowed on X-ray. Treatment makes little difference and the end result is usually a stiff and painful hip with the early onset of osteoarthritis.

RECURRENT DISLOCATION OF THE PATELLA

This is a relatively common condition, typically affecting adolescent girls. The patella dislocates laterally, often as a result of an accident. Subsequently, dislocation occurs relatively easily. The complaint is often that the knee locks in flexion. When this happens it may not be noticed that the patella is dislocated or it may have been 'knocked back' easily, allowing the knee to extend. The knee is usually normal between attacks. The condition may be associated with generalized joint laxity or a mal-

TIBIAL TUBERCLE TRANSPLANT

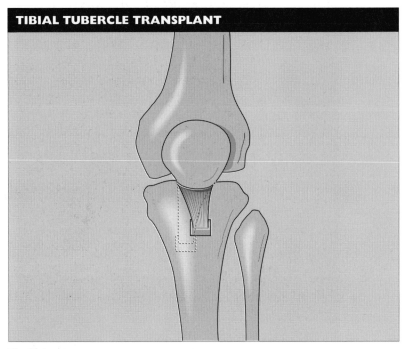

Fig. 28.4

alignment of the tibial tubercle. Rarely, and usually in younger children, it is associated with contracture of the quadriceps muscles, particularly the vastus lateralis. In some cases this appears to have been caused by repeated intramuscular injections for an illness in infancy. In these cases the patella dislocates each time the knee is flexed.

In the ordinary idopathic variety, a useful clinical sign, indeed often the only sign, is a tendency for the patient to be apprehensive when the patella is pushed laterally. 'Skyline' X-rays may show an abnormal tilt of the patella or a defect of the lateral femoral condyle. The patella may be small and placed rather higher than usual.

TREATMENT

The recurrent case is often treated by transplantation of the patellar tendon more medially. If the child is near to maturity this is usually done by transplanting a block of bone bearing the insertion of the tendon to a more medial and distal position on the tibia (Fig. 28.4). The operation is usually successful in preventing dislocation, but there is increasing evidence that it may be followed by osteoarthritis in later life. The younger

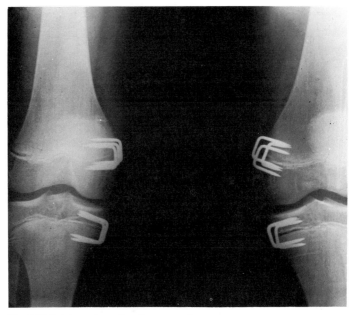

Fig. 28.5 Epiphyseal stapling for genu valgum.

child may require a release of the tight vastus lateralis combined with 'reefing' of the medial capsule.

GENU VALGUM–KNOCK KNEE

Many children have valgus knees when they first walk. These usually start to correct spontaneously by the age of six, provided there is no under-lying cause such as rickets, epiphyseal dysplasia, etc.

Rarely, the condition starts late or persists, is ugly and may predis-pose to osteoarthritis in adult life. If the condition is still troublesome at the age of 11 or 12 it may be corrected easily by inserting staples across the inner side of the femoral or femoral and tibial epiphyses (Blount, Fig. 28.5). These slow down growth on that side and the knee gradually straightens. Slight over-correction is allowed, and the staples are then removed.

TIBIA VARA (BLOUNT'S DISEASE)

A rare condition in which there is a developmental defect of the medial part of the upper tibial epiphysis resulting in a progressive bow-leg deformity. This may be unilateral or bilateral. The deformity may become very severe. It is more common in black children than in white children.

TREATMENT

Osteotomy of the upper end of the tibia is carried out early to correct deformity. This may need to be repeated during growth.

PSEUDARTHROSIS OF THE TIBIA

A condition present at birth or developing in early childhood in which bowing of the tibia occurs, often associated with a cystic defect in the lower third and eventually resulting in a fracture which persistently fails to unite. The cause is unknown, but there is an association with neurofibromatosis and possibly with fibrous dysplasia.

TREATMENT

If the bowing is recognized before the fracture occurs, it may be possible to protect the bone with a plaster-cast or to carry out a bypass bone-graft. The established case is usually very resistant to surgery, although firm internal fixation and bone grafting may secure union. The leg may become grossly shortened and require amputation in late childhood.

PES PLANUS (Fig. 28.6)

There is a wide variation in children and adults in the shape of the foot, ranging from the typical, postural, flat or valgus foot, with its medial border almost touching the ground, to the high arched foot, often with clawed toes. At both extremes of the range, symptoms of aching and pressure may arise. It is always important to exclude an underlying cause such as a paralytic condition or congenital fusion of the tarsal bones. The latter may cause a severe flat foot deformity with powerful peroneal spasm, often called *spasmodic flat foot*. This may require surgical intervention and even fusion of the hindfoot to cure it.

Idiopathic flat foot is usually of little significance. Reassurance and advice on footwear is often adequate. If the shoes are wearing down rapidly on the inner side, a heel seat designed to invert the heel (Fig. 28.7), or stiffening along the inner border of the shoe may be helpful. Only rarely is surgery necessary.

CALCANEAL AND NAVICULAR EXOSTOSES

The posterior-superior part of the os calcis may project medially or

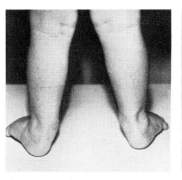
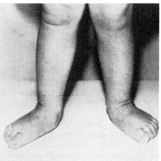

Fig. 28.6 Pes plano-valgus.

HEEL SEAT

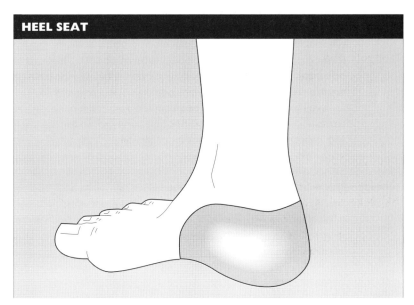

Fig. 28.7

laterally, causing pressure on the shoe. Surgical trimming, avoiding the tendo-achilles, is usually effective.

The navicular is often prominent medially and X-rays may show that there is an accessory bone in the insertion of the tibialis posterior. Pressure on the shoe may be a problem, and surgical removal of the prominence may be necessary, with care not to disturb the insertion of the tendon.

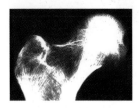

CHAPTER 29

Developmental conditions — the spine

SCOLIOSIS

The word scoliosis means a lateral curve or tilt of a part of the spine. The fact that the spine has several built-in curves means that any sideways tilt will usually also produce some rotation. In a typical scoliosis, the vertebrae are rotated so that the spinous processes describe a more gentle curve than the bodies (Fig. 29.1). If the curve is in the thoracic spine the ribs are distorted by the rotation producing a hump on one side.

It is usual to distinguish between structural and non-structural scoliosis, depending on whether or not the curve is fixed and associated with growth changes in the elements of the spine.

NON-STRUCTURAL SCOLIOSIS

This type of curve may correct on lying down or when the underlying cause is removed, i.e. it may be due to a short leg, a hip deformity, or spasm of the spinal muscles associated with a prolapsed disc, tumour or infection of the spine.

STRUCTURAL SCOLIOSIS

With this type of curve the important feature is the element of rotation, usually best seen when the spine is flexed (Fig. 29.2). With time, deformities of the vertebrae, discs, ligaments and ribs occur.

CAUSES OF SCOLIOSIS

- Congenital and infantile—due to vertebral anomalies and sometimes associated with congenital paralysis, e.g. spina bifida or cerebral palsy.
- Paralytic.
- Neurofibromatosis.
- Idiopathic or adolescent.

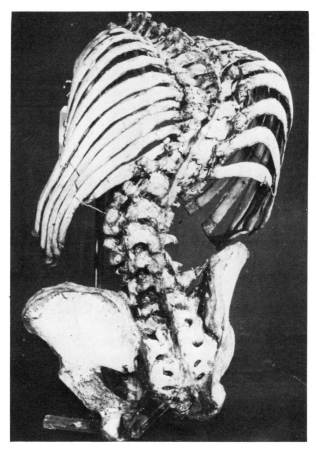

Fig. 29.1 Idiopathic scoliosis.

CONGENITAL SCOLIOSIS

This group is associated with abnormalities of the vertebrae such as hemi- or fused vertebrae. Minor abnormalities are common and usually do not cause scoliosis. The more severe ones may cause a steadily progressive and disabling scoliosis. There is a frequent association with spina bifida and there may also be a paralytic element in such cases.

INFANTILE SCOLIOSIS

In this group the curve develops during the first 3 years without vertebral anomalies. It is commoner in boys and usually convex to the left. There is often plagiocephaly. Approximately 90% resolve spontaneously, but

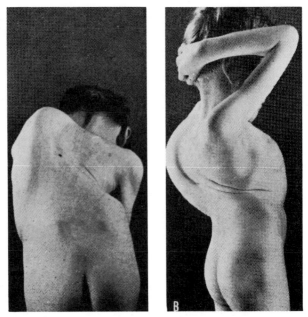

Fig. 29.2 Idiopathic scoliosis showing rib hump.

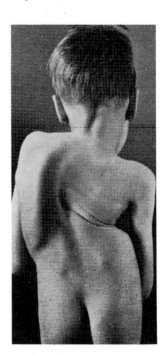

Fig. 29.3 Idiopathic thoracic scoliosis.

10% progress, becoming very severe. It is claimed that measuring the angles which the ribs make with the spine on the two sides may give an indication of the likelihood of progression. The curve is often thoracic or thoraco-lumbar.

ADOLESCENT IDIOPATHIC SCOLIOSIS

In this group the curve may first be noticed at the age of 10 or even earlier. It is commoner in girls and usually convex to the right. The prognosis depends on the age of onset (those arising early having a worse outlook), and on the level of the curve. Lumbar curves rarely constitute a severe cosmetic defect. Thoraco-lumbar curves are rare and of moderate severity. Thoracic curves, especially the upper ones, are the commonest and may become very severe, with appalling deformity. Once a curve has developed, the spine above and below usually develops compensatory curves in the opposite direction (Fig. 29.3). Occasionally,

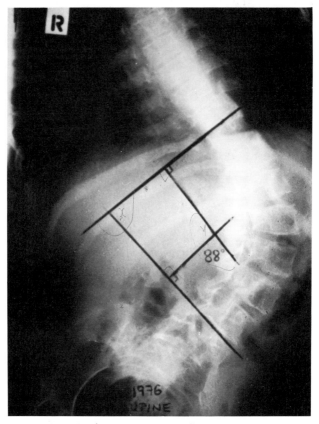

Fig. 29.4 Method of measuring X-rays in scoliosis.

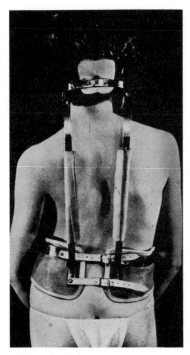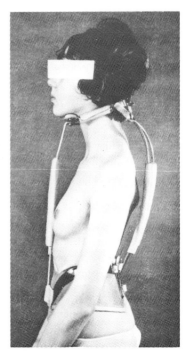

Fig. 29.5 Milwaukee brace.

there are two primary curves in opposite directions, both of these are structural.

CLINICAL PICTURE

The parents usually notice that one of the child's shoulders is held higher than the other or that a rib hump is developing. The curve is often less obvious clinically than radiologically, but viewing the spine in flexion will reveal rotation and a rib hump. Suspending the child by the head may demonstrate that part of the curve is mobile and corrects with gravity. A search should always be made for an underlying cause, such as a neurological condition or neurofibromatosis. X-rays in two planes reveal the extent of the scoliosis and the AP film can be measured to give an index of severity and to follow progress (Fig. 29.4).

MANAGEMENT

The majority of structural scolioses progress, with the exception of most of the infantile cases.

Treatment is extremely difficult, and it is rarely possible to prevent progression completely, although the curve can often be prevented from becoming too severe. The present basis of management is to attempt to

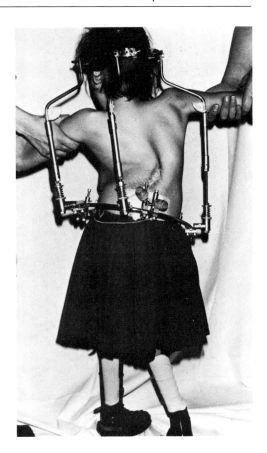

Fig. 29.6 Halo-pelvic traction.

hold the curve by external splintage for as long as possible, then to fuse the spine surgically when the child is old enough to have achieved reasonable growth.

Conservative

Many types of external splint—plaster-casts, braces, traction—devices exist. The most successful has been the Milwaukee brace which exerts pressure under the occiput and chin with a counter pressure on the iliac crests (Fig. 29.5, p. 224). It is clumsy and difficult to fit properly, but can be effective in holding the curve.

Operative

If fusion is contemplated, pre-operative traction or plaster correction, using a plaster jacket wedged open on the concave side (Risser), may be

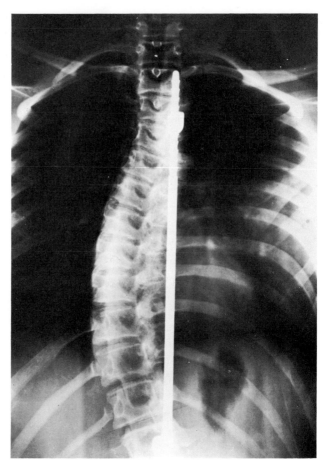

Fig. 29.7 Harrington fixation of spinal fusion.

used to gain as much soft-tissue stretching as possible. A more recent method, allowing the patient greater mobility, is the halo-pelvic traction device (Fig. 29.6).

Following correction, surgical fusion may be carried out from the back, either retaining the pre-operative plaster-cast, or using an internal fixation device. The most popular has been that devised by Harringon, which uses internal rods to hold correction until fusion occurs (Fig. 29.7). A more recent technique fuses the spine from the front by excising the discs and wiring the bodies together to form a solid block (Dwyer). Modern posterior techniques such as those devised by Luque and Cotrel-Dubousset use longitudinal rods and transverse wires to stretch the curve and rotate the vertebrae (Fig. 29.8). These methods rarely give full correction but may prevent the deformity becoming unacceptable. The

COTREL–DUBOUSSET SYSTEM FOR POSTERIOR FUSION

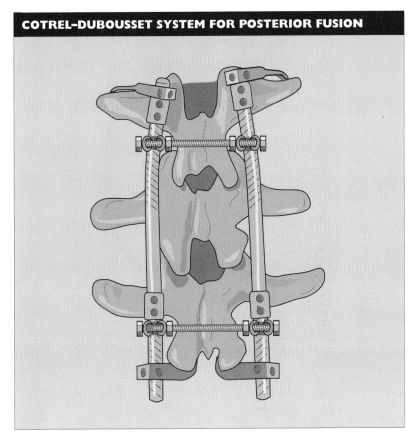

Fig. 29.8 Cotrel-Dubousset fixation system. Courtesy of Athrodex Surgical Ltd.

worst cases are the progressive congenital ones, where fusion may have to be done much earlier, and the paralytic ones, e.g. following polio-myelitis, when the deforming forces may be very great.

ADOLESCENT KYPHOSIS (SHEUERMANN'S DISEASE)

A kyphosis is a curve of the spine which is concave forwards. It may be localized, e.g. following trauma or destruction of a vertebral body by tumour or tuberculosis, or generalized. In Scheuermann's disease the ring epiphyses of the vertebral bodies develop abnormally so the bodies fail to grow properly and become wedge shaped. This results in a long thoracic kyphos producing a round-shouldered stance (Fig. 29.9). Pain is unusual and treatment is rarely necessary. Occasionally, a period of non-weight-bearing in a plaster bed may be advisable during the phase of rapid growth.

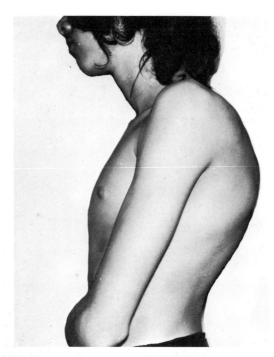

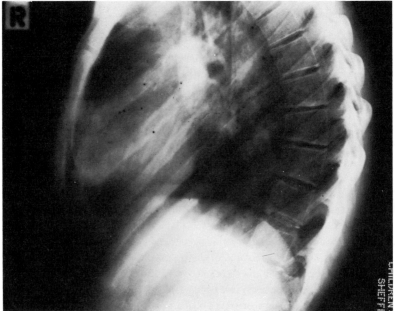

Fig. 29.9 Scheuermann's disease.

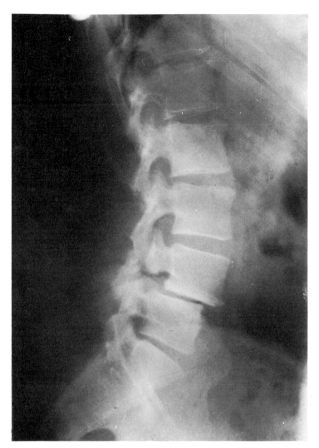

Fig. 29.10 Spondylolisthesis.

SPONDYLOLISTHESIS

In this condition, one vertebra slips forwards relative to the one below—usually L5 on S1 or L4 on L5 (Fig. 29.10). Various types and degrees are possible and, occasionally, lumbar nerve roots may be trapped causing sciatica which may be bilateral.

CAUSES

1 Congenital—usually associated with a long, thin pars-interarticularis (the part of the vertebra lying between the two articular processes) (see Fig. 42.2).

2 Some cases are thought to be associated with stress fractures of the pars-interarticularis, leading to bilateral defects and allowing the upper part of the arch and body to slip away from the lower.

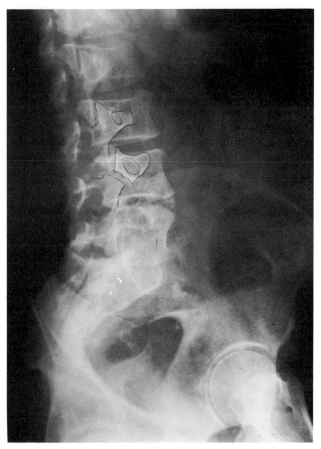

Fig. 29.11 Spondylolisthesis—oblique X-ray to show 'Scottie-dog'.

This produces a characteristic appearance on an oblique X-ray in which the so-called 'Scottie-dog' becomes decapitated (Fig. 29.11). The 'head' of the dog is formed by the articular process and the 'eye' is the pedicle.

3 Definite trauma—causing fractures of laminae, pedicles or articular processes.

4 Associated with disc degeneration, usually at L4, 5 and developing in the elderly patient (see Fig. 29.10).

CLINICAL PICTURE

Most patients present in late childhood or early adult life with low back pain, often with sciatica and sometimes with definite neurological loss in the legs.

The lumbar spine is usually undeformed apart from a definite step in the line of the spinous processes. Straight-leg raising may be reduced due to hamstring spasm.

TREATMENT

This is usually conservative, with a supporting corset. Progression is unusual. In persistent cases or if there is a definite neurological abnormality, laminectomy, followed by intervertebral fusion may be necessary.

In the undisplaced case, usually called *spondylolysis*, associated with backache, it may be possible to pass a screw across the pars-interarticularis on each side giving good stabilization and, hopefully, fusion of the defect (Buck's technique).

CHAPTER 30

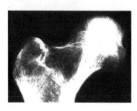

Developmental conditions – epiphyseal conditions

OSTEOCHONDRITIS

Perthes' disease

Sometimes known as Legg–Calve–Perthes disease, this is a disorder of the upper femoral epiphysis in which the growing epiphysis becomes ischaemic and infarcted, and passes through a series of characteristic X-ray changes, eventually healing, with or without distortion of the femoral head. The cause is unknown, but there is evidence that several attacks of ischaemia may occur during the course of the disease.

Clinical features

The condition usually presents at age 7–8, although it may occur at any age from 3 years (or occasionally younger) up to 11 or 12. Boys are affected more commonly than girls and about 15% of cases are bilateral. There is a definite familial tendency and the condition has been described in identical twins. Pain and a limp are the usual presenting features. Pain is often slight and may have been present over several weeks. The clinical signs are usually minor, perhaps slight restriction of movements of the hip, especially internal rotation, associated with some spasm.

The X-ray changes are characteristic and it is often obvious that the condition has been present for time prior to presentation.

Radiology

1 The earliest sign is increased density of the epiphysis and widening of the medial joint space. The changes may occupy all or part of the head (Fig. 30.1), and a lateral film is helpful in judging prognosis.

2 Later, the epiphysis appears fragmented and the head may show signs of flattening (Fig. 30.2). The overlying articular cartilage survives and the head may be more normal in shape than the X-ray suggests. The metaphysis may be widened and show cystic changes.

3 Healing occurs with gradual reabsorption of the dense bone and laying down of normal-looking new bone.

4 Restoration of the bone occurs over the course of several months. The head may be left flattened, widened and with a wider neck (Fig. 30.3).

5 Remodelling may occur until growth ceases. There is evidence that the risk of developing osteoarthritis in later life is proportional to the distortion of the head at the end of the growth period.

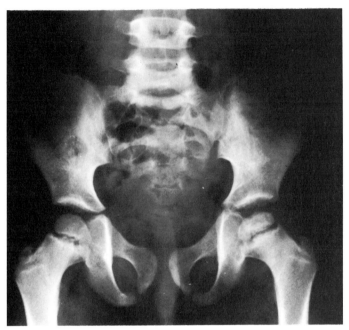

Fig. 30.1 Perthes' disease—early stage with increased density of epiphysis.

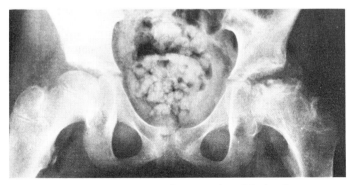

Fig. 30.2 Perthes' disease—showing fragmentation of the head.

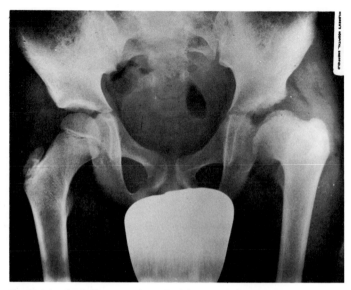

Fig. 30.3 Perthes' disease at the end of the period of reconstruction.

Treatment

There is much argument about treatment and some authorities only treat the child until the immediate symptoms settle—usually over 2–3 weeks. A short period on traction will usually achieve this. Others believe that distortion of the head can be prevented by various measures, conservative and surgical. Many regimes are practised, none of them fully evaluated because of the difficulty of making clinical comparisons. There is a gradually developing agreement that putting the hip in internal rotation and abduction may help to contain the epiphysis within the acetabulum and prevent distortion whilst it is still in the plastic stage.

Conservative

The position of abduction and internal rotation may be achieved either by traction in bed or on an abduction frame, or, without traction, in abduction plasters or an abduction brace. Treatment may be provided in hospital or at home, and some of the regimes allow sufficient mobility to enable the child to attend school.

The value of non-weight-bearing is uncertain; some workers allowing full weight-bearing in plaster cylinders, others insisting on strict bed rest.

Some surgeons abduct and internally rotate the hip then bring the leg down to neutral by carrying out an osteotomy through the inter-trochanteric region. They claim this shortens the period of immobilization and achieves equally satisfactory results.

Prognosis

The prognosis is better in the younger child and when only part of the head is involved. Girls fare worse than boys for any given age. Many of the difficulties centre around treating a condition which quickly becomes symptom-free and is then only manifest as a series of changes on X-rays.

Irritable hip

The child usually presents with pain in one hip or a limp which has lasted for a few days. There may be spasm and restriction of hip movements. With bed rest and observation symptoms usually settle over about two weeks. There are no X-ray changes. Ultrasound investigations may demonstrate an effusion in the joint and if symptoms are severe or fail to settle, this may be aspirated. It is usual to investigate the hip for the possibility of tuberculosis or septic arthritis, but the vast majority settle completely and remain undiagnosed. Rarely, an X-ray taken several weeks later may show the early changes of Perthes' disease.

Other forms of osteochondritis

OSGOOD–SCHLATTER DISEASE

This is a very common condition—usually affecting adolescent boys—in which the epiphysis of the tibial tubercle becomes swollen, and sometimes appears distorted and fragmented on a lateral radiograph. It may be bilateral.

Clinical features

The child presents with pain, accurately localized to the tibial tubercle and with tenderness and sometimes swelling. The knee joint is normal.

Prognosis

Most cases settle spontaneously, although symptoms may recur for up to 2 years.

Treatment

This is rarely necessary, rest for a few days during troublesome periods being sufficient. Occasionally, it is necessary to excise the epiphyseal fragments of bone, shelling them out from the insertion of the patellar tendon.

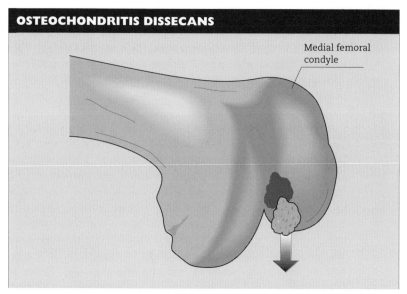

OSTEOCHONDRITIS DISSECANS

Medial femoral condyle

Fig. 30.4

OSTEOCHONDRITIS OF THE NAVICULAR (KOHLER'S DISEASE)

An uncommon condition presenting as pain in the foot in adolescence. The navicular may appear to be flattened and dense on X-ray. Spontaneous resolution is usual.

EPIPHYSITIS OF THE CALCANEUS (SEVER'S DISEASE)

The child presents with pain and tenderness over the posterior aspect of the heel. An X-ray shows increased density of the posterior epiphysis.

Other bones are susceptible to osteochondritis or epiphysitis, e.g. the lunate (Kienbock's disease), the vertebrae, the 5th metatarsal.

OSTEOCHONDRITIS DISSECANS

In this condition an area of bone with its overlying articular cartilage becomes necrotic, gradually separates and may be shed into the joint as a loose body (Fig. 30.4). The cause is unknown, but trauma may play a part in some cases. It commonly occurs in the knee, usually developing on the inner aspect of the medial femoral condyle. It also affects the hips, elbows and ankles. It is occasionally multiple and familial. The patient, usually a young adult, presents with pain and swelling in the joint. A loose body may cause the knee to lock or 'give way'. An X-ray of the knee normally shows the defect—special 'through-knee' views may be necessary to see into the intercondylar notch.

Treatment

This is not always necessary—a simple supporting bandage may be adequate. If the fragment is not completely separated, an attempt may be made to pin it back, in the hope that it will revascularize. An established loose body requires removal.

Prognosis

The short-term prognosis is reasonably good, but if the lesion is extensive, the defect in the joint surface may result in osteoarthritis later in life.

CHAPTER 31

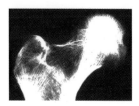

Acute infections – soft-tissue infections

Acute infections are common and often serious. They occur as:

1 localized infections – of soft tissues, of bones and joints; and

2 generalized infections.

SOFT-TISSUE INFECTIONS

Cellulitis

This is a spreading infection of the soft tissues, often caused by a haemolytic streptococcus, less commonly by other organisms. The infected area is painful, hot and oedematous, usually with lymphangitis. There is no localization of the infection or pus formation. The patient is often pyrexial from a marked toxaemia.

TREATMENT

Antibiotic therapy is usually adequate. Penicillin is still the most suitable antibiotic for streptococcal infections, provided the patient is not sensitive to it. Immobilization of the limb in a splint or sling is advisable. Healing is usually complete.

Soft-tissue abscess

Many infections, particularly of wounds and penetrating injuries, with or without a foreign body, eventually become localized to form an abscess.

TREATMENT

Diagnosis can be difficult and often the condition must be differentiated from acute osteomyelitis. The focus is often localized in the diaphyseal region rather than at the metaphysis and there may be spasm of muscles in the affected area. Drainage with antibiotic cover is usually curative. The possibility of a fungal or parasitic infection should be remembered, particularly with tropical soft-tissue abscesses.

Wound infections

Infection of wounds is common, but less likely to occur if adequate wound toilet has been performed with removal of dead or devitalized tissues and foreign material. Post-operative wound infections are often related to excessive tissue damage or to haematoma formation. Infection should be suspected if the patient is pyrexial and the wound is tense, inflamed and oedematous. A swinging pyrexia is classically regarded as indicating a collection of pus.

PROGRESS

The infection may resolve completely, form an abscess, spread locally or become generalized via the circulation and lymphatics.

TREATMENT

Antibiotics may control a developing infection. Natural or surgical drainage is usually necessary if an abscess has formed. A foreign body such as a fragment of soil, clothing or metallic implant may cause a persistent sinus until it is removed.

Tetanus

This is a serious form of wound infection arising from spores of the tetanus bacillus which have been implanted in the wound, often by contamination with soil. The organism is anaerobic and dead tissue is a favourable environment for its growth. Nevertheless, the entry wound may sometimes be no more than a puncture.

CLINICAL FEATURES

The incubation period is from 2 days to 3 weeks. A powerful neurotoxin is produced causing tonic and clonic muscle contractions. These spasms may develop first at the site of infection and quickly and characteristically involve the facial and jaw muscles producing 'lockjaw' and 'risus sardonicus'. There is then gradual spread of muscle involvement and eventually respiratory arrest. The early symptoms may be mild—usually stiffness of the jaw, neck and back muscles. Usually the shorter the incubation time the worse the prognosis.

PREVENTION AND TREATMENT

Active immunization with toxoid is now usually provided from school age. Following any penetrating injury occurring more than 5 years after active immunization, a booster dose is given. If the interval is more than 10 years, a new course is started and 250 units of human tetanus immunoglobulin is also given. Adequate wound toilet with excision of dead tissue is an important preventive measure. Treatment of the established case requires the anaesthetic facilities of an intensive care unit.

Gas gangrene

An uncommon condition caused by the anaerobic bacillus *Clostridium welchii*, occasionally by other clostridia. It usually occurs in wounds contaminated by soil and manure, especially if necrotic tissue is present. It causes gas to form in the tissues with a red discoloration of the skin, a foul smelling discharge, and spreading gangrene. The toxin is potentially lethal, but anti-serum and early wide excision of dead muscle or amputation may be life-saving. Hyperboric oxygen has been advocated but its value remains uncertain.

ACUTE GENERAL INFECTIONS

Septicaemia and pyaemia

Acute septicaemia and pyaemia occasionally complicate infections which are initially well-localized.

Poliomyelitis

Poliomyelitis is one of the few virus infections of orthopaedic importance. It is now rare in many countries but occurs sporadically. It starts as an acute intestinal infection, the organisms occasionally spreading to the anterior horn cells of the spinal cord, leading to rapid necrosis of these cells with resulting paralysis. Occurring primarily in children and young adults, it normally begins as a meningitic illness and the paralysis occurs quickly over the next few days.

The paralysis is typically patchy, but may be very extensive. Muscles which have been recently exercised seem to be particularly vulnerable. The lower limbs tend to be affected more than the upper, and muscles supplied by several cord segments are rarely paralysed completely. There is no sensory loss. The paralysis quickly reaches a maximum, then recovery occurs to a variable extent over the next few months.

TREATMENT

In the acute stage, rest with splintage of joints to avoid contracture is all that can be done. Respiration may need to be supported. Following this, physiotherapy and re-training are needed.

PRINCIPLES OF TREATMENT

- To avoid contractures by physiotherapy and muscle rebalancing.
- To utilize remaining muscles to best effect.
- To stabilize joints, either by muscle rebalancing, orthoses, or surgical fusion.
- To maintain and maximize the patient's ability and function.

The main orthopaedic interest lies in rehabilitation.

The function of paralysed muscles can sometimes be replaced by tendon transplantation, using a functioning muscle which can be spared from another site (p. 399). Muscle imbalance can also be corrected by weakening the stronger group, e.g. by tendon lengthening or denervation.

Orthoses are widely used in the after-treatment of poliomyelitis (p. 412).

As in other paralytic conditions, a severely paralysed limb may fail to grow at the same rate as the opposite one, and surgical lengthening of tibia or femur may be needed. An alternative procedure is to shorten the longer leg by surgical arrest of epiphyseal growth. This can be achieved by implanting wire staples across the epiphyses.

Rubella

Rubella and other virus infections such as measles occasionally cause an acute polyarthritis or synovitis. Symptoms are rarely severe and complete recovery is usual with no residual joint damage.

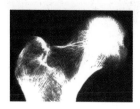

Acute infections – bone and joint infections

ACUTE OSTEOMYELITIS

This is a common condition, and is usually caused by *Staphylococcus pyogenes*, but occasionally by other organisms, e.g. streptococcus, pneumococcus, salmonella and *Escherichia coli*.

It occurs mainly in children. Poor living conditions predispose to it, and there may be an obvious primary focus of infection such as a boil, sore throat, etc.

There is often a history of preceding injury and it may be that some patients develop infection in a subperiosteal haematoma.

PATHOLOGY

The infection usually starts in the vascular metaphysis of a long bone or in the centre of a short bone. Common sites are the lower end of the femur and upper end of the tibia, either end of the humerus, radius and ulna, and the vertebral bodies. Because of the confined space and tension, tissue necrosis occurs readily and an abscess may form within the bone. The pus usually breaks out under the periosteum, stripping it up and eventually penetrating to point on the surface (Fig. 32.1).

Large areas of bone may become necrotic, making penetration by antibiotics difficult and forming 'sequestra' or hidden areas of dead and infected bone. These may act as foreign bodies, maintaining the sepsis in chronic form. If the centre of the shaft becomes infected the nutrient artery may thrombose leading to sequestration of the whole shaft.

In this case, if the patient survives, the sequestrated shaft may become surrounded by a shell of new bone, with holes through which pus may continue to find its way to the surface, forming persistent sinuses. This shell is called an involucrum. With improved management this complication is now rarely seen.

Clinical features of acute osteomyelitis

• Acute onset with high fever and malaise.

ACUTE OSTEOMYELITIS

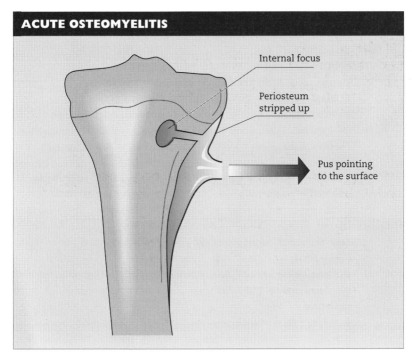

Internal focus

Periosteum
stripped up

Pus pointing
to the surface

Fig. 32.1

- Pain which is usually localized to the metaphyseal region of the bone.
- Swelling and reluctance to move the joints of the affected limb.
- Localized tenderness and heat over the site of infection.
- In later cases, if not controlled by antibiotics, oedema develops over the site of pus formation. When the pus eventually breaks through the periosteum fluctuation may be felt, but this is a late sign.

Swelling of nearby joints is usually due to a 'sympathetic' effusion. Occasionally, especially if the metaphysis is intracapsular, the joint itself may become infected.

The condition is not uncommon in neonates and is difficult to diag-

INVESTIGATIONS

- The white cell count and ESR are usually raised.
- Blood should be taken for culture before antibiotics are administered.
- An X-ray may show no changes in the early stages. Two to three weeks later, an area of porosis, perhaps with subperiosteal new bone formation may be seen. Sequestration, i.e. the separation of dense, dead bone occurs much later.

nose, often remaining almost silent. The baby usually fails to thrive and cries when the limb is moved.

TREATMENT

This is urgent. If the condition is suspected:

1 Blood is taken for culture.

2 A combination of antistaphylococcal and broad spectrum antibiotics is then started. Fucidin and erythromycin make a popular combination. These may be given parenterally if the child is too ill to take oral medication.

3 The limb should be splinted, e.g. in a Thomas' splint, sling or plaster back-slab.

PROGRESS

The antibiotics usually control the septicaemia and fever quite quickly.

1 If given early enough, the antibiotics may control the infection and complete healing may then take place with reabsorption of small sequestra.

2 Pus formation may already have occurred by the time treatment has started. In this case, the temperature usually starts to swing after first settling on antibiotic treatment. The pain and swelling persist. Localized oedema of the skin is a useful sign of pus formation. Fluctuation is often difficult to detect.

3 If pus is suspected, surgical drainage is necessary. Pus may break through the periosteum or this may need to be incised. If no pus is found, the bone may be drilled but this is usually unnecessary.

4 Following drainage, splintage is maintained and antibiotics continued or changed according to the culture. If the condition then settles, a total of 6 weeks' antibiotic therapy is usually recommended. The ESR is a guide to recovery during this period. The majority of children are cured by this regime and recurrence is unusual. Occasionally, full control is not achieved and the condition becomes chronic (Chapter 33).

OSTEOMYELITIS OF THE SPINE

This may be difficult to diagnose and is often less acute than with other sites. Fever with bone pain and muscle spasm are usual. Walking may be difficult and painful. The disease typically affects the vertebral bodies, but may affect the posterior elements.

Diagnosis may need blood culture and aspiration or drainage of pus from a paravertebral abscess. Cord symptoms are rare but serious.

Acute osteomyelitis of the spine occasionally occurs in adults, often in association with urinary tract infection.

TREATMENT

This relies on antibiotics and surgical drainage where necessary, with rest in a plaster bed or frame until symptoms subside and healing is occurring, when mobilization can gradually be allowed.

ACUTE SUPPURATIVE ARTHRITIS

This is a serious and damaging condition, which arises:

1 From progression of osteomyelitis, usually in joints where the metaphysis is intracapsular – especially the hip and upper end of radius. Occasionally, in older children spread occurs through the epiphyseal plate into the epiphysis and then into the joint itself. Osteomyelitis of the acetabulum may be difficult to distinguish from septic arthritis.

2 From haematogenous spread, particularly in infants, where multiple joint infections may occur and be relatively silent. The prime focus is usually in the lungs. In adults, gonococcal arthritis may follow genitourinary infection.

3 In rheumatoid joints especially in patients on steroids. The infection may arise by haematogenous spread or by direct implantation from an intra-articular injection, particularly if a steroid drug has been injected.

4 Following penetrating injuries.

PATHOLOGY

The infection is usually staphylococcal but may be by other organisms. The synovium becomes inflamed and thickened, fluid is increased and quickly becomes purulent. Muscle spasm and softening of ligaments and capsule may allow dislocation (especially of the hip in an infant – Smith's arthritis). Pus eventually ruptures through the capsule and points, but by then the articular cartilage is usually severely damaged. In the hip the increased pressure may cause ischaemic necrosis of the femoral head.

Repair occurs with much fibrosis and often bony ankylosis.

CLINICAL FEATURES

The patient is usually very ill with high fever and rigors due to septicaemia. The joint is acutely painful and swollen and is hot and very tender. There is almost always extreme muscle spasm, often allowing no movement of the joint or the limb. The differential diagnosis is from osteomyelitis with a sympathetic effusion, rheumatic fever, rheumatoid arthritis or Still's disease (usually multiple joints), Reiter's syndrome, and gout.

RADIOLOGY

There may be no X-ray changes in the early stages. Later, sub-periosteal new bone may become visible with generalized peri-articular porosis. Pathological subluxation or dislocation may occur and this may be difficult to diagnose in the infant whose epiphyses are not yet ossified.

MANAGEMENT

To establish a diagnosis, the joint should be aspirated on suspicion. The organisms may be identified by culture of blood and the joint aspirate. If the aspirate is merely turbid, antibiotic therapy alone may be adequate. (Erythromycin and fucidin are an acceptable combination.) The joint should be immobilized on a splint or sling. If the aspirate is frank pus, open operation should be carried out, draining the pus and irrigating the joint with antibiotics, then closing the skin. Unlike other sites of pus formation it is not usual to leave a drain into the joint unless the sepsis is very severe and the joint is likely to be totally destroyed. In these circumstances, some authorities advise continuous irrigation with antibiotics for several days.

A decision has to be made, depending on how much damage has already occurred in the joint, whether to aim for movement or bony ankylosis. Either splintage in a position of function is continued or movement is encouraged once the sepsis is eradicated.

The antibiotic therapy is usually continued for 6 weeks.

A badly damaged and painful joint may require surgical fusion later.

Septic arthritis arising secondary to penetrating injuries and open wounds is usually less destructive, and although drainage may be required, a mobile joint may often be preserved.

CHAPTER 33

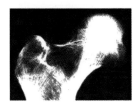

Chronic infections

CHRONIC PARONYCHIA

This is a persistent nail fold infection usually caused by a fungus or by repeated irritation, e.g. with detergents. It does not suppurate and usually responds to anti-fungal agents given locally or systemically.

CHRONIC INFECTIONS OF THE NAILS

These are often fungal and result in discoloration and deformities of the nail. They can be eradicated by oral anti-fungal agents.

CHRONIC PYOGENIC OSTEOMYELITIS

This is an uncommon, localized bone infection arising from one of the situations listed below.

1 After trauma to bone, e.g. compound fracture or penetrating injury. Bullet wounds with much contamination are particularly liable to result in pyogenic osteomyelitis.

2 By haematogenous spread—usually from an unidentifiable source. The infection may take the form of a cavity in the bone with surrounding sclerosis, giving rise to intermittent attacks of pain—Brodie's abscess. It may contain pus but organisms are not always cultivated.

3 As a result of inadequately treated acute osteomyelitis. In the typical case the infection is perpetuated by necrosis of bone, often resulting in sequestra ranging in size from a few millimetres to almost the whole shaft. The living bone becomes thickened and honeycombed and may surround the sequestrum completely, preventing its discharge (involucrum).

4 As a complication of surgery, particularly when foreign material is implanted. The infection usually results in failure of the implant.

CLINICAL COURSE

The disease is characterized by 'flares' of infection with pain and swelling, and often pus formation, alternating with periods of quiescence—sometimes lasting several years. Occasionally, particularly following penetrating injuries, compound fractures and replacement arthroplasty, a sinus may form and discharge continuously. Often when the discharge stops the condition becomes acute until the resulting abscess is drained.

INVESTIGATIONS

X-rays demonstrate the abnormal bone texture with thickening and diffuse cavity formation (Fig. 33.1). A sequestrum usually shows up as a localized mass of bone, denser than its surroundings.

Culture of the pus from a persistent sinus usually yields mixed organisms from secondary infection. The ESR is usually raised and the white cell count shows a moderate leucocytosis.

TREATMENT

This is difficult and consists of the following.

I Treating acute episodes with the appropriate antibiotic which is usu-

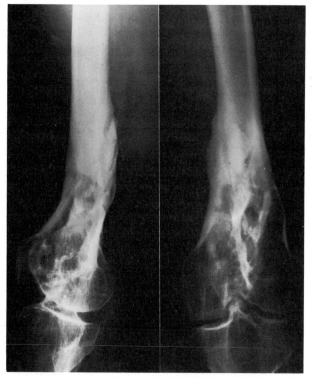

Fig. 33.1 Chronic osteomyelitis following a compound fracture.

ally known from previous culture. Surgical drainage may be necessary.
2 Attempts at eradication. This is often impossible, but long-term antibiotics combined with excision of sequestra and opening up of poorly draining cavities may be successful. For the extensively involved bone the procedure of 'guttering', which involves opening the medullary cavity widely and allowing the wound to granulate and heal from the bottom, used to be popular. Newer methods involve opening the bone widely, scraping out cavities and closing the defect with muscle on a vascular pedicle or a split skin or pedicle skin graft. There is interest in removing the infected segment completely and closing the gap by performing an osteotomy some distance away and transporting the healthy bone to fill the gap using an Ilizarov frame and bone lengthening techniques (p. 80).

Chronic osteomyelitis occurring as a complication of replacement arthroplasty presents formidable problems and is becoming increasingly common (p. 362).

3 Amputation may occasionally be the most satisfactory way of relieving symptoms.

COMPLICATIONS

- Secondary infection elsewhere caused by haematogenous spread.
- Pathological fracture (uncommon).
- Amyloidosis.
- Squamous carcinoma developing in a sinus tract.

TUBERCULOSIS OF BONES AND JOINTS

Two strains of tubercle bacillus are responsible, human and bovine. The latter has been eliminated from the UK, but is occasionally seen in immigrants.

Bone and joint tuberculosis usually occurs in the later stages of the generalized disease. The initial infection is either via the respiratory tract or the intestine, and the bacilli reach the spine or limbs by blood spread.

INCIDENCE

When tuberculosis was common, infection usually occurred in children. In most cases the infection was minor and healed, leaving the child immune. Now, in the developed countries infection is rare, many adults remain tuberculin negative, and, apart from immigrants, the highest incidence is in old people. There is evidence, however, of a resurgence of the disease worldwide.

PREVENTION

In the UK, the disease has been eliminated to the point where generalized immunization of children with BCG vaccine is no longer considered necessary and only particular groups such as medical staff and definite contacts are immunized. The disease is still very common, however, in the underdeveloped world and is increasingly being seen in patients with HIV infection. Drug resistance is an increasing problem.

PATHOLOGY

The prominent features are listed below.

1 Destruction of bone and articular cartilage by tuberculous granulation tissue with areas of healing by fibrosis.

2 Thickening of synovial membrane which becomes studded with tubercles and extends as a pannus under the edges of the articular cartilage, destroying it.

3 Abscess formation, especially in spinal tuberculosis. The pus tracks along tissue planes, particularly within the psoas sheath in association with spinal infections and may point some distance from the original site, e.g. in the groin. Spread can occur through cartilaginous epiphyses and end-plates and across the intervertebral discs.

4 In the healing phase fibrosis occurs. The joint may remain mobile or may develop a fibrous or bony ankylosis.

CLINICAL FEATURES

Infection of bone alone is unusual, occasionally occurring in metacarpals, phalanges, ribs or greater trochanter. Usually, the infection involves both bone and joints:

1 starting in the metaphysis as in acute osteomyelitis and spreading to the joint, especially when the metaphysis is intracapsular; or

2 starting in the synovial membrane.

In both cases the whole joint and bone ends are quickly affected.

X-ray appearances

1 Osteoporotic changes around the joint may be the first sign.

2 Erosion of the joint surfaces with decreased joint space.

3 Destruction of bone (and intervertebral discs).

4 Soft-tissue shadows representing abscesses, e.g. the 'bird's nest' shadow of a para-vertebral abscess which is almost always present in spinal tuberculosis.

INVESTIGATIONS

1 The ESR is usually raised and is an index of progress.

2 Moderate lymphocytosis is usual.

3 The tuberculin (Mantoux or Heaf) test is positive in all except early cases (who rarely have bone and joint TB). The test is usually positive at 1 in 10 000 dilution. Very occasionally, a patient with widespread 'miliary' tuberculosis may be tuberculin negative.

4 Biopsy of lymph glands may show typical tuberculosis, but biopsy of bone or synovium is usually more reliable, allowing histological examination, culture and guinea-pig inoculation for final confirmation.

5 Bacilli may be cultured from sputum or urine.

TREATMENT

The modern trend is towards conservative treatment. Sanatorium treatment is no longer considered necessary. Infection is always generalized and drug therapy has revolutionized treatment. It can usually be started before waiting for final confirmation of the diagnosis. It must be emphasized, however, that because of the risks of encouraging the emergence of drug resistant strains, it is absolutely essential that drug therapy be controlled by careful sensitivity testing of the organisms.

1 The currently recommended regime uses rifampicin, isonazid and pyrazinamide, usually starting with all three drugs and reducing to two on the basis of the sensitivities. A 6 month course would be usual for pulmonary TB, but longer periods may be required in the case of bone and joint disease, particularly of the spine. Rifampicin is expensive but very effective. Pyrazinamide may often be stopped after 2 months. Isonazid is neurotoxic.

2 Streptomycin remains a useful drug, but has the disadvantages that it has to be given parenterally and may cause deafness and vestibular disturbances.

3 Thiacetazone has the advantage of being inexpensive, which is of importance in developing countries. It may produce a rash in patients with AIDS. Ethambutol may be used, but it is known to cause ophthalmic symptoms and blindness, so that monitoring by an ophthalmologist is desirable.

There is disagreement about the value of draining tuberculous abscesses and clearing out cavities. Studies in Africa and the Far East suggest that conservative measures may be adequate, i.e. drug therapy with rest and immobilization in the early stages and gradual joint movement later. Bony fusion used to be the aim of orthopaedic management and may still be best for the badly damaged joint.

Tuberculosis of the hip (p. 359)

This is usually seen in children. It causes a limp with generalized malaise and aching pain. There is gradual destruction of the joint which becomes

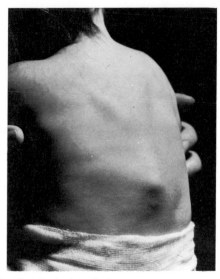

Fig. 33.2 Gibbus in spinal tuberculosis.

drawn into adduction and flexion. The head of the femur is easily destroyed and dislocation may occur. Abscesses and sinuses may form around the joint. The differential diagnosis includes Perthes' disease, transient synovitis, Still's disease, slipped epiphysis.

TREATMENT

This relies on chemotherapy and traction initially. When the spasm subsides, if joint destruction is not too severe, gradual mobilization is allowed. Abscesses may need surgical drainage.

Tuberculosis of the spine–Potts' disease

The spine is a common site for tuberculosis in children and adults, the disease usually occurring in the thoracic or cervical regions. It tends to start in the vertebral end-plate and spreads to the adjacent disc.

SYMPTOMS

Pain and malaise with loss of weight, as in most tubercular infections, is often accompanied by wasting of the back muscles, but with spasm and restriction of spinal movements. There is often a localized kyphos or 'gibbus' (Fig. 33.2), and pain on percussion. There may be cord or root compression.

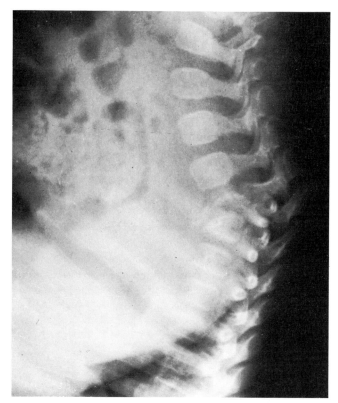

Fig. 33.3 Lateral X-ray showing spinal tuberculosis.

X-rays

These show destruction of vertebrae and intervertebral discs and a paravertebral abscess shadow (Fig. 33.3). On an abdominal film the outline of the psoas may be obscured by the abscess.

Differential diagnosis

The differential diagnosis is from neoplasia, pyogenic osteomyelitis, myeloma. Needle or surgical biopsy and culture is usually necessary to establish the diagnosis.

TREATMENT

This is primarily drug therapy. Authorities differ on the need for drainage of abscesses and removal of necrotic material. In the thoracic region this can be done, if desired, through an antero-lateral approach to the spine, removing the posterior part of several ribs. The approach can also be made by removing the proximal end of one or more ribs and the transverse processes (costo-transversectomy), or through the pleural cavity. Abscesses which are pointing should certainly be drained. Whether treatment is conservative or surgical, initial immobilization in a plaster bed is usual, followed by a spinal support until stability is achieved, usually by the affected vertebral bodies fusing together.

Tuberculous paraplegia–Pott's paraplegia

This may occur at any level, but is usually thoracic. It occurs at two stages of the disease process:

1 early paraplegia, mainly due to abscesses and necrotic debris; and

2 late paraplegia, probably partly mechanical due to bone destruction with angulation, and partly vascular.

Either type may or may not recover. The present trend is to rely on conservative treatment initially, with immobilization on a plaster bed and antibiotics. If recovery does not occur in the first few weeks, or if there is deterioration, the spine may be decompressed by draining the abscess, and the segments fused surgically.

SINUSES

A sinus is a blind track communicating with an epithelial surface such as the skin or an internal organ. The track itself may be lined with epithelium. Chronic infection may play a part in the persistence of a sinus, sometimes secondary to the underlying pathology. A sinus may form for several reasons.

1 Congenital. These usually represent the persistence of an embryological structure, e.g. a branchial or thyroglossal sinus.

2 Foreign body. This may be material which is foreign to the body, or dead tissue which may behave as a foreign body, particularly if infected. A bony sequestrum is an example of this. Healing will rarely occur, once infection is established, until the foreign material is removed. This is particularly a problem with infected prostheses.

3 Chronic infection. Such chronic conditions as tuberculosis, fungal infections, etc. may produce a chronic sinus after the abscess has discharged or been drained.

4 Neoplasia. Rarely, a sinus may communicate with a neoplastic mass. A long-established chronic sinus may itself develop secondary neoplastic changes.

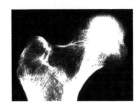

CHAPTER 34

Neoplastic conditions – general principles

The borderline between true neoplasms, i.e. groups of cells which continue to proliferate indefinitely in an uncontrolled fashion, and those which proliferate for a time, eventually becoming mature, is a blurred one. It is convenient to distinguish the second group as hamartomata.

The true tumours are usually subdivided into benign and malignant but, again, the distinction is not always clear either from the histological or behavioural point of view.

TUMOURS OF ORTHOPAEDIC INTEREST

These fall into two groups: (1) metastatic tumours – usually deposited in bone, these are the commonest tumours of the skeletal system; and (2) primary tumours.

METASTATIC TUMOURS

Bone is a common site for the deposition of secondary tumours – usually of epithelial origin.

Most epithelial tumours and occasional sarcomata can metastasize to bone. Soft-tissue metastases in the limbs are much less common. Metastases from the prostate may reach the bone by venous spread and are common in the lumbo-sacral spine and pelvis. Breast metastases are similarly common in ribs, thoracic vertebrae and clavicles. Arterial spread may result in deposition anywhere in the skeleton, particularly the flat bones, vertebrae and proximal ends of femur and humerus.

PRIMARY SITES

The commonest primary sites are:
- breast
- bronchus
- thyroid
- kidney
- prostate.

Radiological appearances

There is usually a circumscribed area of radio-lucency which may extend through the cortex. Pathological fracture is common.

Metastases from a carcinoma of the prostate and occasionally the breast are usually bone forming—producing islands of dense, sclerotic bone, occasionally with patches of rarefaction.

CLINICAL FEATURES

1 Deep-seated pain is the usual problem, frequently being the first warning that the patient has a neoplasm. The primary site may or may not be obvious.

2 Occasionally a swelling or fracture may be the presenting feature.

INVESTIGATIONS

The primary may have to be sought in the usual way. A suspected bony metastasis may be revealed by scanning the area after injection of a radio-isotope (e.g. strontium or technetium), which is taken up selectively in the tumour area. Extensive metastases tend to elevate the serum alkaline phosphatase level because of the associated bone destruction and re-formation. Metastases from a prostatic neoplasm cause a rise in the serum acid phosphatase level (which is rarely raised by the primary alone).

Management

The presence of bony metastases usually means a poor prognosis for life.

1 Severe bone pain can be incapacitating, but may respond to local radiotherapy or occasionally to chemotherapy. Surgical excision is rarely justified, but amputation may sometimes be necessary to relieve the pain.

2 Pathological fractures are normally best treated by internal fixation to enable the patient to mobilize early. With local radiotherapy and firm fixation, union often occurs. In certain situations prosthetic replacement of the diseased bone may provide the best symptomatic treatment.

3 Certain tumours respond to hormone therapy, e.g. breast carcinoma may respond to oophorectomy, androgen or steroid treatment, and prostatic carcinoma with secondaries has a fairly good prognosis when treated with oestrogens. Breast carcinoma is now commonly treated with anti-oestrogen drugs, of which tamoxifen is the best-known.

4 Despite the presence of metastases, it may still be worth treating the primary lesion if it is causing or is likely to cause local symptoms.

PRIMARY NEOPLASMS

Connective tissue cells		Mesenchymal cells	
Collagenous tissue	Neuroma Fibrosarcoma Angioma	Fat	Lipoma Liposarcoma
	Aneurysmall bone cyst Angiosarcoma	Muscle	Leiomyoma Leiomyosarcoma Rhabdomyosarcoma
Cartilage	Enchondroma		
	Chondrosarcoma Chondroblastoma	Synovium	Synovioma
		Marrow	Myeloma Ewing's tumour
Bone	Osteoid osteoma Osteoma Osteosarcoma Osteoclastoma		Non-Hodgkin's lymphoma Hodgkin's disease Leukaemia

Table 34.1

PRIMARY NEOPLASMS—GENERAL CONSIDERATIONS

Bones are made up of many tissues: bone, cartilage, fibrous tissue, blood vessels, marrow elements, etc., and since tumours can arise from most of these tissues and from muscle, fat, nerve sheaths, synovium and skin, the range of tumours of the locomotor system is wide.

CLASSIFICATION

Any classification of primary neoplasms is likely to be unsatisfactory in that the precise tissue of origin is often uncertain, mixed cell tumours are common, and different areas of a given tumour may contain different types of tissue. A simple classification is given for reference and as an aid to memory (Table 34.1). It is not meant to be exhaustive, but contains the commonest tumours likely to be encountered. All are relatively rare but make up about 20% of tumours found in young people.

SITE

Some tumours affect the metaphyses of long bones. Osteoclastoma arises within the site of the original epiphysis after the closure of the plate. The vertebral bodies are frequently the sites of myelogenic tumours.

EFFECTS ON BONES

Most tumours stimulate bone resorption, and consequently show up as translucent areas on X-ray. The cortex may be expanded by resorption from the inside and deposition from the outside. Alternatively, the tumour may break through the cortex into the soft tissues. When this occurs, the periosteum is usually elevated from the bone and a triangle of new bone is produced in the angle where it leaves the shaft—Codman's triangle (Fig. 34.1).

Some tumours stimulate bone formation so that dense areas appear in the zone of translucency. Cartilage tumours are often characterized by having a spongy trabecular or honeycomb appearance. Pathological fractures are common and may heal despite the presence of the tumour.

CLINICAL FEATURES

Most tumours present as localized swellings either in bone or in the soft tissues. Pain associated with such a swelling is often an ominous symptom

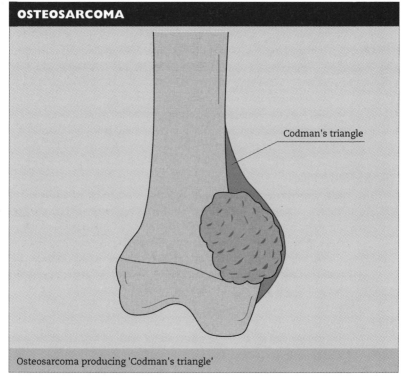

OSTEOSARCOMA

Codman's triangle

Osteosarcoma producing 'Codman's triangle'

Fig. 34.1

suggesting rapid growth. The pain is typically non-mechanical, i.e. not related to activity and often wakes the patient at night. It is usually the presenting feature of an osteosarcoma. The swelling may be well localized, or ill-defined. In malignant conditions, the swelling is often warm with distended blood vessels overlying it. There may be some reduction of movement in the nearby joint.

INVESTIGATIONS

X-rays in several planes are essential—often the appearances are sufficiently characteristic to suggest the diagnosis, but they should never be relied upon alone for decisions on treatment.

The ESR is often raised and biochemistry disturbed, e.g. the serum calcium and alkaline phosphatase may be raised by increased bone turnover. Abnormalities of the serum proteins are found in myelogenic tumours.

Diagnosis usually rests finally on biopsy. For accuracy, this should include a reasonable-sized, representative piece of tissue. In some cases the whole lesion may be easily excised. Punch biopsy is rarely adequate, but aspiration of marrow may be sufficient in the diagnosis of myeloma, secondary neoplasms etc. The sternum is a useful site for marrow aspiration. The biopsy should be taken by the surgeon who will be responsible for the definitive treatment because the siting of the incision may be important if limb salvage is to be attempted or amputation is required.

TREATMENT

Accurate diagnosis is essential for rational treatment.

Surgery

Most benign and many malignant tumours can be excised completely. This often necessitates wide excision and bone-grafting, or occasionally the insertion of a prosthesis. Some tumours are highly malignant with a very poor prognosis and wide excision or amputation will only be curative if metastases have not occurred. Even then recurrence is likely. Amputation may be necessary even in the presence of metastases to relieve local symptoms.

Radiotherapy

Some tumours are radio-sensitive, e.g. Ewing's tumour, and non-Hodgkins lymphoma of bone. In other cases radiotherapy may be used for palliation or to help union of a fracture.

Cytotoxic drugs

The use of modern cytotoxic drugs, in elaborate regimes often involving lethal doses, and using 'rescue' procedures with antagonists, has greatly improved survival times for some tumours. The side effects are often severe, but the method shows great promise in the treatment of neoplasms such as osteosarcoma and Ewing's sarcoma which were until recently almost universally lethal.

CHAPTER 35

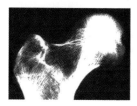

Neoplastic conditions – primary neoplasms

PRIMARY SKELETAL TUMOURS

Soft-tissue tumours

These can arise from any tissue within the body. Their incidence is approximately 60 per million per year (3000 per year in the UK) of which half occur in the musculoskeletal system. There are no specific clinical features suggesting malignancy in any lump, but the following are highly suggestive:

1 any lump larger than 5 cm;
2 any lump that is increasing in size;
3 any lump that has recently become painful;
4 any lump deep to the fascia; and
5 any lump that has recurred after previous excision.

Soft-tissue sarcomata tend to metastasize via the blood stream to the lungs. Local control is essential and relies upon surgical excision with a wide margin around the tumour. 'Shell-out' procedures are unacceptable and result, almost inevitably, in local recurrence. Amputation may sometimes be necessary for large tumours. Despite these measures, metastases occur in 50% of patients and in these cases the outlook is bleak. Radiotherapy can be used to help local control following surgical excision.

Neoplasms derived from collagenous tissue – specific features

NEUROMA

This is not usually a tumour but a reaction to damage of a nerve. It consists of a round swelling on the end or side of the nerve, made up of fibrous tissue and nerve sheath elements. It may be painful and require excision.

True neuromata usually arise from the endoneural connective tissue or from the Schwann cells (Schwannoma). They may be multiple as in neurofibromatosis and occasionally become malignant—neurofibrosarcoma.

FIBROMA

Tumours which could be described as true benign fibromata are rare and often represent hamartomata. The 'desmoid' is a slow-growing tumour, consisting of dense fibrous tissue, usually affecting the rectus sheath but also found in the limbs, particularly in relation to the major nerves and muscle aponeuroses. It is non-metastasizing. It frequently occurs during pregnancy and may be hormone dependant. Treatment consists of wide excision, but local recurrence is usual.

FIBROSARCOMA

This is usually a slowly growing soft-tissue tumour of muscle, tendon, ligament or periosteum. Metastasis usually occurs late but the tumour often recurs locally. The recommended treatment is wide surgical excision.

HAEMANGIOMA

Most of these tumours are hamartomatous lesions of small size which grow slowly. A haemangioma in a vertebral body may cause complete collapse of the body. Lymphangiomata occur occasionally and are usually soft semi-cystic lesions with a tendency to recur after excision.

HAEMANGIOSARCOMA

These are rare soft-tissue tumours, some of which regress spontaneously—others metastasize.

ANEURYSMAL BONE CYST

This is a lesion which has some of the characteristics of a tumour, but is probably non-neoplastic and may be a complex arterio-venous malformation. It produces spongy blood-filled cyst-like cavities in bone—usually near the ends but not in the epiphysis. It slowly expands the bone, eventually breaking through the cortex (Fig. 35.1). It usually occurs in the second decade, and is often painful. Treatment is by curettage, with or without bone-grafting. Radiotherapy may be useful for inaccessible or inoperable cases. The prognosis is usually good.

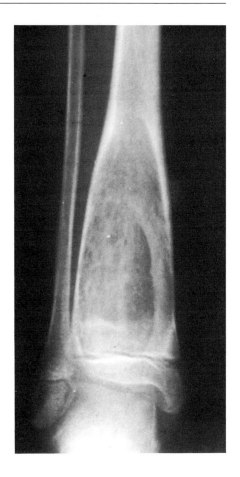

Fig. 35.1 Aneurysmal bone cyst.

Neoplasms derived from cartilaginous tissue

ENCHONDROMA

A hamartomatous mass of cartilage cells arising in the metaphysis of a cylindrical bone, usually in childhood or adolescence. It may expand the bone or break through the cortex. It can usually be excised without recurrence. It usually occurs in the hands or feet. If seen in a flat bone it is more likely to be a chondrosarcoma.

Multiple enchondromatosis—see p. 206.

OSTEOCHONDROMA

A solitary lesion of similar type to that found in multiple osteochondromatosis (p. 206).

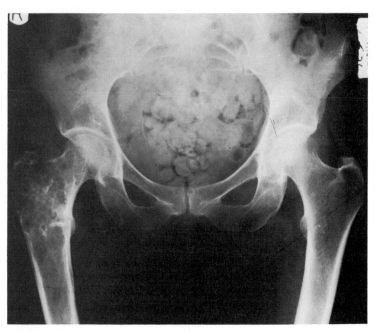

Fig. 35.2 Chondrosarcoma.

CHONDROSARCOMA

A tumour which arises from chondroblasts and can produce only chondroid and collagen—not bone. It is rather more common in males. It typically affects the bones of the trunk and the proximal ends of long bones. It is unusual under the age of 30. Two types are seen—one arising within the bone and the other on the surface, sometimes in an osteochondroma. Benign chondromata in the digits rarely become malignant. The tumour may cause pain and a slowly increasing swelling, perhaps over a period of 10 years. Radiologically, it is represented by a translucent area which may expand the bone (Fig. 35.2) and is often crisscrossed by spicules of calcification. It metastasizes, but complete excision, if necessary by amputation, is frequently curative, with a 50% 5-year survival rate. If the tumour is entered during excision, recurrence is more likely, so if the diagnosis seems likely, excision biopsy is preferable to opening the tumour.

CHONDROBLASTOMA

A rare tumour affecting the epiphyses of adolescents. It causes pain and grows slowly. It is usually benign, but should be excised adequately.

Neoplasms derived from bone tissue

OSTEOID OSTEOMA

A curious lesion causing chronic pain characteristically relieved by aspirin and appearing on X-ray as an area of dense sclerosis with a central translucent nidus. It can occur in any bone and multiple X-ray views may be necessary to reveal the characteristic appearance. Occasionally CT and isotope bone scanning may be helpful. The lesion is almost certainly not a tumour—histology shows osteoid and some new bone proliferation at the centre of a sclerotic area. Curettage usually cures the condition which is, in some cases, self-limiting.

OSTEOMA

A hamartomatous growth from the surface of a bone. It is intramembranous in origin and frequently occurs on the skull or face. It can be cured by excision.

OSTEOSARCOMA

This is a malignant neoplasm arising from bone cells which are undifferentiated and capable of forming bone, cartilage and collagenous tissue. It is the most commonly occurring primary tumour of bone, with an incidence of 3 per million population. It usually occurs under the age of 30, in boys more than girls and in cylindrical bones.

In older patients, typically over 50, it tends to occur in flat bones as well as long bones, and is then usually associated with Paget's disease.

In young patients the commonest bone affected is the femur (50%). The upper tibia and the upper end of the humerus are also common sites. It almost always affects the metaphysis.

Clinical features

Pain is the dominant feature—usually preceding the onset of a swelling and often waking the patient at night. The child may limp. The tumour grows rapidly and may become hot and congested with dilated vessels in the overlying skin. It usually grows eccentrically, elevating the periosteum with a resultant deposition of sub-periosteal bone (Codman's triangle). It eventually breaks through the cortex and fungates in the soft tissue. The patient becomes debilitated and often feverish. Metastasis to the lungs tends to occur early.

Radiological features

The typical feature is a destructive lesion in the metaphysis—usually translucent and often with reactive periosteal new bone or rays of

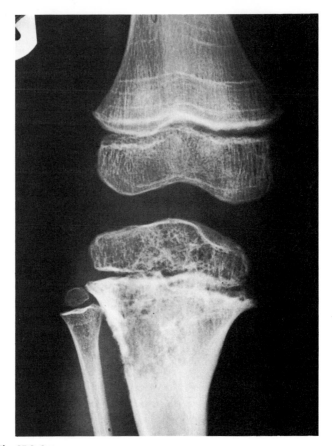

Fig. 35.3 Osteosarcoma.

ossification within the expanding tumour ('sunburst effect'). A soft-tissue mass may be apparent. Areas of calcification may occur, but are less evident than in chondrosarcoma (Fig. 35.3).

Investigations

The ESR is usually raised, as is the alkaline phosphatase. Bone scanning is useful for demonstrating more proximal or multiple lesions. Magnetic resonance imaging (MRI) and CT scanning have proved to be of value in assessing the extent of spread, particularly within the soft tissues.

Histologically, these tumours are pleomorphic with obvious malignant cells showing mitoses, but often with areas of bone, cartilage and fibrous tissue, which may confuse the diagnosis. The tumour is usually highly vascular, but there may be extensive necrosis. This variation in histological pattern makes accurate diagnosis difficult and considerable experience is required in interpreting the sections.

Treatment

Surgical biopsy is essential. When the diagnosis is confirmed, treatment now almost always commences with chemotherapy. This has the advantage of immediately treating the micro-metastases which are almost certainly present by the time of diagnosis (but rarely detectable even with CT scanning of the lungs). Another advantage is that the primary tumour will often show some shrinkage. After 6–9 weeks, surgery is carried out. Limb salvage can often be achieved i.e. resecting the tumour-bearing bone and surrounding soft tissues, the limb being reconstructed with a custom-built prosthesis and artificial joint if necessary. Survival appears to be no worse than after amputation and the procedure offers better palliation for those patients who already have pulmonary metastases. If the tumour is too extensive at the time of diagnosis and there is a poor response to chemotherpy, amputation may still be necessary. For patients with metastases at diagnosis, the prognosis is poor, but for those without detectable metastases, there is now a cure rate of 60%.

Osteosarcoma arising in Paget's disease is one of the most malignant tumours known and survival for 2 years is very unusual with any form of therapy.

OSTEOCLASTOMA (GIANT CELL TUMOUR)

The origin of the osteoclast is not known for certain. It is a characteristic of osteoclast tumours that they form multinucleated giant cells.

Clinical features

The tumour affects young adults within 10–20 years after fusion of the epiphysis—usually at the lower end of the femur or upper end of the tibia—occasionally in the cylindrical bones of the hands and feet. It starts in the metaphysis, extends into the original site of the epiphysis and expands the bone eccentrically. It usually grows slowly and maintains a shell of thin cortex (Fig. 35.4).

Pathology

Microscopically, the tumour consists of spindle cells and giant cells, usually with a collagenous stroma. Metastasis is unusual and late.

Treatment

Excision is usually possible, but prosthetic replacement of the joint surface may be necessary.

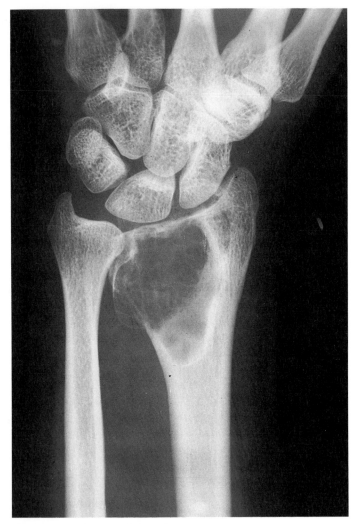

Fig. 35.4 Osteoclastoma of the radius.

Neoplasms derived from fat tissue

LIPOMA

This is a very common, slowly growing soft tumour, usually occurring in the superficial fascia or in muscle. It is encapsulated and recurrence after complete excision is unusual.

LIPOSARCOMA

This tumour usually occurs in the 5th decade, affecting the fat of the buttock, thigh and occasionally shoulder region. It grows slowly but invades widely. Pain is rare.

Treatment

Wide excision is necessary, but recurrence is usual and metastases may occur. Hindquarter amputation may be necessary for buttock or upper thigh tumours.

Neoplasms rising from muscle cells

LEIOMYOMA AND LEIOMYOSARCOMA

These are rare smooth muscle tumours, occasionally occurring in the limbs.

RHABDOMYOSARCOMA

This is a tumour of striated muscle usually arising over the age of 50. Wide excision is necessary to prevent recurrence or metastases.

NEOPLASMS ARISING FROM SYNOVIAL TISSUE–SYNOVIOMA

Giant-cell tumours of the tendon sheath are sometime called *synoviomata* and are benign.

Synovial sarcomata are malignant tumours which have nothing to do with synovium or joints. They have a typically biphasic histological pattern with spindle cells and cells which look like synovium. They arise in the soft tissues in the limbs, predominantly in young people. There is often a long history of a lump which may rapidly increase in size. It is often soft or cystic and may be confused with a simple ganglion. All such swellings should be sent for histological examination. Metastases to the lungs occur frequently, but may take many years to occur.

Treatment

This is surgical, with wide excision.

Tumours arising from recticulum or marrow elements— myeloma (plasma cell myeloma)

This originates in the haemopoietic tissue of red marrow. It is occasionally solitary, but usually multiple when first diagnosed. It almost always occurs over the age of 40, and tends to affect the pelvic girdle and the vertebrae.

Diagnosis

It is a neoplasm of plasma cells which normally produce gamma globulins—these become elevated in the serum and detectable in the urine. Electrophoresis of serum enables accurate protein fractionation to be carried out, giving characteristic protein curves. About 69% of cases of myeloma produce excessive amounts of globulin. One of these, 'Bence-Jones' protein, is a light-chain globulin which passes the glomeruli and can be demonstrated by testing the urine. It is found in less than one half of patients with myeloma.

Excess uric acid may be excreted and amyloid is often deposited in the tissues. Kidney insufficency occurs in about two-thirds of patients.

Clinical and radiological features

Bone pain is the usual complaint, often in the spine or pelvic region. On X-ray the lesions are typically circumscribed and osteolytic—giving a punched out appearance, particularly in the skull and pelvic bones. Diffuse osteoporosis may also occur and vertebral bodies may collapse.

Pathology

The tumour cells resemble plasma cells and diagnosis is not usually difficult.

Treatment

The disease is essentially a diffuse one so that local excision is rarely appropriate except for the solitary lesion. Whole body irradiation and newer methods of cytotoxic therapy have increased the survival time considerably.

EWING'S SARCOMA

A malignant tumour arising in bone marrow in patients under the age of 30. About two-thirds of the tumours occur in cylindrical bones, but the older the patient the more likely is the tumour to arise in a flat bone because it develops from red marrow. It is not confined to the ends of long bones—a useful diagnostic point.

Clinical features

Pain is the outstanding feature, with tenderness at the site of the lesion. The tumour tends to invade and penetrate the cortex without expanding it very much. Occlusion of nutrient vessels may cause bone necrosis. Fever and leucocytosis are common, probably because the tumour tends to become necrotic.

Radiological features

The most striking feature is bone destruction and often a soft-tissue swelling. There may be some periosteal bone formation (Codman's triangle). Occasionally, there are onion-skin layers of new bone formation around the lesion.

Diagnosis

Biopsy is essential. Occasionally, the centre of the tumour may be necrotic and liquefied, resembling pus. The tumour consists of round cells of uniform appearance—usually with areas of degeneration.

Treatment

The tumour is highly malignant and metastasizes early, usually within 6 months. Chemotherapy, followed by surgical excision where possible, has become the treatment of choice and survival times have improved considerably for a tumour which has long been considered to have a mortality rate as high as 95%. Radiotherapy is valuable for inaccessible sites, for inoperable tumours and for palliation

NON-HODGKIN'S LYMPHOMA

This is a destructive bone tumour of adults, rather like Ewing's sarcoma, both radiologically and histologically, but with a better prognosis. Chemotherapy has again improved the survival rate.

HODGKIN'S DISEASE AND LEUKAEMIA

Both of these conditions may cause deposits in bone, especially vertebrae, as part of the generalized disease. Cytotoxic therapy is now producing increasingly long survival times.

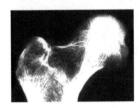

CHAPTER 36

Paget's disease

This disease, described by Sir James Paget in 1879 and named by him 'osteitis deformans', is not easy to categorize. Its cause is unknown, but characteristic inclusion bodies can be found in the bone cells suggesting a viral origin. It is one of the commonest bone diseases, affecting in Great Britain as many as 4% of the population.

DISTRIBUTION

Great Britain and western Europe have the highest world incidence. It is also common in the eastern states of the USA and eastern Australia where it is almost confined to migrants of British descent. It is almost unknown in Africa and the Indian subcontinent. There are regional variations in the UK, northern England having the highest incidence.

PATHOLOGY

The main feature of Paget's disease is a disordered architecture of the bone.

1 The Haversian systems are not produced in their usual alignment along lines of stress and the microscopic appearance becomes a 'patchwork' of disorganized trabeculae.

2 The bone is sometimes hard, sometimes soft, and deformities are common especially in weight-bearing bones.

3 Long bones become thickened, especially the cortex, and the distinction between cortex and medulla becomes lost. The trabeculae are coarsened and exaggerated.

4 The skull can become enormously thickened (Fig. 36.1), sometimes with areas of osteolysis (osteoporosis circumscripta).

5 The bones are vascular and bleed freely.

6 Fractures are common in the long bones and are characteristically transverse. The femur and tibia are the commonest sites for fractures.

7 'Pseudo' or stress fractures are also common in bones which are bowed. These are cracks with surrounding sclerosis, which may eventually progress with minimal violence to a true fracture (Fig. 36.2).

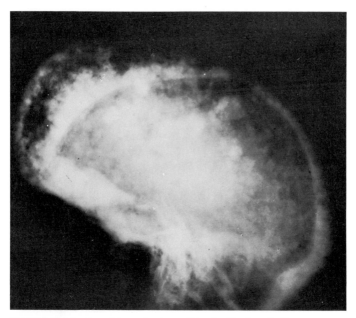

Fig. 36.1 Thickening of the calvarium of the skull in Paget's disease.

8 The vertebrae may be widened, with coarse trabeculae. Some vertebrae are almost always affected, as is the skull.

9 The condition may affect a single bone and may remain localized or may be widespread.

CLINICAL FEATURES

Paget's original description has hardly been modified over the last 100 years. His patient was a kyphotic individual with an enlarged skull, a simian posture with wide pelvis, bowing of femora and tibiae, and varus femoral necks. He developed deterioration of vision and hearing due to foraminal compression caused by thickening of the bones of the skull. He required a progressively increasing size in hats as his skull enlarged, and he eventually died from a sarcoma (Fig. 36.3).

1 Most patients remain completely symptomless and the condition is never diagnosed.

2 Bone pain is a relatively common presenting symptom. It can affect any bone, particularly the tibia, and it can become disabling. Headache is a rare feature of Paget's disease of the skull.

3 Some patients complain of deformity of a long bone usually either the tibia or femur. The radius may also become bowed, but rarely the ulna, and this may result in restriction of pronation and supination of the forearm.

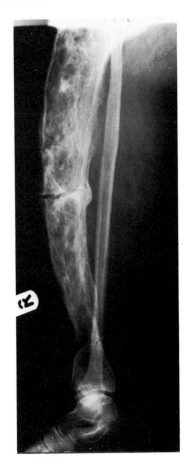

Fig. 36.2 Paget's disease showing deformity of the tibia and pseudo-fractures.

4 Many patients present with one of the complications, particularly a pathological fracture.

Complications

1 Pathological fractures are common and, of course, painful. They sometimes originate as a pseudo-fracture. A sudden increase in pain in the limb is usually representative of either a fracture or the development of a sarcoma.

2 Osteoarthritis—this frequently occurs in joints affected by Paget's disease, especially the hip. It can be difficult to distinguish the pain of arthritis from that of the Paget's disease. Joint replacement surgery can be difficult and dangerous.

3 Sarcoma—this occurs in less than 1% of patients, but is invariably highly malignant and is rapidly fatal. It may be an osteo-, chondro-, or

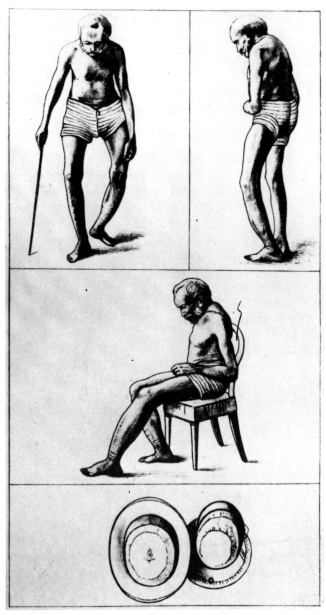

Fig. 36.3 Paget's original patient.

fibrosarcoma. It is usually metaphyseal but may occur in the skull or vertebrae.

4 Paraplegia—this may be due to collapse or spreading of a vertebra or to vascular changes affecting the spinal cord. It is an uncommon complication.

5 Compression of cranial nerves leading to deafness or visual disturbances.

DIAGNOSIS

This rests on the clinical and X-ray appearances coupled with a considerably raised alkaline phosphatase. Biopsy is rarely necessary unless a sarcoma is suspected. A bone scan using Tc-labelled diphosphonate will usually detect the disease before it becomes visible on X-ray. The main differential diagnosis is prostatic metastases in bone.

MANAGEMENT

The treatment of bone pain has been made possible by the development of two groups of drugs:
- thyrocalcitonin;
- bisphosphonates.

Calcitonin

Calcitonin is produced by the thyroid gland and has been shown to have a specific effect on osteoclastic resorption of bone. It gives dramatic relief from pain, coupled with a restoration of the biochemistry and radiological appearances towards normal. In Paget's disease it produces a marked lowering of serum calcium which may be used as a test. Its main use in therapy is to relieve chronic pain. The most useful preparation is salmon calcitonin which must be given by daily injection. After several months a plateau is reached in the response and the drug may often be stopped for a while without return of symptoms, although biochemical relapse is rapid.

Diphosphonates or bisphosphonates

This group of drugs reduces bone resorption by mechanisms which remain unknown. They are useful for relieving pain, although the long-term affects are not fully evaluated. Disodium etidronate (EHDP) is now available for general use and is given orally. Other members of the group are still under trial.

Apart from pain relief, treatment is usually directed to the management of fractures, although there is some evidence that deformity may be preventable. Fractures, particularly of the femur and tibia, may not always heal readily and internal fixation is often preferred. Surgery may be difficult and dangerous because of the hardness of the bone and the risk of haemorrhage. Sarcomata are resistant to any treatment and this can only be palliative.

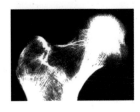

CHAPTER 37

Degenerative conditions – disorders of collagenous tissues

This group of conditions is characterized by deterioration in the structure and strength of those tissues which contain a high proportion of collagen i.e. ligaments, tendons, fascia, intervertebral discs. The cause is unknown, but this type of pathology becomes more common with ageing, and in some respects has features suggesting an accelerated ageing process. Inflammation is not a major feature, but may occur as a reaction to injury or spontaneous rupture and be part of the healing process.

INTERVERTEBRAL DISC DEGENERATION

The young intervertebral disc consists of a well-demarcated nucleus pulposus and annulus fibrosus. Starting in early adult life, changes occur in the matrix chemistry, with the proportions of the mucopolysaccharide constitutents becoming altered in such a way that the water-binding properties are diminished. In addition, the fibrous content of the nucleus increases until in old age the disc consists almost completely of a collagen feltwork. In consequence, the disc loses its elasticity and ability to act as a shock absorber and the disc space becomes narrowed and distorted. These changes occur in everyone with age, but in some individuals the changes seem to progress more rapidly and must be regarded as pathological. In the early stages of this degenerative process the changes may occur unevenly within the disc and considerable stresses may be set up. Such stresses, coupled with a localized weakness of the annulus, may allow nuclear material to burst through the annulus, particularly during lifting or straining—this condition is usually called disc prolapse.

INTERVERTEBRAL DISC PROLAPSE

For the reasons described above, this condition tends to occur when some degree of degeneration has occurred, but before the disc is completely converted to collagen, usually between the ages of 30 and 45, although it may occur outside these limits. The degenerative process seems to affect the more mobile parts of the spine, i.e. lumbar and cervical and it is in these areas that disc prolapse is most common.

The prolapse can either occur through the annulus or through the end-plate into the vertebral body, the latter producing acute low back pain and eventually showing on X-ray as a translucent area close to the disc — a so-called Schmorl's node.

Most disc prolapses occur posteriorly and the posterior ligament in the midline tends to direct the material postero-laterally where it may press on the nerve root as it lies within the foramen and cause root symptoms and signs.

Rarely, a central posterior prolapse may occur causing pressure on the spinal cord or central roots of the cauda equina and in these cases severe paralysis may occur with disturbed bladder function.

Lumbar disc prolapse

PRESENTATION

1 The condition often occurs in fit young adults. It may occur acutely when lifting a heavy weight or whilst straining. The patient often complains that his back 'went' or became locked so that he was unable to straighten. Acute pain is felt in the lower back, sometimes radiating to the buttock or down the leg, although the latter symptom is often delayed. Less commonly, the first symptom is leg pain without significant lower back pain. The onset is often less acute than this and not definitely related to stress. The pain may come on gradually over several hours either in the back or the legs or both.

2 The most common levels for a disc prolpase are L5I–SI and L4–L5. Root pressure at this level causes radiation down the back of the leg as far as the outer border of the foot or the dorsum of the foot i.e. sciatica. Prolapse at a higher level may affect the roots of the femoral nerve with radiation down the front of the thigh.

3 Radiation to the buttock is common and may occur without root pressure. It is thought to be referred from the ligaments of the spine.

CLINICAL SIGNS

1 The patient is often in severe pain and may stand and walk with difficulty. He or she is often more comfortable standing with the spine flexed and every movement is carried out carefully to protect the back. With the patient standing, it may be evident that the lumbar lordosis is flattened, and that there is considerable spasm of the erector spinae. There may be a tilt of the spine to one or other side (sciatic scoliosis) (Fig. 37.1).

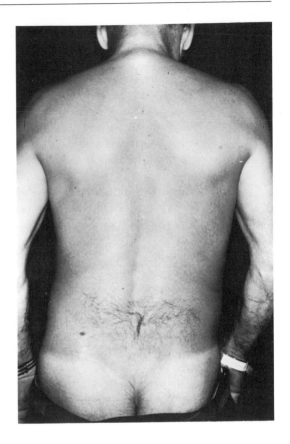

Fig. 37.1 Sciatic scoliosis.

2 There is usually tenderness over the lower spinous processes and often over the sacro-iliac joint and sciatic nerve on the affected side.

3 Movements are usually restricted in all directions, especially flexion. If the patient attempts to touch his toes his finger tips may not reach his knees. Lateral flexion is often freer on one side than on the other, usually being greater towards the side to which the spine is tilted.

4 The patient may climb on to the couch with difficulty. Lifting the leg with the knee straight may cause increased pain down the leg and hamstring spasm, restricting the movement to only a few degrees i.e. a positive 'straight leg raising' test. Dorsiflexing the foot may make this worse. Hip movements are usually free.

5 There may be neurological signs, depending on which root is affected.

A prolapse at L4–L5 tends to compress the L5 root, causing weakness of dorsiflexion of the ankle and particularly the extensor hallucis longus and a patch of sensory loss over the dorsum of the foot. The ankle jerk is usually present.

A prolapse of L5–S1 usually affects the S1 root with pain down the back of the calf to the outer side of the foot where there may be anaesthesia. There may also be weakness of the peronei, toe flexors, calf and tibialis posterior. The ankle jerk is usually lost.

A higher prolapse may cause neurology in the femoral nerve territory with diminution of the knee jerks. Stretching the femoral nerve by extending the hip and flexing the knee may also be painful and cause quadriceps spasm—positive 'femoral stretch' test.

In many cases the neurological signs are minor and must be sought carefully.

MANAGEMENT

There is considerable disagreement as to the best treatment for this condition, and many regimes ranging from manipulation to vigorous exercises are practised.

1 In the acute case rest for the spine is essential. Many patients settle with complete bed rest on a firm mattress and with analgesics. Opinions vary as to how long this should continue, but after a few days in most cases the symptoms settle sufficiently to enable the patient to mobilize with or without a supporting spinal corset.

2 In less severe cases the patient may manage with a firm lumbar support—preferably of rigid polythene or similar material, although some orthopaedic surgeons recommend a plaster-cast which is not so easily discarded.

3 Those patients who fail to settle may require a period of traction in bed with weights attached by skin extensions to the legs. The vast majority settle on this regime over a 2 week period. A light corset is then advisable for about 3 months with protection from heavy lifting or straining.

Whatever method of conservative treatment has been used, recurrence of symptoms is common and may lead to the need for surgery.

Most surgeons advise a CT or preferably MRI scan prior to surgery, to confirm the diagnosis and level of prolapse. If neither of these is available, myelography can be used.

The traditional operation consists of cutting a window in the ligamentum flavum and laminae and removing the prolapsed disc material. Results in the appropriate case are generally good.

MICRODISCECTOMY

This is a minimally invasive technique which involves approaching the disc with instruments which are introduced percutaneously and visualized through a telescope. The disc material is ground up and removed by suction.

INDICATIONS FOR SURGERY

- An absolute and urgent indication is the development of bladder symptoms, either retention of urine or difficulty with micturition.
- Almost as urgent is the development of extensive muscle weakness.
- Other indications are relative, e.g. failure to settle with conservative treatment, repeated attacks, much time lost from work, etc.

CHEMONUCLEOLYSIS

Chymopapain is a proteolytic enzyme which can be used to dissolve disc material by catalysing rapid hydrolysis of the non-collagenous ground substance of the nucleus pulposus. It has been used in the management of disc prolapse which has failed to respond to conservative treatment but has not gained widespread acceptance. It is administered by direct injection into the affected disc, under X-ray control. Serious neurological signs are regarded as a contraindication to this treatment. Complications are said to be few, but anaphylaxis occasionally occurs.

CERVICAL DISC PROLAPSE

PRESENTATION

The patient is usually a young adult and the condition often occurs as a result of a sudden twisting movement. It tends to be under-diagnosed. There is acute pain and spasm in the neck muscles. The pain often radiates over the shoulder and down the upper arm. There may be paraesthesiae and weakness in the arm and fingers.

CLINICAL SIGNS

- The neck is held stiffly and twisted to one side, with obvious spasm of the sternomastoid and sometimes trapezius—'wry neck' or acute torticollis.
- There is usually tenderness down one side of the spine and over the neck muscles.
- All neck movements are restricted, especially lateral flexion and rotation.
- Neurological signs are relatively uncommon, but depending on the level, which is usually lower cervical, there may be anaesthesia down the outer border of the arm, the thumb and index, or the inner border of the arm, the ring and little fingers, with loss of biceps or triceps jerks. Occasionally, weakness of hand movements may occur.

TREATMENT

Most patients settle spontaneously with analgesics. A firm surgical collar is often helpful and the persistent case may benefit from intermittent traction on the neck and heat treatment in the Physiotherapy Department. Symptoms rarely last more than 3 weeks.

Surgery is very seldom required, but may be necessary if there is persistent root pressure with significant neurological loss.

SPONDYLOSIS

Disc prolapse may be an acute event in the course of continuing degeneration of the disc. As the disc becomes more narrowed and fibrotic, the mechanism of the intervertebral joint becomes disturbed and the postero-lateral articulations, which are true synovial joints, may develop secondary osteoarthritis.

The complex of disc degeneration and secondary osteoarthritis of these joints is known as spondylosis. This usually causes symptoms in the cervical and lumbar regions.

Symptoms arise from:

1 the disc itself;

2 the stresses on the ligaments;

3 the osteoarthritic joints; and

4 pressure on local nerve roots. Pressure arises from the formation of:

(a) osteophytes along the margins of the disc forming a ridge which may press on the nerve roots in the lumbar region and spinal cord in the cervical region; and

(b) osteophytes around the intervertebral foramina compressing the nerve roots.

CLINICAL FEATURES

Chronic or intermittent pain is the usual feature, either in the neck, occipital region or lower back. Acute exacerbations are usual and there may be radiating pain and neurological symptoms in the arms or legs. There is often tenderness over the affected vertebrae. Movements are usually limited to some extent, especially during acute episodes. There may be neurological signs, although these are relatively uncommon.

In the cervical spine, considerable narrowing of the foramina is necessary before root compression begins to occur. Occasionally, a bony ridge may cause cord compression resulting in long tract neurological signs, with spasticity in the legs.

RADIOLOGY

The X-ray changes are characteristic—usually narrowing of the disc

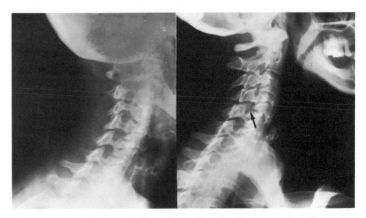

Fig. 37.2 Cervical spondylosis–oblique view showing narrowing of an intervertebral foramen on one side.

space, lipping of the edges of the body and often sclerosis of the postero-lateral joints with encroachment by osteophytes on the foramen, seen best on an oblique view of the spine (Fig. 37.2). Symptoms often bear little relation to the severity of the X-ray abnormalities.

MANAGEMENT

These can be very resistant conditions to treat.

1 Reassurance and simple symptomatic treatment are often sufficient–a collar or lumbo-sacral support is usually helpful, with graded exercises to maintain movement, heat and shortwave treatment during acute attacks. Sleeping position and thickness and consistency of mattress and pillows are important considerations.

2 Manipulation, either with or without anaesthesia, often gives symptomatic relief, but is better avoided if neurological signs are marked.

3 Periods of traction either intermittently or in bed can settle acute exacerbations.

4 Rarely, surgery to decompress roots or cord may be indicated. Surgical fusion of affected segments is rarely helpful because the condition usually affects many segments or even the whole spine.

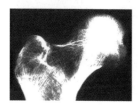

CHAPTER 38

Degenerative conditions — other disorders of collagenous tissues

Several of the conditions described below may occur simultaneously or at intervals in the same patient. They seem to form part of a syndrome of degenerative conditions affecting collagenous tissues.

CAPSULITIS OF THE SHOULDER (ROTATOR CUFF SYNDROME)

ANATOMY

The shoulder can be thought of as a double joint, i.e. that between the glenoid and the head of the humerus, and that between the upper end of the humerus, covered by the rotator cuff of muscles, and the under-surface of the acromion and the acromio-clavicular joint. The intervening sub-acromial bursa forms a secondary joint cavity (Fig. 38.1).

PATHOLOGY

In older individuals a degenerative process seems to affect the collagen of the tendinous rotator cuff and may produce symptoms in several ways. These sometimes follow an injury to the arm which has led to a period of immobilization of the shoulder.

1 The cuff may rupture over part or the whole of its extent.

2 The cuff may become acutely inflamed, perhaps as a result of a strain or partial rupture.

3 The area of inflammation may be associated with localized deposition of calcium, in which case the symptoms are usually much more severe. The lesion may be visible on an AP X-ray as a calcified area lying just above the greater tuberosity.

4 The acromio-clavicular joint may become osteoarthritic and form osteophytes which may abrade the underlying rotator cuff.

Clinical features

If the cuff ruptures, the ability to abduct the shoulder is usually lost completely. There is tenderness around the upper end of the humerus.

ANATOMY OF THE SHOULDER REGION

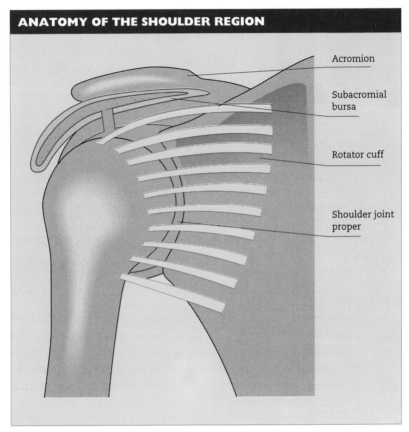

Acromion

Subacromial bursa

Rotator cuff

Shoulder joint proper

Fig. 38.1

There may be extensive bruising and it may be possible to feel the rent in the cuff by palpating just below the acromion.

In 2, 3 and 4 above, the usual symptoms are pain in the shoulder, mainly in the region of the deltoid insertion, but in some cases radiating down the arm.

❙ There is tenderness localized over the affected area, usually just below the acromion. Occasionally, this is localized over the origin of the biceps — *bicipital tendinitis*. Lesions affecting the anterior or posterior parts of the rotator cuff on the whole have a good prognosis and tend to respond well to local steroid injections. If there is significant osteoarthritis of the acromio-clavicular joint this is usually tender and thickened. Lesions of the superior part of the cuff and capsule are often associated with degeneration of the acromio-clavicular joint and are more likely to give rise to long-continued chronic symptoms and may require surgery.

2 Abduction is usually possible to 30 degrees; beyond this, the greater tuberosity begins to impinge on the undersurface of the acromion and is painful because of the bursal irritation. Occasionally, it may be possible to abduct the shoulder passively beyond 120 degrees, and the patient may then be able to continue the movement upwards — 'painful arc'.

3 Depending on which part of the rotator cuff is affected, internal or external rotation of the shoulder may be limited.

Investigations

Apart from demonstrating calcification, as above, and osteoarthritis of the acromio-clavicular joint, X-rays of the shoulder are not usually very helpful. Arthography has been used to demonstrate tears in the cuff, but is likely to be superseded by MRI scanning.

Arthroscopy of the shoulder is becoming more widely used and can demonstrate many of the pathological findings mentioned above.

Management

These conditions tend to become chronic and, although they usually settle with time, forced exercises can perpetuate them.

Acute

In the acute stage, rest in a sling is advisable, with mild analgesics. The course of the condition can often be shortened by one or more injections of hydrocortisone into the tender area or, usually more effectively, into the subacromial bursa. Twenty-five milligrams of hydrocortisone with local anaesthetic is usually adequate, but synthetic steroids can also be used. Once symptoms begin to settle, a course of active and passive exercises usually enables full shoulder movement to be regained.

Acute calcification can sometimes be dispersed by passing a wide-bore needle into the tender area, with considerable immediate relief of pain.

Surgery for an acute rupture is of debatable value, although an extensive rupture may be better repaired. Arthroscopic techniques of repair are being explored and show considerable promise. Conservative treatment is usually along the same lines as for acute tendinitis, with a period of rest initially, followed by active and passive therapy, to restore movements. The recovery period is often protracted.

Chronic

In the very chronic or wrongly treated case, the bursa may become thickened and fibrotic, and the shoulder becomes stiffer and stiffer until eventually only scapular movement is left — 'frozen shoulder'. The fully established frozen shoulder is best treated by rest until movement begins to return, when physiotherapy can again be attempted. Occasionally, in the resistant case, a manipulation under general anaesthesia may succeed in breaking down some of the adhesions and fibrosis. This must be followed by carefully supervised physiotherapy in an attempt to preserve the movements gained. It is, however, an imprecise and unpredictable form of treatment and some authorities recommend surgical exploration of the rotator cuff and capsule. Various surgical procedures are available, some of them being carried out arthroscopically. Shaving of the under surface of the acromion, acromionectomy, with or without excision of the outer end of the clavicle, and osteotomy of the glenoid have all been recommended. Reasonable movements may then be regained with physiotherapy.

TENNIS ELBOW

This is a very common condition affecting tennis players and people whose work involves much gripping and twisting of the forearm, such as car mechanics and bricklayers. It is thought to be a degenerative condition, but there is little pathological evidence for this. There have also been suggestions that the condition may be due to a localized entrapment of the radial or posterior interosseous nerve, but the evidence for this seems unconvincing.

Clinical features

The condition affects the origin of the extensor muscles of the wrist, particularly the extensor carpi radialis brevis and typically causes chronic pain on the outer side of the elbow radiating down the outer border of the forearm, especially when gripping. Tenderness is accurately localized over the front of the lateral epicondyle. Extending the elbow and simultaneously pronating the forearm and flexing the wrist and fingers exacerbates the pain. There are no X-ray changes.

Management

The condition almost always settles spontaneously, but may last many months. Rest and local hydrocortisone injections relieve symptoms in about 70% of patients. Rarely, surgery may be indicated, the usual procedure being to detach the whole or part of the common extensor origin from the lateral epicondyle, but results are unpredictable.

TENOSYNOVITIS

A condition in which a tendon sheath becomes inflamed and often distended with fluid. The cause sometimes appears to be trauma, particularly associated with repetitive movements. It usually affects the flexor or extensor tendons of the thumb or fingers where they cross the wrist within a synovial sheath. The area is tender and movements of the tendon cause pain, often radiating to the appropriate digit and sometimes associated with crepitus. The symptoms are usually chronic, unlike those associated with suppurative tenosynovitis.

Treatment

A change of occupation may be sufficient to relieve the symptoms, otherwise a period of 2–3 weeks' immobilization in a plaster-cast, extended to prevent thumb or finger movements is usually curative.

DE QUERVAIN'S TENO-VAGINITIS

This condition is due to thickening of the tendon sheaths of the abductor pollicis longus and extensor pollicis brevis where they cross the radial styloid. The cause is unknown, but repeated movements, e.g. repetitive gripping may be responsible for some cases.

Clinical features

The patient complains of pain at the site, made worse by gripping and by extending the thumb. Forced flexion of the thumb whilst the wrist is deviated to the ulnar side also causes pain. There is localized tenderness and often a swelling over the radial styloid.

Treatment

A hydrocortisone injection may give rapid relief or, alternatively, a period of 2–3 weeks in a plaster-cast, including the thumb, may also cure the condition. Resistant cases can usually be cured by slitting open the sheath surgically, making sure that all the tendinous strips are completely freed.

TRIGGER FINGER

This is a similar condition affecting the sheath of the flexor tendon and causing the tendon to 'snap' as it passes through. Alternatively, the patient may be unable to extend the finger actively from the fully flexed position. A nodule is usually palable at the site of thickening, opposite the head of the metacarpal. The condition occurs occasionally in young babies, almost always affecting the thumb ('clasped thumb').

Treatment

The condition may resolve spontaneously. Steroid injections into the sheath may be effective, but if this fails, the condition can be readily cured by longitudinal division of the tendon sheath, ensuring that the tendon runs freely. Either of the above conditions may be an early manifestation of rheumatoid arthritis.

REPETITIVE STRAIN INJURY (RSI)

This term is used to describe a variety of ill-defined conditions thought to be caused by repetitive movements and stresses. Many types of occupation involve such activities, particularly production line techniques such as trussing chickens, folding cardboard boxes, etc.

Some of the conditions described above may develop as a result of repetitive work and are accepted as 'Prescribed Diseases' for the purpose of Industrial Compensation, but in many cases the patient's complaints are not accompanied by definite physical signs of the type which would be expected from a condition such as tenosynovitis. In such cases, the suspicion of malingering may arise. The subject is mainly of medicolegal importance because of the possibility of industrial injury claims against the employee.

DUPUYTREN'S CONTRACTURE

This is an ill-understood condition affecting the collagenous tissue of the palmar fascia. There is frequently a family history. It is occasionally related to cirrhosis of the liver and rarely to epilepsy. It affects middle-aged men much more commonly than women.

Clinical features

1 The characteristic feature is a very slowly progressing flexion contracture of the fingers and thumb. It is usually bilateral but may be more severe on one side.

2 The palmar fascia feels thickened and nodular and tends to pucker the overlying skin. Definite bands can be felt running along the sides of the fingers due to thickening of the lateral extensions of the fascia.

3 The proximal interphalangeal joint is usually most affected, together with the metacarpo-phalangeal joint.

4 Thickened pads may develop over the knuckles and occasionally nodules may occur on the medial side of the sole of the foot.

Treatment

Progression may be delayed by steroid injections into the palmar fascia. Usually, surgery is necessary for the established contracture and this involves careful dissection of the whole of the affected area of fascia. Skin closure can be difficult but the skin usually heals well. Recurrence is not unusual. Occasionally, a finger may be better amputated if deformity is very severe.

PLANTAR FASCIITIS (painful heel syndrome)

A condition occurring usually in late middle age and characterized by chronic pain under the heel. Usually, the only physical sign is tenderness at the attachment of the plantar fascia on the undersurface of the os calcis. There may be an obvious 'spur' at this point of attachment, visible on a lateral X-ray. These spurs are, however, common and not necessarily significant in the pathology of this condition.

Treatment

The condition frequently responds to an injection of hydrocortisone and local anaesthetic, repeated if necessary on two or three occasions at intervals of three weeks. A Sorbo pad in the heel of the shoe also helps to relieve symptoms. The condition is self-limiting and usually subsides after several months.

GANGLION

This presents as a cystic swelling occuring in relation to a joint or tendon sheath. Ganglia are particularly common on the dorsum of the hand and wrist and around the ankle. Small ganglia on the palmar aspect of the fingers may be very tense and can feel like a small pea.

The typical ganglion arises insidiously and may vary in size. It is often painless, but may cause local aching. It is fluctuant and trans-illuminant. It is filled with a gel which is thought to be derived from synovial fluid. It is believed to arise by a protrusion of synovium or synovial fluid through a microscopic split in the capsule or fibrous sheath, the opening acting as a flap-valve. This accounts for its tendency to vary in size or to disappear, and also for the fact that it occasionally develops after trauma to the wrist or foot.

Treatment

A ganglion may be dispersed by a blow or pressure. It may also be aspirated. Recurrence is usual following these manoeuvres, and surgical removal may be necessary. A disc of fibrous sheath or capsule (presumably bearing the flap-valve) should be excised with the ganglion if recurrence is to be avoided.

RUPTURE OF TENDONS

BICEPS BRACHII

The long tendon usually ruptures within the shoulder joint. There is acute pain and the belly of the muscle becomes abnormally prominent. The tendon does not usually heal but symptoms subside and function returns to normal.

QUADRICEPS FEMORIS

This may rupture above or below the patella. Diagnosis is usually easy as the gap may be palpable and with an infrapatellar rupture the patella is obviously high. Active extension of the knee is lost. Operative repair is usually advised, followed by a period of protection and gradual movement.

TENDO ACHILLES

This usually ruptures during sport such as badminton. The patient feels as though he has been kicked behind the ankle. A gap is usually palpable and plantar flexion of the ankle is lost. Squeezing the calf muscle normally causes passive plantar flexion of the foot when the tendon is intact, but not when it is completely ruptured.

Treatment

The results of surgical repair differ very little from those of conservative treatment. In either case, the ankle is immobilized in plantar flexion for 3 weeks, followed by a further 3 weeks with the ankle in neutral, after which mobilization is allowed.

HAND TENDONS

Spontaneous rupture of hand tendons usually occurs as a complication of rheumatoid arthritis. Surgical repair may be possible.

CHAPTER 39

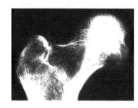

Degenerative conditions of articular cartilage

Degenerative changes commonly occur in hyaline articular cartilage, culminating in the fully developed condition of osteoarthritis, often called osteoarthrosis because it is essentially a non-inflammatory condition.

The precise point at which degeneration can be called true osteoarthritis is difficult to establish. The earliest change in the cartilage, i.e. the development of minute splits and softening of the surface, probably does not always progress to fully-established arthritis.

OSTEOARTHRITIS

This is a disease of synovial joints in which the articular cartilage becomes split, fissured and softened, and gradually wears away, sometimes down to underlying bone. The subchondral bone then becomes thickened and eburnated and there is proliferation of new bone around the edges of the articular surface, leading to the formation of osteophytes. Secondary changes occur in the capsule and ligaments and the joint becomes stiffened and painful.

Pathology

The changes appear to begin in articular cartilage with softening and splitting known as fibrillation. Research is proceeding vigorously into the causation of the condition. Attempts are being made to answer the following two questions.
- Are the changes preceded by changes in the underlying bone?
- Is the disease primarily one of cartilage?

UNDERLYING BONE CHANGES

1 Changes in bone density can often be demonstrated in osteoarthritic joints.

2 The bone often shows marked haemodynamic changes, particularly affecting the venous circulation.

3 The bony architecture is often abnormal as a result of previous trauma or disease.

4 The bone often shows trabecular fractures and cysts, although usually late in the condition.

PRIMARY CARTILAGE DISEASE

Most of the indications point in this direction, and there are two main possibilities:

1 the changes may be essentially biochemical; or

2 the changes may be essentially mechanical.

BIOCHEMICAL

1 The collagen may be affected—this seems unlikely as collagen is relatively inert and there are no collagenases in osteoarthritic joints. It is possible, however, that abnormal synthesis may be a factor.

2 The proteoglycan matrix may be abnormal. Changes in proteoglycan ratios can be demonstrated in osteoarthritic cartilage and these may affect water-binding capacity and hence mechanical strength. Hormones are known to affect proteoglycan metabolism, e.g. osteoarthritis is particularly prone to occur in acromegalic patients.

MECHANICAL

The collagen might wear or disrupt, allowing proteoglycan matrix to leak out. This could occur as a result of:

1 fatigue failure, perhaps due to defective lubrication; or

2 abrasive wear—caused by high spots or incongruities in the joint.

The importance of synovial fluid in maintaining cartilage requires further study. Some incongruity between the joint surfaces is necessary for fluid circulation.

Pathogenesis

Certain facts are known about the pathogenesis of cartilage degeneration.

1 Previous damage to and distortion of the joint by disease or trauma is a frequent predisposing factor.

2 Weight-bearing joints are affected more than non-weight-bearing—especially the hip and knee (but seldom the ankle).

3 The condition is age related, although early changes in articular cartilage can be demonstrated in adolescents.

4 Immobilization may cause changes which regress when movement is restored.

5 Direct damage to articular cartilage may cause widespread changes throughout the matrix.

Not all these changes progress, but the changes which occur over weight-bearing areas or high spots probably do progress to true osteoarthritis.

If there is pre-existing distortion of the joint, the osteoarthritis is known as secondary. If there is no obvious underlying cause, the osteoarthritis is known as primary.

Rarely, a patient presents with widespread osteoarthritic changes in many joints—a condition which is almost certainly due to metabolic abnormalities in the cartilage.

Clinical features of osteoarthritis

(see under relevant joints)

Any joint which has been damaged by disease or trauma may begin to show osteoarthritic changes several years later, the usual interval being about 5–10 years. In the absence of previous pathology, the hip and knee are the commonest joints affected, as also are the spinal joints as part of the complex known as spondylosis (p. 282).

1 Pain is the usual presenting feature—usually slowly increasing in severity as the joint stiffens. The pain is usually exacerbated by exercise, but the joint often feels stiff after rest. Pain-disturbed sleep is an important index of severity.

2 Stiffness may make tasks such as putting on stockings difficult, but is not usually in itself a major cause of complaint.

3 Deformity tends to develop partly as a result of muscular spasm—the stronger muscle groups overcoming the weak, and partly as a result of capsular and ligamentous contracture, together with distortion of the joint surface. Deformity can interfere with function, particularly gait. At the hip there is often a flexion and adduction contracture which shortens the limb and may stress the spine.

4 Osteophytes occasionally break off and act as loose bodies.

The principal physical signs are:

• moderate synovial thickening and bony enlargement of the joint due to osteophytes and occasional effusions during acute episodes;

• tenderness around the joint;

• restriction of movements which may become almost total, although fusion does not occur;

• muscle spasm and pain on attempting movements beyond the 'limit'

• crepitus on movement;

• fixed deformities; and

• abnormalities of gait or upper limb function.

> ## RADIOLOGICAL SIGNS
>
> - Narrowing of the joint space—the most important sign.
> - Osteophyte formation around the edges of the joint.
> - Subchondral bone sclerosis.
> - Subchondral cysts and trabecular fractures.
> - Pre-existing pathology may be evident.

Other investigations are usually negative.

Management

CONSERVATIVE

The condition is a slowly progressive and painful one, and most patients can be managed conservatively for many years.

1 Analgesics are usually the mainstay of treatment. Anti-inflammatory analgesics are of less help in osteoarthritis than in rheumatoid arthritis.

2 Protection of the joint, e.g. the patient may benefit by losing weight, and a stick or other support may be helpful.

3 Change to a lighter occupation.

4 Physiotherapy, i.e. intermittent heat treatment or short-wave diathermy, with supervised exercises to maintain movements.

SURGICAL

The severe case may eventually come to surgery, particularly when sleep is disturbed or work has become impossible. There are various surgical possibilities, and each patient needs to be assessed carefully before a decision is made.

1 Arthroscopic lavage

Clearing out of debris, osteophytes, cartilage fragments, etc., sometimes with partial synovectomy, can be a useful palliative procedure, especially for the knee.

2 Osteotomy

For certain joints an osteotomy, usually below the joint, e.g. through the inter-trochanteric region for the hip and through the upper tibia for the knee, can relieve pain dramatically. The mechanism of its action is unknown but is thought to have a vascular basis. It is somewhat unpredictable, although the effects may last for several years. It is usually reserved for joints with a reasonable range of movements.

3 Arthrodesis (p. 400)

This can be the most certain way of relieving pain, especially in the young person. It always causes some disability, but if sound it will stand up to heavy stresses over many years.

4 Arthroplasty (p. 400)

This is the age of the arthroplasty; many artificial replacements being available for almost every joint. The hip and knee have received most attention and very satisfactory pain relief and function can now be attained.

Many factors need to be considered in deciding which surgical treatment is best for each patient. These include age, occupation, general mobility, psychological make-up, severity of symptoms and the condition of other joints. The final decision will usually involve balancing the risks of the procedure against the likely advantages.

CHONDROMALACIA

This is a degenerative condition of the articular cartilage, usually seen in adolescents and young adults and usually affecting the patella. Its cause is unknown. The articular surface of the patella becomes soft, roughened, fibrillated and wears away. It causes pain and recurrent effusions and often the knee 'gives way' unexpectedly.

It can be diagnosed by the fact that pressure over the patella causes pain, the undersurface is tender and there is a characteristic rough crepitus on moving the joint.

TREATMENT

The condition often settles spontaneously after a number of years, but persistent cases can be difficult to treat. Shaving off the rough cartilage surface can be helpful, as also can re-aligning the patellar tendon by transplanting the tibial tubercle or, less drastically, by releasing the lateral aponeurosis and capsule. Severe cases may need excision of the patella, although this is not always curative because of changes in the underlying femoral condyles. Osteoarthritis is a common late end-result.

CHAPTER 40

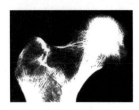

Metabolic diseases of bone and bleeding disorders

In addition to its supporting function, bone acts as an important organ in controlling the metabolism of calcium and phosphate in the body.

The skeleton contains 98% of the body's calcium. The daily turnover of calcium can be represented diagrammatically (Fig. 40.1). Calcium is interchanged between the body-pool, the gut, kidneys and bone, and in normal circumstances the amount excreted balances the amount taken in by the diet. Many factors influence this system.

1 Parathyroid hormone. This is a polypeptide and its output is determined by the serum calcium level, increasing when the calcium level is low. It restores the calcium level to normal by increasing tubular reabsorption from the kidney and mobilizing calcium from the bones.

2 Calcitonin. This hormone is produced by the C-cells of the thyroid gland. Its precise role is disputed, but it inhibits bone resorption and is secreted in response to a raised serum calcium.

3 Vitamin D. Cholecalciferol is a fat soluble vitamin contained in many fatty foods, notably milk and fish-liver oils, and is also synthesised in the skin by the action of sunlight. It is converted to 25-hydroxycholecalciferol in the liver by the addition of an OH radical and is further converted in the kidney to 1,25-dihydroxycholecalciferol (1,25-DHCC). Other conversions are also possible in the kidney, although 1,25-DHCC appears to be the main metabolically active one. The active vitamin affects:

(a) the gut—increases calcium absorption;

(b) the bone—it indirectly affects both bone deposition and resorption; and

(c) the muscle—muscle weakness occurs in vitamin D deficiency.

Increased levels of 1,25-DHCC tend to increase both calcium and phosphate levels in the serum. Because the active metabolites are produced in the kidney, renal failure may produce the effects of vitamin D deficiency, and this can only be overcome by giving large doses of cholecalciferol or, alternatively, giving the more active metabolites.

In vitamin D deficiency, the parathyroids are stimulated to restore the calcium levels—secondary hyperparathyroidism.

CALCIUM POOL

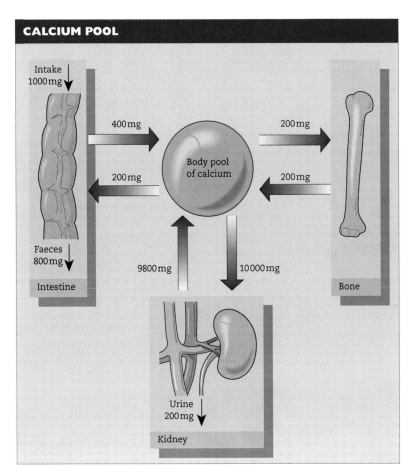

Intake
1000 mg

400 mg

200 mg

Body pool
of calcium

200 mg

200 mg

Faeces
800 mg

9800 mg

10000 mg

Intestine

Bone

Urine
200 mg

Kidney

Fig. 40.1

These and many other factors influence bone formation and deposition. Imbalance between them causes either increased or decreased bone mass. The understanding of these bone changes has been confused by the use of imprecise terms. The classification below is that suggested by Aegeter and Kirkpatrick.

BONE LOSS

Bone loss (with decreased radiological density and usually thinning of the cortex) can be due to:
1 decrease in osteoid formation (osteopenia);
2 decrease in mineralization of osteoid (osteomalacia); or
3 increase in removal of bone by osteoclasts (osteolysis).

Osteopenia

DIETARY CAUSES

Deficient intake of vitamins or essential proteins may occur in the malabsorption syndromes, and rarely from a true dietary deficiency, e.g. scurvy.

Scurvy—vitamin C deficiency

This has become rare and only occurs in the fully developed form in children between the ages of 6 months and 1 year, although old people may have a subclinical deficiency. Vitamin C is necessary for collagen synthesis and osteoid deposition, especially at the growing ends of bones.

Pathological Features

In the long bones the zone of provisional calcification occurs as usual and appears on X-ray as a dense band at the epiphysis with an adjacent lucent band representing deficient osteoid formation. The epiphysis is ringed with a zone of calcification. Capillaries are abnormally fragile, causing soft-tissue haemorrhages, often under the periosteum at the ends of long bones and in the soft tissues. These particularly affect the gums and skin. Fractures and epiphyseal displacements are common, and unite with enormous amounts of callus. Wounds may be slow to heal.

Treatment with ascorbic acid is rapidly curative.

ENDOCRINE CAUSES

Cushing's syndrome or steroid therapy

Both of these cause a generalized osteopenia, often with crush fractures in vertebrae. Steroid therapy over a long period may also cause ischaemic necrosis of epiphyses notably the femoral head. This is becoming a problem in patients who have had renal transplants, and have been given steroids for immunosuppression.

Hyperthyroidism

Detectable osteopenia occurs uncommonly.

DISUSE ATROPHY

Bone formation is responsive to mechanical stress, and a period of immobilization in a plaster-cast or of enforced bed rest may lead to localized or generalized osteopenia.

OSTEOGENESIS IMPERFECTA

See Chapter 27.

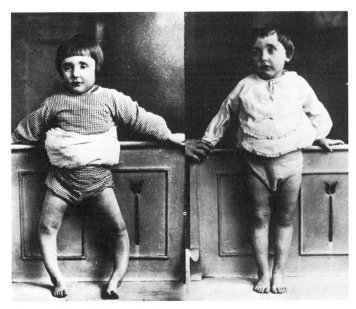

Fig. 40.2 Rickets–before and after treatment.

Osteomalacia

RICKETS

This is a childhood form of osteomalacia. Its effects are due to failure of osteoid to ossify from lack of vitamin D. Dietary deficiency has now become rare except in economically deprived countries, particularly where there is also deficient exposure to sunlight.

In growing bones the failure of ossification leads to widening of the epiphyseal lines, and generalized demineralization. The epiphyses are widened and have a 'cupped' appearance, usually best seen on an AP radiograph of the wrist.

Clinical features

Symptoms usually start about the age of one. The child is small and fails to thrive, it develops deformities such as bowing of the femora and tibiae, a large head and deformity of the chest with thickening of the costochondral junctions (ricketty rosary) and a transverse sulcus in the chest caused by the pull of the diaphragm (Harrison's sulcus) (Fig. 40.2).

Investigations

The serum calcium is usually normal, the phosphate is low and the alkaline phosphatase is raised.

Treatment

Ordinary doses of vitamin D are curative.

RENAL RICKETS AND VITAMIN D RESISTANT RICKETS

As described above, renal disease may interfere with vitamin D metabolism, diminishing the production of the more active derivatives. This may result in malabsorption and abnormal utilization of calcium and phosphate, with secondary parathyroid stimulation and consequent further demineralization. The effects are complex and not fully understood.

Certain types of renal tubular insufficiency may result in reduced reabsorption of phosphate causing hypophosphataemia and secondary bone demineralization.

Both the above types of rickets are resistant to normal doses of vitamin D, but may respond to enormous doses or to the more active metabolites such as 1,25-dihydroxycholecalciferol. Large and repeated doses of phosphate may be valuable in the second type.

The orthopaedic problems are the same as those of ordinary rickets, with similar bone deformities and also a tendency to fragmentation and slipping of the femoral head, resulting in coxa vara.

The deformities of all types of rickets may be corrected if necessary when the disease is under control. Prophylactic pinning of the slipping femoral neck may be useful in renal rickets, although the prognosis for life is poor.

ADULT OSTEOMALACIA

The changes are mainly those of softening of the bones. The effects on the growing epiphyses do not apply in the adult so that deformities are not usually severe. The condition is probably more common than is usually thought, particularly in older people who may have dietary deficiency and do not receive sufficient sunlight.

In Britain, the condition is commonly found in Asian immigrants whose diet may be deficient and may also encourage calcium deficiency, for example, phytic acid in the flour used to make chappatis combines with calcium to make it unabsorbable.

Clinical and radiological features

1 Generalized bone pain with occasional exacerbations usually in the spine due to crush fractures.

2 Anorexia, weight loss, muscle weakness, sometimes bony deformity.

3 X-rays show diffuse osteoporosis, pathological vertebral wedging and pseudo-fractures, which are translucent zones with surrounding sclerosis, usually running at right angles to the margin of the bone (Looser's

zones). They are well seen in the vertebral border of the scapula and the ischio-pubic ramus.

Diagnosis

Serum calcium and phosphate may be lowered. Alkaline phosphatase is raised. Iliac crest bone biopsy is useful and shows the typical un-mineralized osteoid 'seams' lying against normally calcified areas.

Treatment

Vitamin D in normal doses or, more effectively, a more active metabolite, is usually rapidly curative.

Osteolysis

Here, the loss of mineralized bone is due to osteoclastic resorption in excess of deposition. The most potent factor producing this is over-activity of parathyroid secretion.

HYPERPARATHYROIDISM

Three types are recognized:

1 Primary hyperparathyroidism, due either to generalized hyperplasia of the parathyroid or to an adenoma.

2 Secondary hyperparathyroidism, usually in response to renal disease or as a sequel to osteomalacia or malabsorption. The hormone acts to restore serum calcium and phosphate levels by causing demineralization.

3 Tertiary hyperparathyroidism is the expression used to describe the situation where the constantly stimulated gland of secondary hyper-parathyroidism develops an autonomous over-secretion so that even if the underlying cause is eliminated, the gland may still over-secrete.

In primary hyperparathyroidism the serum calcium in blood and urine is raised and phosphate lowered. In secondary hyperparathyroidism calcium may be normal or even low, and phosphate levels vary, depending on the renal pathology.

PRIMARY HYPERPARATHYROIDISM (VON RECKLINGHAUSEN'S DISEASE)

This is characterized by generalized skeletal porosis and the development of cystic lesions filled with soft brown connective tissue. These usually occur in the long bones, but are not always present. Because of these cysts the disease is sometimes called osteitis fibrosa cystica.

Clinical features

These consist of generalized bone pains, indigestion, weakness and

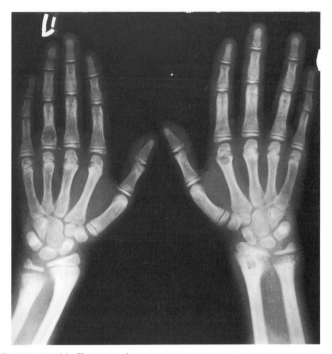

Fig. 40.3 Osteitis fibrosa cystica.

anorexia. Fractures and deformities complicate the condition. Renal calculi may occur and eventually renal failure.

Radiological features

There is generalized porosis and characteristic localized lesions, which are usually well circumscribed in long bones. These may be widespread or few in number (Fig. 40.3). A lateral radiograph of the skull may show a characteristic 'pepper pot' appearance which is virtually diagnostic.

Resorption of the lamina dura of tooth sockets and thinning of the cortical bone in phalanges also occurs.

DIAGNOSIS

This rests on high serum calcium, low phosphate and raised alkaline phosphatase. Bone biopsy may be helpful.

TREATMENT

In the primary case, the parathyroid adenoma may be excised. Generalized hyperplasia, if it is primary, may require removal of two or more of the glands.

Osteoporosis

As commonly used, this term is based on clinical and radiological findings rather than on pathology. It is most common in old age and particularly in post-menopausal women, although men are not immune.

Its causes probably include dietary deficiency, lack of stress on bones, both of which cause osteopenia or osteomalacia, and hormonal changes which may act by influencing the effect of parathyroid hormone and therefore allowing osteolysis. In other words all the mechanisms of reduction of mineralized bone mass may apply.

CLINICAL FEATURES

It usually affects women over 60 and to a lesser extent men of the same age. Occasionally, symptoms become marked at or soon after the menopause. The clinical features are bone pains, lassitude, and acute back pain due to pathological vertebral fractures. The gradual development of a kyphosis and loss of height are the main features. Hip fractures in the aged are almost certainly related to osteoporosis.

DIAGNOSIS

All patients should be screened biochemically and radiologically to attempt to exclude the specific disorders listed above.

In typical senile or post-menopausal osteoporosis the X-rays show generalized loss of density of bones and thinning of the cortices from within. The bones may have a 'ghostly' quality. Vertebrae may be wedged or the discs may protrude into the bodies ('ballooning' of the disc) (Fig. 40.4). Kyphosis is usual and stress fractures may occur.

It is now possible to assess the degree of osteoporosis by measuring bone density using a dual-energy X-ray absorptiometric device known as the DEXA Scanner and this is currently being used as a screening technique to detect patients at risk, particularly post-menopausal women.

HISTOLOGICAL FEATURES

The Haversian canals are widened and the trabeculae are thin and sparse. The bone which is present is usually adequately mineralized, but there may be occasional 'osteoid seams'. There is evidence that not only is there a decreased quantity of mineralized bone in osteoporosis, but the quality of the ossified matrix may also be abnormal.

TREATMENT

Treatment and prophylaxis are controversial. It is usual to give the patient an orthopaedic support for the spine, to encourage exercise and

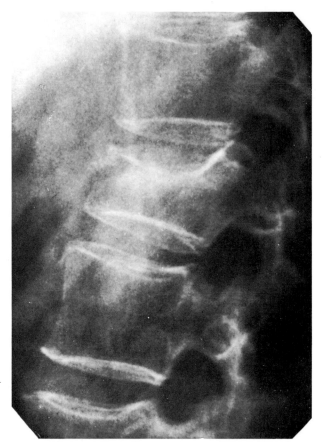

Fig. 40.4 Osteoporotic spine with crush fractures.

to give dietary supplements of calcium, vitamin D, and proteins, although the effects of the latter are probably marginal. Oestrogen therapy, often called 'hormone replacement therapy' (HRT), is now accepted as a useful method of prophylaxis for peri- and post-menopausal women identified by screening as being particularly at risk. Compliance is often poor, particularly if a formulation which causes post-menopausal bleeding is used, and there have been fears of precipitating breast and uterine cancer.

Androgen therapy has also been tried with little proven benefit. High fluoride levels in drinking water are associated with a lower incidence of osteoporosis so fluoride therapy has been advocated, but has been shown to be associated with a high incidence of hip fracture. Newer forms of treatment have included calcitonin and bisphosphonates which have been shown to reduce the risks of osteoporotic fractures. Many forms of treatment can be shown to influence the biochemistry of osteoporotic patients, but it is difficult to prove that they influence the condition of the bones or that they alleviate symptoms.

COAGULATION DEFECTS

HAEMOPHILIA AND RELATED DISORDERS

Haemophilia is the most important of the genetically determined defects of the blood clotting mechanism causing orthopaedic problems. In classical haemophilia, Factor VIII and in Christmas disease, Factor IX is deficient in the plasma. Haemophilia is a sex-linked recessive disease affecting males only, except on the rare occasions when a marriage between a male patient and a carrier female may produce a female child with the disease. In about one third of the patients the disease appears to occur spontaneously. The level of Factor VIII may vary from time to time, and the patient may at some times be below the danger level for bleeding and at other times above. Below 1% of normal, most patients are at risk of developing joint haemorrhages.

Clinical features

The disease may be suspected if there is a history of prolonged or severe bleeding from minor injuries, with a tendency to develop extreme bruising or swelling. Small wounds such as pinpricks may not bleed abnormally, but extraction of a tooth may be followed by a dangerous haemorrhage.

Haemorrhages tend to track along fascial planes and fill tissue compartments and may result in nerve compression or vascular occlusion. Bleeding within the iliacus sheath is a common example of this phenomenon, and is often accompanied by paralysis of the femoral nerve. Median and ulnar palsies are also relatively common, usually associated with bleeds into the forearm muscular compartments.

The main orthopaedic problems are those relating to the development of acute haemarthroses and large intra-muscular collections. These occur spontaneously in severe haemophiliacs and are a frequent reason for hospital admission. The knee, elbow and ankle are the commonest joints involved. There may be a definite injury, but in many cases the bleeding appears to be truly spontaneous and may occur during sleep, although even here minor trauma cannot be ruled out. Haemarthroses tend to be more common in young patients, particularly adolescents.

Recurrent bleeding in the same joint is common and leads to gradual destruction of the articular cartilage, with internal fibrosis and a tendency to develop contractures.

The haemarthroses are usually extremely painful and accompanied by severe muscle spasm. The joint is distended, except in those patients where repeated bleeds have produced so much fibrosis that distension is impossible. There is usually a local increase in temperature, and tenderness over the synovium. In chronic cases the range of movement may be diminished, with almost total destruction of the joint.

Large soft-tissue collections of blood may fail to reabsorb and may, indeed, increase in size, forming cysts which may compress surrounding structures and even penetrate bone.

Diagnosis

The patient is often aware of his condition and may have similarly affected relatives. Those patients presenting for the first time require a full and detailed haematological investigation of the clotting factors to assess the precise nature of the defect and its severity.

Treatment

The mainstay of treatment is replacement of the defective factor by transfusion. This usually relieves the pain dramatically.

The factor can be supplied in several forms:

1 Fresh frozen plasma. This can be given as an out-patient procedure, but is most effective within 4 hours of the onset of bleeding. A dose of 12 mg/kg body weight will restore the Factor VIII level to 15–20% and control the bleeding.

2 Cryoprecipitate. This material is a cold precipitate of fibrinogen containing considerable Factor VIII activity (but not Factor IX). It can be reconstituted to give a potent preparation.

3 Freeze-dried human AHG (Factor VIII) concentrate. This can be stored for long periods.

4 Animal anti-haemophilic globulin.

The use of some of these products has been complicated by the transmission of HIV infection to the patients and all blood products are now appropriately treated and screened.

A restoration of 15–20% factor level is adequate for most minor to moderate bleeds. Levels of 30% or more may be needed for severe bleeds or bleeds in dangerous situations. At this level of cover, almost any surgical procedure can be carried out.

Other aspects of treatment

It is usual to splint the limb which has developed the haemorrhage to prevent further bleeding. Large haemarthroses may be aspirated, with the patient covered by Factor VIII therapy. This appears to reduce the risk of permanent damage to the articular cartilage by the blood in the joint. Cover is needed until bleeding has obviously stopped. After this, the blood usually reabsorbs and the joint becomes comfortable to move. At this point, mobilization can be started, but it is normally necessary to give a further period of cover, particularly if physiotherapy or manipulation is necessary to regain movements. The chronically damaged knee is very prone to repeated bleeds and a caliper or splint may be tried in the hope of diminishing the need for hospitalization and preventing unnecessary damage to the joint.

Nerve palsies are usually treated conservatively, although a severe bleed into a closed fascial space may need surgical decompression.

Joint contracture may be treated by the usual orthopaedic techniques, including surgery, provided adequate cover is available.

It should be remembered that, after severe bleeding, transfusion of blood may be necessary for replacement of blood volume, independently of factor replacement. Some patients eventually develop inhibitors in the plasma, and no longer respond to Factor VIII concentrate. At this point risks from fatal bleeding are much intensified, and many die eventually from renal complications.

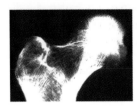

CHAPTER 41

Inflammatory rheumatic conditions

The inflammatory rheumatic conditions form a heterogeneous group in which the common factor is inflammation affecting synovial membranes of joints and tendon sheaths, bursae and entheses (ligamentous insertions).

There have been many theories about the aetiology of these conditions, including chronic or acute infection, stress, hypersensitivity, or disturbances of collagen metabolism.

There is a clear genetic predisposition, although the mechanisms by which the genotype and the environment interact are not yet understood. Infection, with either bacteria, mycoplasmas or viruses, as yet not definitely identified, remains a possibility. These various factors perhaps initiate a sequence of synovial and articular cartilage changes, in turn mediated by lysosomal enzymes and continued by secondary immunological phenomena, including auto-immunity.

Certainly, immunological disturbances can readily be demonstrated and many humoral antibodies have been identified in this group of conditions.

PATHOLOGY

The synovial membrane appears to be the target organ and is usually found to be chronically inflamed, with thickening and increased vascularity of the synovium which forms fronds and villi.

1 There is an infiltration of vascular synovium around the periphery of the articular cartilage, forming a dull red pannus which appears to destroy the cartilage from the edges.

2 Ligaments become softened and the joint becomes lax, particularly if there is a considerable effusion.

3 Bone erosion may lead to sub-articular cysts and in severe cases ankylosis may occur.

Microscopically, the synovium is infiltrated by masses of lymphocytes and, to a lesser extent, polymorphs and there are areas of 'fibrinoid' necrosis with granulation tissue and repair fibrosis.

Many tissues other than synovium are affected, but not all collagenous tissues suffer. In some of the inflammatory rheumatic conditions, lesions can be found in skin, lungs, abdominal viscera, muscles, heart and blood vessels, and in the nervous system. The skin may be thin and loses its elasticity, and so-called 'rheumatoid nodules' are frequent.

RHEUMATOID ARTHRITIS

This is a common disease usually occurring in middle age and in women more than men. It usually presents with slowly increasing stiffness and aching in the small peripheral joints, particularly of the hands, and may progress to cause severe incapacity and deformity.

CLINICAL FEATURES

The mode of presentation, the joints affected, and the subsequent progress are very variable.

The disease may begin in one or several joints and may progress rapidly with almost continual acute inflammation in the joints, or it may begin insidiously with morning stiffness only, perhaps progressing in semi-acute exacerbations each involving more and more joints. Occasionally, the first manifestation of the disease may be a carpal tunnel syndrome or isolated tenosynovitis. The hands, wrists and knees are usually involved, but most joints can be affected, including those of the spine.

There is often weight loss, weakness and loss of appetite, and, rarely, there may be mild fever during the acute attacks.

Eventually, the joints become obviously inflamed, swollen with fluid and synovial thickening, restricted in movement and often with ligamentous laxity, allowing deformities such as the characteristic ulnar deviation of the fingers (Fig. 41.1) to develop.

The joints are tender and feel 'boggy', and there may be much muscle spasm. Tendon sheaths also swell, particularly in the hand, and cause pain on finger movements. Occasionally, the infiltrated tendons rupture producing secondary deformities and loss of function. Destruction of joint surfaces may also contribute to deformity in late cases.

Remissions occur, usually temporary, but occasionally the disease appears to burn out. The deformities are, of course, permanent. Secondary osteoarthritic changes are very common.

RADIOLOGICAL CHANGES

The earliest change is usually a diffuse porosis around the joint due to the effects of cytokines, with increased vascularity. Later, the joint space may

RHEUMATOID ARTHRITIS

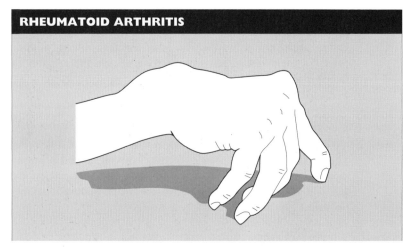

Fig. 41.1 Rheumatoid arthritis affecting the hand.

become narrowed and destruction of the joint surface may be obvious (Fig. 41.2). Subluxation and dislocation are common and occasionally ankylosis occurs.

DIAGNOSIS

The clinical picture is usually clear, but early or mono-articular cases may be difficult to diagnose. The ESR is usually raised and sometimes the white cell count is increased.

Agglutination tests such as the sheep cell and latex tests eventually become positive in at least 70% of cases. They are not often helpful in diagnosis, but tend to relate to severity.

Synovial biopsy may be useful in excluding infective conditions such as tuberculosis, but rarely in distinguishing between the various rheumatic conditions.

MANAGEMENT

The disease is chronic and usually slowly progressive so that management is a combination of medical, social and psychological measures.

Medical

During the acute stages, rest and a helpful environment appear desirable, but their effects are uncertain. Bed rest may be needed, but retaining mobility is important. Local measures include splinting painful joints followed by passive exercises when the pain becomes less, with long-term active exercises to maintain mobility. Wax baths and hydrotherapy all have a place.

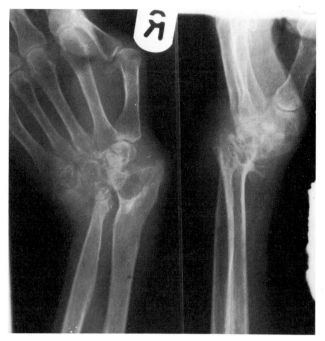

Fig. 41.2 Rheumatoid arthritis affecting the wrist joint.

Systemic therapy

This has become the mainstay of medical treatment which is usually best controlled by experienced rheumatologists with appropriate surgical help.

1 Salicylates, aspirin or sodium salicylate, have been popular, but are now little used in rheumatoid arthritis. They relieve pain and have anti-inflammatory properties. Approximately six grams a day may be necessary, and at this level gastro-intestinal and auditory disturbances are common.

2 Other anti-inflammatory drugs. There are many of these on the market and they are often classified as non-steroidal anti-inflammatory drugs (NSAIDs). Phenylbutazone and indomethacin have been popular and effective, but the former has been withdrawn because of its toxicity. The propionic acid derivatives have the advantage of being less toxic than the salicylates and indomethacin, but in general are less effective, although they can be longer-acting.

3 Steroids, usually prednisolone, may be necessary to make life tolerable for some patients, but they have severe side effects if used over long periods. There is some evidence that low doses of prednisolone given early in the disease may modify the course of the condition, but there is general agreement that high or long continued dosage is harmful.

4 So-called 'second-line' drugs are considered to have disease-modifying properties. These include gold, penicillamine and methotrexate. There is a current trend favouring early diagnosis, whenever possible, and the use of these drugs to modify the course of the condition before serious damage to the joints occurs.

Physiotherapy is usually invaluable in maintaining activity and function.

Surgery

Surgery has gradually offered more and more to the rheumatoid patient but careful selection of patients is essential.

1 Synovectomy, i.e. removing the diseased synovium, can give excellent relief of pain, but there is conflicting evidence as to whether it slows down joint destruction. The knees and the joints of the fingers are best suited to this procedure.

The synovium regrows in 3–4 weeks, but the rheumatoid process appears to be delayed, sometimes for several years. Synovectomy of tendon sheaths may prevent tendon rupture.

2 Repair of ruptured tendons and capsular procedures may restore active movement to the fingers.

3 Joint fusion. Certain joints such as the wrist benefit from fusion, but for most joints arthroplasty is more likely to give good function. Fusion of adjacent vertebrae may be necessary in the cervical spine when subluxation threatens cord damage.

4 Arthroplasty. A wide range of procedures is available, using the same prostheses as those for osteoarthritis. The results are often better than with osteoarthritis because the functional demands of the patient are less, but the risk of sepsis, particularly in patients on steroids, is considerable. Surgery is usually performed when the disease is well controlled by systemic therapy.

Social and supportive measures

These are all important in maintaining morale and independence. The patient's work may need to be modified, and appliances and home circumstances designed to cope with disability. Nevertheless, many patients do not reach this degree of severity and of those who do, most remain surprisingly independent.

STILL'S DISEASE

The disease in children is the equivalent of the adult condition and is characterized by its systemic effects. It is much less common than the adult form.

The term *juvenile chronic arthritis* includes Still's disease and a number of less well-defined conditions, some of which may be mono-articular or may have minimal joint involvement—so-called *pauciarticular*.

CLINICAL FEATURES

The onset is often insidious, but may be acute. Fever, lymph gland involvement and anaemia are usually present in addition to the joint pains and stiffness. Uveitis occasionally occurs.

The main joints affected are the knees, ankles, wrists and occasionally the spine. The degree of pain varies, children occasionally presenting with chronically swollen joints which are painless and functioning normally.

Deformities occur, as in the adult form, and there is a more marked tendency to ankylosis, especially in the cervical spine. Epiphysial growth may be disturbed.

RADIOLOGICAL FEATURES

As in the adult rheumatoid, these may not be striking in the early stages. The changes are essentially the same, although much less marked. The carpus is usually affected and fusion of the wrist may occur.

DIAGNOSIS

The ESR is usually raised, but serological tests are usually negative, except in the pauciarticular form. Pericarditis and a history of preceding streptococcal infection favours the diagnosis of rheumatic fever, although this is now rare in the UK. In the mono-articular case the distinction is usually from osteomyelitis or suppurative arthritis.

TREATMENT

The same local and general measures are needed as in the adult. Salicylates have been the most popular drugs, but naproxen and ibuprofen are now the drugs of choice, although steroids may be needed for the severe case.

Physiotherapy is important in maintaining joint movements, particularly when the disease is beginning to settle.

Surgery is rarely needed, and synovectomy, although occasionally used, is usually followed by a very long period of rehabilitation.

After the disease has subsided, surgery may be helpful in restoring joint movement by dividing tight contractures, adhesions, etc. Occasionally, osteotomies may be necessary to correct severe deformities.

PROGNOSIS

The outlook is good: 60–75% of patients recover fully, although this may take several years. A few patients become severely disabled and death may occur from visceral involvement.

POLYMYALGIA RHEUMATICA (PMR)

This is a form of rheumatic disease usually occurring in patients over the age of 60. It is rare under 50 years of age. It affects women more than men and is characterized by aching pain and stiffness in the muscles of the neck, shoulder girdle and occasionally in the back and pelvic girdle. In approximately 20% of cases it is associated with arteritis of the cranial vessels and sudden blindness due to occlusion of the retinal artery is a constant risk.

DIAGNOSIS

This is essentially clinical, but the ESR is usually considerably raised and biopsy of the temporal artery may reveal the associated arteritis.

TREATMENT

High doses of steroids, e.g. 50–60 mg of prednisolone per day is recommended for cranial arteritis, but lower doses, i.e. less than 20 mg per day are adequate for PMR. The disease usually subsides over a period of months or years.

ANKYLOSING SPONDYLITIS

This is a very definite entity in the rheumatic spectrum. The histocompatibility antigen HLA-B27 is detectable in about 90% of patients with the disease. This has also been found in associated conditions such as anterior uveitis and Reiter's syndrome.

CLINICAL FEATURES

The disease, which is essentially an enthesitis, tends to affect young adults — males more than females. It usually starts with pain and stiffness in the lumbar region and over a period of months or years this gradually extends to involve the whole spine and the manubrio-sternal joints.

The characteristic feature is ossification of the ligaments of the spine and the intervertebral discs so that the spine is converted into a solid rod, usually with a gradually increasing kyphos (Bamboo spine, Fig. 41.3). In severe cases the patient may not be able to raise his head to see in front of him. Other joints may be involved, particularly the larger joints, with rheumatoid-like symptoms and signs and a tendency to severe stiffness. The sacro-iliac joints are affected as a necessary prerequisite for the diagnosis and the radiological appearances of irregularity and marginal sclerosis with eventual fusion are very characteristic. Plantar fasciitis (p. 291), Achilles tendinitis and tenderness over bony prominences are common.

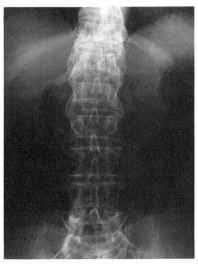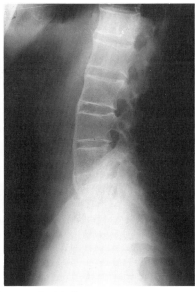

Fig. 41.3 Ankylosing spondylitis producing intervertebral fusions.

Fibrosis of the lungs and aortitis also occur and iridocyclitis is an occasional accompaniment. The ESR is usually, but not always, raised. Tests for rheumatoid factor are negative.

TREATMENT

It is rarely possible to influence the pathological course of this condition. Phenylbutazone is useful in relieving painful joint symptoms and backache, but because of its toxicity it should only be considered if other NSAIDs have failed. It is now licensed only for hospital use for this condition.

Physiotherapy, particularly exercises to maintain joint movement, may be helpful in early cases, and a period of rest in a corrective plaster shell may be needed if deformity is progressing quickly. Severely deformed patients may require a corrective osteotomy of the spine. The disease usually progresses slowly, but its activity may eventually lessen, leaving the patient with residual problems which may need such measures as joint replacement.

ACUTE SYNOVITIS (MONOARTHRITIS OR THE 'ACUTE PAINFUL JOINT')

Patients frequently present with a swollen painful joint, with an obvious effusion and often with synovial thickening. The knee is the most commonly affected. Many of these represent the earliest manifestation of rheumatoid disease, but investigations should be carried out with the following possibilities in mind:

1 rheumatoid arthritis;

2 Reiter's syndrome (or septic arthritis due to gonococcus);

3 psoriasis (which produces an arthropathy very similar to rheumatoid arthritis);

4 ulcerative colitis;

5 ankylosing spondylitis;

6 tuberculosis; and

7 gout.

REITER'S SYNDROME

The synovitis or arthritis is associated with non-specific urethritis and conjunctivitis. The disease is either sexually transmitted or associated with bacillary dysentery.

CLINICAL FEATURES

The arthritis may be acute or of gradual onset and may be widespread or mono-articular. The ophthalmic symptoms and urethritis may occur separately. Plantar fasciitis and Achilles tendinitis may be a feature. The arthritis is usually self-limiting, but recurrence is common. The ESR is usually raised. Rheumatoid factor tests are negative. HLA-B27 antigen is present in over 70% of cases. In the chronic case, periostitis is a common feature. Sacro-iliitis occurs as in ankylosing spondylitis.

TREATMENT

The urethritis, which may be non-specific or related to chlamydial infection, may be treated with antibiotics, but is difficult to eliminate. Chronic joint symptoms are treated by rest in the acute phase, with physiotherapy and anti-inflammatory drugs as necessary.

PSORIATIC ARTHRITIS

About 5–10% of patients with psoriasis suffer from a polyarthritis of rheumatoid type. Usually, the small joints of the hands and feet are affected. Distal interphalangeal joints may be involved and there may be large joint, sacro-iliac or spondylotic changes.

This is a sero-negative arthritis; the disease may be asymmetrical with little periarticular osteoporosis and the skin lesions are characteristic.

TREATMENT

This is similar to that for rheumatoid arthritis, but the prognosis is usually better.

GOUT

This is a metabolic disease characterized by the deposition of urates in the tissues, hyperuricaemia and, in about 10% of cases, increased excretion of uric acid in the urine. It is a common disease affecting men in 95% of cases and postmenopausal women. The arthritis usually affects the distal joints of the hands and feet and the knees. It particularly (and characteristically) affects the metatarso-phalangeal joints of the great toes.

CLINICAL FEATURES

The disease is chronic, but characterized by acute attacks in which the affected joints, usually single, become severely painful, swollen, often red and impossible to move. This usually settles spontaneously in less than three weeks. The joint may be gradually damaged by repeated attacks. Other features include the formation of gouty tophi — collections of urate drystals in the soft tissues, especially in the ear lobes, hands and feet.

Over the years, the condition gradually becomes more generalized. Any form of trauma, including surgery, may precipitate an attack, as may alcohol, certain antibiotics, and purine-rich foods such as liver. Blood dyscrasias such as myeloid leukaemia and polycythaemia are also pre-disposing factors. Renal complications such as stone formation are well-recognized and, rarely, renal failure may lead to deterioration and death.

INVESTIGATIONS

The X-ray appearance may be typical, with well-demarcated, rounded erosions close to the joint margins, usually in the hands. Joint destruction may be seen later.

The most useful investigation is the serum uric acid which is usually well above normal, although occasionally isolated readings may be within normal limits.

TREATMENT

Two drugs are useful for treating the acute attack:

1 colchicine which is very specific and may be used as a therapeutic test, it is, however, toxic and unpleasant to take; and

2 phenylbutazone, which usually relieves symptoms very quickly, but is not now advised; Indomethacin may be used instead.

Most patients are also treated with a drug such as allopurinol which lowers the serum uric acid in the anticipation of preventing further attacks. Nevertheless, acute attacks may be precipitated by allopurinol or probenecid if given without NSAID cover.

PSEUDOGOUT

A condition which is, in some respects, similar to gout, but usually less acute and in which the crystals deposited in the affected joint are of calcium pyrophosphate rather than uric acid. A common feature is calcification of the menisci of the knees, although this is rather non-specific. There is usually evidence of osteoarthritis. No specific treatment is known, but NSAIDs are usualy helpful in relieving symptoms.

SECTION 4

Regional orthopaedics

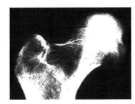

CHAPTER 42

The spine and trunk

The spine is an elastic rod, the movement between two vertebrae being slight, but the overall movement considerable. The mobile parts of the spine normally have a lordotic curve, i.e. convex forwards, and the fixed parts, i.e. thoracic and sacral, a kyphotic curve (Fig. 42.1).

The marrow of the vertebral bodies retains its blood-forming capacity throughout life and vertebrae are, therefore, subject to blood-borne diseases and diseases of the haemopoietic system. Being cancellous, they unite readily after fracturing. Ossification occurs from a single centre in the body and a 'ring' epiphysis for each end plate. It is these latter which develop abnormally in Scheuermann's disease (p. 227).

The neural arches are formed by the pedicles, laminae and spinous processes (Fig. 42.2). They ossify from a centre on each side and it is the failure of these to fuse which makes minor degrees of spina bifida so common in the lumbar region.

The ligaments — flavum, supraspinous, interspinous and anterior and posterior are essential for the stability of the spine.

The intervertebral discs account for almost one-third of the total height of the spine. They are disrupted more readily by trauma in the cervical than in the other regions of the spine.

The posterior articulations are true synovial joints formed by the articular processes of two vertebrae. Their shape governs the stability of each region. In the cervical spine they are horizontal and allow considerable rotation; in the lumbar spine they are vertical and permit flexion and extension much more than rotation (pp. 82–3). They are true synovial joints and are subject to the appropriate diseases, notably osteoarthritis.

The ribs prevent significant movement in the thoracic spine, but the shock-absorbing function of the discs is still important.

EXAMINATION OF THE SPINE

❚ *Inspection*. The patient should be seen standing or sitting and the posture of the spine, its shape and any exaggerated or abnormal curves noted. A localized kyphos or gibbus may be visible, usually in the thoracic region. Any lateral curvature must be tested for fixity by flexing the spine.

THE SPINE

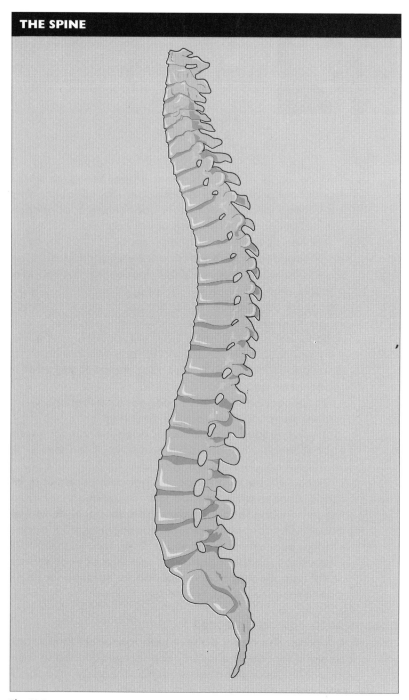

Fig. 42.1

TYPICAL THORACIC VERTEBRA

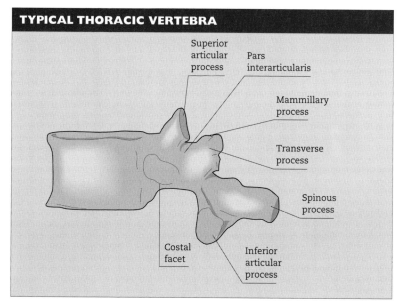

Superior articular process

Pars interarticularis

Mammillary process

Transverse process

Spinous process

Costal facet

Inferior articular process

Fig. 42.2

Spasm of the erectors is common in painful conditions and may produce a tilt.

2 *Palpation*. Running the fingers down the spinous processes will detect a localized kyphos or a gap in the ligaments. Occasionally, a 'step' in the spine may help to diagnose a subluxation or spondylolisthesis (p. 229).

Tenderness is often a valuable sign and should be localized accurately. Deep tenderness may be elicited by thumping the spine with the border of the clenched fist and may be a sign of vertebral body disease.

In the cervical spine, tenderness is often felt over the side of the neck and over the trapezius muscle.

Temperature differences are rarely felt in spinal disease.

3 *Movements*. All movements should be tested. The mobile areas of the spine normally move smoothly. In certain conditions the movement may become more localized, with obvious fixed areas. Limitation of movement may occur in one direction and not in others. Rotational movements are particularly prone to restriction.

4 *Measurement* is rarely of value in diagnosis of spinal conditions, except that overall height may diminish progressively in certain diseases, notably osteoporosis. Radiological measurement is valuable in scoliosis.

5 *Neurology*. Full neurological assessment of arms and legs is essential in examining any spinal condition. Thoracic lesions may cause girdle pains and anaesthesia around the trunk.

6 Circulatory disturbances may be relevant, e.g. an aortic aneurysm may be a cause of chronic back pain.

7 Lymphatic glands should be palpated, e.g. an acute torticollis may arise secondarily to inflamed neck glands and many neoplastic conditions affecting the spine may cause enlargement of glands.

8 A full general examination, particularly of the abdomen, breasts and urinary system is always indicated.

SPINAL CONDITIONS

CONGENITAL CONDITIONS

Klippel–Feil syndrome (p. 200).
Congenital torticollis (p. 200).
Spina bifida (p. 197).
Congenital scoliosis (p. 199).

DEVELOPMENTAL CONDITIONS

For example:
Scheuermann's disease (p. 227).
Spondylolisthesis (p. 229).
Idiopathic scoliosis (p. 223).
Infantile scoliosis (p. 221).

TRAUMA

See Chapter 12.

INFECTIVE CONDITIONS

Acute infections

1 Osteomyelitis not infrequently affects vertebral bodies, rarely the neural arch. The thoraco-lumbar junction is a frequent site.

2 *Extradural abscess.* The signs and symptoms may be similar to those of acute osteomyelitis, sometimes with definite neurology.

3 *Acute discitis.* An infective condition affecting the intervertebral disc. It may occur primarily, usually in children, or as a complication of surgery for disc prolapse in adults. The symptoms and signs are similar to those of osteomyelitis. On X-ray the disc may look normal initially, but later becomes ill-defined and destroyed and eventually fusion of the two bodies occurs.

Treatment

Antibiotics and a period of bed rest are usually adequate.

Chronic infections

1 *Tuberculosis* (p. 249).

2 *Chronic osteomyelitis*—often a slowly progressing form of acute osteomyelitis.

NEOPLASTIC CONDITIONS

1 *Metastases*. All parts of the spine are commonly affected by metastasizing carcinoma—erosion and collapse of bodies tends to occur. The neural arches are occasionally affected. A bone scan may reveal the lesion before X-ray changes occur.

2 *Primary*. Most primary lesions are of haematological origin, e.g. myeloma, leukaemia. Osteosarcoma and fibrosarcoma occur occasionally, notably in Paget's disease.

METABOLIC CONDITIONS

Almost all metabolic bone conditions produce spinal changes, usually with softening and collapse of bodies and development of a kyphos—localized or generalized.

DEGENERATIVE CONDITIONS

Disc degeneration and osteoarthritis of the posterior intervertebral joints, the combination being known as spondylosis (p. 282), are common in both cervical and lumbar regions.

SPINAL STENOSIS

Narrowing of the spinal canal may occur in several ways. The canal may be congenitally small or abnormal in shape—usually triangular. Trauma, spondylolisthesis, osteophytes, and disc prolapse may all produce local narrowing. In some individuals, narrowing of this type, usually in the lumbar region, may compress the cauda equina and produce a characteristic syndrome of pain of claudication type but extending down the back of the legs in the sciatic nerve distribution. This is markedly related to exercise and to posture. There may be neurological signs although these may only be detectable after exercise. The condition occurs in middle age. Computed tomography or, preferably, MRI scanning may be diagnostic. For the appropriate case surgical decompression is likely to relieve the symptoms.

RHEUMATIC CONDITIONS

1 Rheumatoid arthritis and Still's disease affect the spine in most well-established cases. The cervical spine appears to be most vulnerable and in the adult, erosion of posterior joints and softening of ligaments may allow subluxation of one vertebra on the next, usually producing neurological changes and at the higher levels, occasionally, sudden death. Rheumatoid disease of the neck is usually painful and, because of its dangers, fusion is usually advised if there is any tendency to subluxation. In Still's disease the tendency is to spontaneous fusion of adjacent segments.

2 Ankylosing spondylitis (p. 316). In this condition the spinal changes are progressive and serious. The sacro-iliac joints are also affected early and sclerosis of these joints is often visible on X-ray.

Chronic back pain

Pain in the neck and back are both very common and in the UK currently account for over 80 million days lost from work per year, a steadily increasing figure. There is, nevertheless, a 90% chance that an acute attack of back pain will settle sufficiently to allow a return to work within 6 weeks. If this does not occur, the pain is likely to become chronic and after a 6 month absence from work, the chances of the patient returning to the same job fall to 50% and after 2 years' absence there is little likelihood of a return to any form of work.

Recent interest in spinal disorders has made it possible to diagnose an increasing range of pathological conditions, some of them affecting the posterior facet joints and often causing root compression. The MRI scanner is proving to be of great value in this respect. However, many patients cannot be accurately diagnosed and are presumed to be suffering from ligament strains, 'fibrositis', 'lumbago', sacro-iliac strain or ill-defined muscle strains. Virtually nothing is known about the pathology of these conditions, which are often complicated by psychological factors, particularly if compensation for an injury is involved. The term 'simple back pain' has been suggested as a convenient non-specific diagnostic label.

1 A characteristic feature is usually chronic, disabling pain in the neck and shoulders, or low back and buttock. The pain is of a mechanical nature in that it varies with physical activity and with time.

2 Palpation often elicits muscle spasm and tender spots or nodules in the fascia or muscles of shoulder or pelvic girdle.

3 Movements are usually moderately limited, although may be more free if the patient's attention is distracted.

4 Neurological examination is usually normal.

5 Many patients are overweight, fail to take exercise and have a poor posture; correction of these factors may be important in relieving symptoms.

There is little doubt that pain can be referred to various parts of the shoulder, pelvic girdle and buttocks from ligamentous strains in the spine, and the condition usually called 'sacro-iliac strain' seems to be a definite entity with localized tenderness and pain on stressing the joint. Nevertheless, lack of knowledge of pathology makes the problem of back pain a difficult one, and many forms of treatment may be unsuccesful or actually harmful.

A practical approach to the problem is to assess the patient when first seen by taking a careful history and carrying out a full clinical examination, and to categorize the condition into:

1 simple back pain;

2 nerve root pain; and

3 possible serious spinal pathology.

Simple back pain implies no root compression and no evidence of serious spinal pathology such as tumour or infection.

Nerve root pain implies a root distribution of symptoms and signs and is commonly caused by a disc prolapse, spinal compression, surgical scarring or an underlying neurological condition.

Serious spinal pathology should be suspected if the symptoms last for longer than 6 weeks or if the pain is non-mechanical in character, the patient is unwell or losing weight, there is structural deformity of the spine, widespread neurology or a history of malignancy or infection.

MANAGEMENT

Evidence of acute spinal cord or cauda equina compression is a justification for *immediate* referral by a General Practitioner to a surgeon experienced in spinal conditions.

The patient suspected of having serious spinal disease should have X-rays of the spine, and ESR and further investigations as necessary.

The patient categorized as having simple back pain or single non-progressive nerve root pain need not have an immediate X-ray and should be managed conservatively. Symptomatic treatment usually makes use of simple analgesics, NSAIDs, physiotherapy, heat, massage and exercise. Occasionally, manipulation is helpful, but should be avoided if there is nerve root pain. Prolonged bed rest is harmful and is better avoided if possible or kept to a maximum of 3 days. Patients with nerve root pain may require longer periods of bed rest and progress is usually slower. Psycho-social management is important and every effort should be made to keep the patient with simple back pain at work.

Surgery has little place to play in the management of spinal conditions unless the diagnosis is clear-cut and the patient has been fully assessed, both physically and psychologically.

A summary of the early management of back pain is given below.

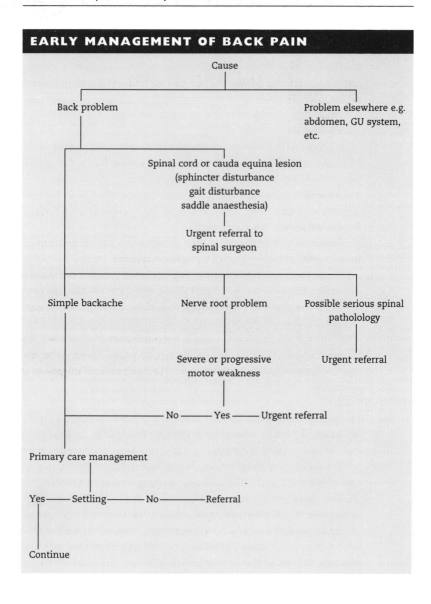

EARLY MANAGEMENT OF BACK PAIN

Cause

Back problem   Problem elsewhere e.g.
                                abdomen, GU system,
                                etc.

Spinal cord or cauda equina lesion
(sphincter disturbance
gait disturbance
saddle anaesthesia)

Urgent referral to
spinal surgeon

Simple backache   Nerve root problem   Possible serious spinal
                                                     patholology

                         Severe or progressive   Urgent referral
                         motor weakness

                    No ——— Yes ——— Urgent referral

Primary care management

Yes ——— Settling ——— No ——————— Referral

Continue

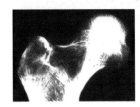

CHAPTER 43

The shoulder and upper arm

Movements of the shoulder are shared between the shoulder joint proper, i.e. between humerus and scapula, and movement of the scapula on the chest wall.

Normally, during abduction there is a smooth integration between these movements, but in pathological conditions, one may predominate over the other, e.g. stiffness at the shoulder joint may mean that the only possibility for abduction is at the scapulo-thoracic joint. On the other hand, stiffness or ankylosis of the sterno-clavicular joint may virtually eliminate scapular movements.

The rotator cuff muscles surrounding the upper end of the humerus and the capsule of the shoulder are important for stabilizing the shoulder and producing rotation, while the deltoid provides most of the power of abduction.

CLINICAL EXAMINATION

1 *Inspection.* The patient should be observed standing or sitting in a comfortable position and the levels of the shoulders noted, together with the presence or absence of swellings or wasting. Deltoid wasting accompanies many shoulder conditions, as does wasting of the posterior scapular muscles.

2 *Palpation.* The landmarks are the tip of the acromion, the sterno-clavicular joint, the coracoid process and the spine of the scapula. The greater tuberosity of the humerus is also normally palpable. Tenderness is commonly found over the trapezius area, and in capsulitis may be localized to the greater tuberosity. Increase in temperature and boggy swelling may accompany infective conditions or rheumatoid arthritis.

3 *Movements.* Abduction, flexion, internal and external rotation should be tested (Fig. 43.1). Abduction should be observed from behind to distinguish the various components of this movement. External rotation is tested with elbow pressed into the side of the body. A useful rapid test is to ask the patient to put his hand behind his neck and behind his back. The patient may avoid attempting external rotation when the joint is unstable, e.g. in recurrent dislocation. The shoulder can sometimes be

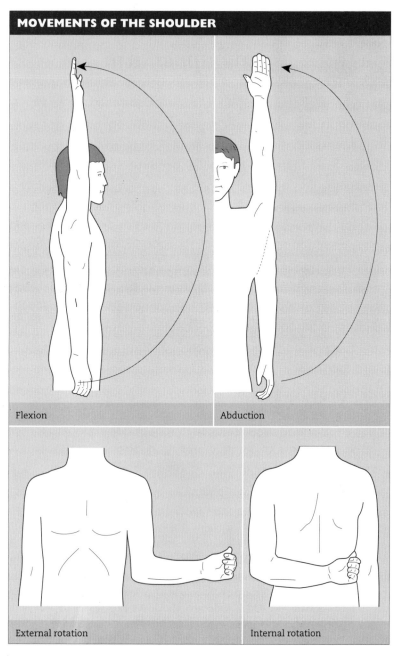

Fig. 43.1

'telescoped' upwards and downwards, usually following a paralytic condition such as a stroke.

4 *Measurement.* The girth of the upper arm may be an index of deltoid or biceps and triceps wasting.

5 *Neurology.* Damage to the axillary nerve may produce a patch of anaesthesia over the belly of the deltoid. Other shoulder conditions may be associated with brachial plexus injury. Many shoulder conditions cause pain indistinguishable from that due to cervical pathology, so a full neurological examination of the arm is always indicated.

6 *Circulation.* The blood supply in the arm may be impaired in certain shoulder conditions which cause pressure on the axilla. Axillary vein thrombosis is an uncommon condition, usually affecting young men and causing swelling and discoloration of the whole arm.

7 *Lymphatics.* The lymphatic glands in the axilla or supraclavicular fossa may be enlarged from shoulder disease, particularly infective conditions.

CONDITIONS AFFECTING THE SHOULDER

CONGENITAL

Sprengel's shoulder (p. 179).

TRAUMA

See Chapter 14.

Recurrent dislocation (p. 100).

DEVELOPMENTAL CONDITIONS

Rarely, recurrent dislocation is due to a developmental defect of the glenoid or humeral head. Constitutional laxity is also an occasional cause.

INFECTIVE CONDITIONS

Acute infections

The upper end of the humerus is an occasional site for the development of osteomyelitis. Shoulder movements are usually restricted. Pus may collect under the deltoid or in the axilla. Suppurative arthritis of the shoulder is rare and usually occurs in babies or as a complication of rheumatoid arthritis. The sterno-clavicular joint is also occasionally the site of acute pyogenic arthritis.

Chronic infections

Tuberculosis may affect the shoulder. It is usually accompanied by severe muscle wasting and stiffness of the joint.

NEOPLASTIC CONDITIONS

Secondary neoplasms are not uncommon in the upper end of the humerus, especially from breast carcinoma. Primary neoplasms are rare, but osteosarcoma and osteoblastoma may occur at this site.

DEGENERATIVE CONDITIONS

The shoulder joint is not commonly affected by osteoarthritis which is usually of the secondary type following injury. The joint is not weight-bearing and symptoms are rarely severe enough to warrant surgery. Arthrodesis of the shoulder can be a useful procedure provided scapular movement is adequate. Shoulder prostheses are being developed, but are not yet entirely satisfactory.

Capsulitis (p. 285)

This is a very common condition. The shoulder is prone to stiffness following a period of immobilization, e.g. in a sling, and physiotherapy is always advisable in older people as the stiffness is very difficult to overcome later.

Bicipital tendinitis (p. 286)

Biceps rupture (p. 292)

RHEUMATIC CONDITIONS

Rheumatoid arthritis may affect the shoulder or sterno-clavicular joints, also occasionally the acromio-clavicular joint. Wasting and stiffness with pain are usual and the shoulder may become unstable.

The usual therapeutic measures are helpful. Surgery is rarely needed, but prosthetic replacement or an excision arthroplasty can be beneficial. Excision of the sterno-clavicular joint can also give reasonable pain relief and improve function in the appropriate case.

CHAPTER 44

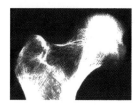

The elbow region

The elbow is a stable joint which is prone to stiffness following injury, even when the injury is relatively minor.

ANATOMY

The elbow joint itself functions as a simple hinge, its stability depending on the close fit of the trochlea in the trochlear notch of the ulna. The superior radio-ulnar joint functions as part of the hinge and also as the rotation point for pronation and supination of the forearm.

The epiphyseal centres of the lower humerus appear between the ages of 2 and 12 (Fig. 44.1). Fractures of the condyles in children often separate off much larger fragments than the X-ray appearances would suggest.

EXAMINATION OF THE ELBOW

1 *Inspection.* Deformity should be noted. Flexion deformities are common and may follow even minor injuries. Trauma to the elbow may result in disturbance of growth on either side causing cubitus valgus (increased carrying angle) or cubitus varus (decreased carrying angle). Increasing cubitus valgus carries the risk of ulnar nerve damage due to traction (p. 38). Wasting of the biceps and triceps is common in many elbow conditions.

2 *Palpation.* The bony landmarks are the olecranon and the two epicondyles. In the flexed position these form the points of an equilateral triangle (Fig. 44.2). The radial head can be palpated below the lateral epicondyle and is often slightly tender in the normal individual.

3 *Movements.* The normal elbow range is from 0–150 degrees; pronation and supination 90 degrees each from the mid position—note that the mid-prone position rather than the anatomical position is usually taken as zero. It should not be possible to tilt the forearm medially or laterally in full extension.

OSSIFICATION CENTRES AT THE ELBOW

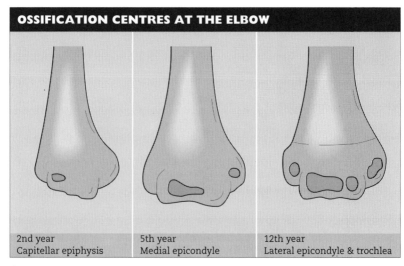

2nd year	5th year	12th year
Capitellar epiphysis	Medial epicondyle	Lateral epicondyle & trochlea

Fig. 44.1

LANDMARKS AT THE ELBOW

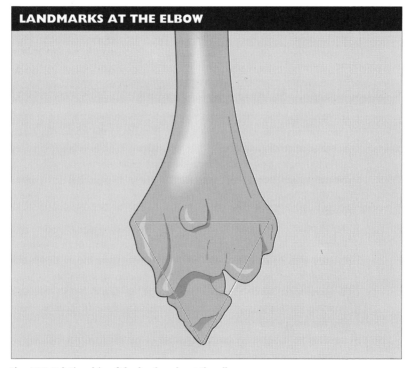

Fig. 44.2 Relationship of the landmarks at the elbow.

CONDITIONS AFFECTING THE ELBOW

CONGENITAL

Congenital dislocation of the radial head occurs very rarely, normally forwards, and may be associated with other congenital malformations. Treatment is rarely necessary, but occasionally removal of the radial head in early adult life may be helpful.

TRAUMA

See Chapter 15.

INFECTIVE CONDITIONS

Osteomyelitis

This occasionally affects the lower end of the humerus or upper end of the radius and ulna. Suppurative arthritis is uncommon in the elbow except in association with rheumatoid arthritis.

Chronic infections

Tuberculosis of the elbow is rare and is usually associated with considerable muscular wasting. If ankylosis seems inevitable, splintage in a functional position is necessary. In a right-handed person, flexion of at least 90 degrees is necessary in the right elbow to enable the patient to feed easily. If both elbows are stiff, one should be fixed at just over 90 degrees and the other at 20–30 degrees to enable toilet functions to be performed.

NEOPLASMS

Metastases may occur in any of the bones around the below, but primary tumours are rare.

DEGENERATIVE CONDITIONS

Tennis elbow (p. 288)

Golfer's elbow

A very similar condition to tennis below, but affecting the medial side, with tenderness over the medial epicondyle and pain on hyperextending the fingers and wrist.

Olecranon bursitis

Acute

This usually occurs in people whose occupation involves leaning on the elbows. The bursa fills with blood and becomes acutely swollen and inflamed. Rarely, the bursa is infected and fills with pus.

Treatment
Aspiration may be necessary if the bursa is very tense. If pus is aspirated, drainage and antibiotic therapy are indicated.

Chronic

The bursa is chronically distended with fluid and there is a tendency for the exudate which contains fibrin to form small nodules or 'melon-seed bodies'. These are usually tender, but pain is not usually a prominent feature of chronic olecranon bursitis.

Treatment
Aspiration drains straw-coloured fluid which is not infected. This rarely cures the condition and excision of the bursa may be necessary if it continues to cause symptoms.

Osteochondritis dissecans (p. 236)

The bony fragment may separate from the capitulum or trochlea and become free as a loose body, causing intermittent pain, locking and swelling. The condition is often bilateral and may go undiagnosed until osteoarthritis supervenes later in life.

Osteoarthritis

The elbow is not infrequently found to be osteoarthritic in a patient who has few symptoms, but simply limitation of range in the joint. Pain eventually becomes troublesome. The patient is usually a man in his late 30s or 40s and the condition is often bilateral, but often with symptoms on only one side.

Treatment

Conservative treatment is usually adequate. Occasionally excision of loose bodies or the radial head may be helpful.

RHEUMATIC CONDITIONS

The elbow is frequently affected by rheumatoid arthritis. The joint is gradually destroyed and may become unstable. All the joint surfaces are affected, particularly the humero-radial.

Clinical features

Pain and swelling are usual features, with synovial thickening and often a considerable effusion. Stiffness is not usually severe.

Treatment

The usual conservative measures are indicated, physiotherapy being particularly important in retaining movement.

Surgery

1 Synovectomy is possible and is usually combined with excision of the radial head.

2 Arthrodesis is almost never indicated.

3 Excision of the joint surfaces may give a reasonable arthroplasty. Interposition of a flap of fascia may provide a more stable joint. Elbow prostheses are being increasingly widely used and can give very satisfactory relief of pain with useful function.

CHAPTER 45

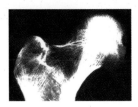

The forearm, wrist and hand

THE FOREARM

The upper end of the radius is a component of two joints—the elbow joint, where it contributes to the hinge mechanism, and the superior radio-ulnar joint, where it provides for pronation and supination.

Both the hinge movements of the elbow and rotation of the forearm are usually still possible when the radial head is excised, but some stability to varus and valgus stressing is lost. Stability of the lower radio-ulnar joint depends on the integrity of the triangular cartilage attached to the ulnar styloid process and the distal margin of the ulnar articular surface of the radius. This structure is also a component of the wrist joint.

THE WRIST

The wrist joint proper is the articulation between the distal surface of the radius, the triangular ligament and the proximal row of carpal bones—scaphoid, lunate and triquetral. This joint allows palmar and dorsiflexion and ulnar and radial deviation. Rotation is prevented by the fact that the complete articular surface is oval (Fig. 45.1).

Further palmar and dorsiflexion is permitted at the joints between the proximal and distal rows of carpal bones. The metacarpals of the fingers, with the exception of the fifth, move very little at their bases, but the thumb metacarpal, which articulates only with the trapezium, has a considerable range.

The metacarpo-phalangeal joints of the fingers allow considerable abduction and adduction in addition to flexion and extension, but the interphalangeal joints are simple hinge joints, with a collateral ligament on each side.

EXAMINATION OF FOREARM, WRIST AND HAND

I *Inspection*. The patient should be watched as he or she uses the arm and hand for activities such as handling objects, gripping and writing. A

THE PROXIMAL SURFACE OF WRIST JOINT

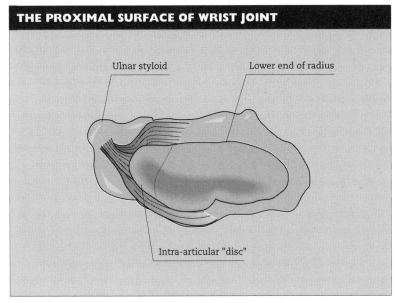

Ulnar styloid

Lower end of radius

Intra-articular "disc"

Fig. 45.1

careful look-out should be kept for 'trick' or compensatory movements, devised (often unconsciously) by the patient to overcome deficiencies. A typical example is the use of an adjacent finger to flex down a finger which lacks active flexion (Fig. 45.2).

Deformities should be noted and carefully analysed. Some deformities are almost diagnostic, e.g. the 'dinner fork' deformity of a Colles' fracture, and the 'mallet' or 'boutonnière' deformities of the finger. Ulnar deviation of the fingers at the metacarpo-phalangeal joints is a common manifestation of rheumatoid arthritis.

Wasting of individual muscle groups may be one of the first signs of neurological loss, e.g. the wasting of the thenar muscles in median nerve compression. Wasting of the interosseous muscles, best seen in the first dorsal muscle between thumb and index, indicates an ulnar nerve or lower brachial plexus lesion (Fig. 45.3).

2 *Palpation.* Landmarks at the wrist are the styloid processes of radius and ulna, the former normally lying more distally than the latter. The pisiform on the ulnar side and the scaphoid tubercle at the base of the thumb define the medial and lateral limits of the carpal tunnel.

Swellings are common in the wrist and hand; their extent and exact position in relation to the surrounding tissues should be determined. Most cystic swellings in this region are ganglia and these are usually *transilluminant.*

USE OF TRICK MOVEMENTS

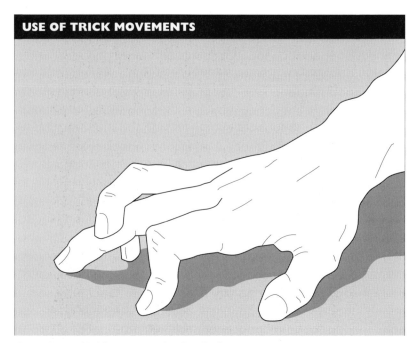

Fig. 45.2 Use of 'trick movements' to flex the finger.

Tenderness should be elicited carefully, and its exact position noted in relation to joints, ligaments, bones, tendons, etc.

Increased temperature is usual in infections of the hand and fingers. In these conditions oedema is common and this normally collects on the dorsum of the hand, even when the infection is in the palm.

3 *Movements.* The ranges of pronation and supination are usually measured from the mid-prone position, taking this as 0 degrees, rather than the anatomical position of full supination. Rotation through 90 degrees is usually possible in both directions. Wrist flexion and extension vary considerably between individuals. Approximately 90 degrees in both directions is normal. Dorsiflexion can be easily compared on the two sides by asking the patient to place his palms together in a 'praying' position and then elevate his elbows. Palmar flexion is similarly tested by placing the back of the hands together and dropping the elbows (Fig. 45.4). Radial and ulnar deviation are usually about 20 degrees, ulnar deviation being slightly greater.

At the metacarpo-phalangeal joints the range of flexion increases slightly from index to little finger. The range of flexion at the thumb metacarpo-phalangeal joint varies considerably from individual to individual, from a few degrees to 90 degrees (always compare both sides if

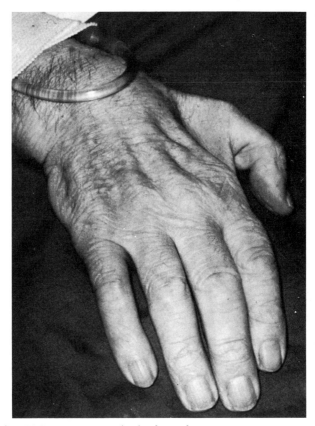

Fig. 45.3 Interosseous wasting in ulnar palsy.

TESTING WRIST MOVEMENTS

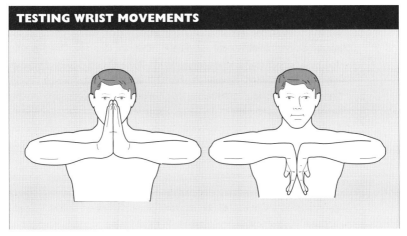

Fig. 45.4

pathology is suspected). The proximal interphalangeal joints of the fingers flex somewhat beyond 90 degrees, and the distal joints somewhat less than 90 degrees. Movements of the thumb relative to the palm are difficult to classify, but movement of the first metacarpal in a plane at right angles to the palm is usually called abduction and adduction, and movement in the plane at right angles to this is called flexion and extension. Internal rotation movements of the metacarpal are described as opposition. This classification corresponds to the names of the various muscles moving the thumb.

4 *Measurement* of the forearm is rarely helpful except in assessing muscle wasting.

5 *Neurological examination.*

MOTOR FUNCTION

The functions of the hand and fingers are complex, and muscle groups and individual muscles should be tested systematically. A knowledge of the normal anatomy and physiology is essential. The following rules are helpful.

I Pronation is produced mainly by the pronator quadratus and pronator teres muscles (median nerve, C6, 7). Supination is a stronger movement produced principally by the biceps and supinator muscles (musculo-cutaneous and posterior interosseous nerves, C5, 6).

2 The wrist flexors can be tested by asking the patient to flex the wrist and palpating the radial and ulnar flexor tendons (radialis, median nerve, C6, 7), (ulnaris, ulnar nerve, C8, T1).

3 All joints of the fingers are flexed by flexor digitorum profundus (median nerve to index and middle fingers, ulnar nerve to ring and little (C8, T1)). Apart from the index, the profundus cannot flex individual fingers when the others are held extended. It is tested by asking the patient to flex the terminal interphalangeal joint whilst the proximal interphalangeal joint is held extended.

4 The proximal interphalangeal joints are flexed by the flexor digitorum superficialis (sublimis) (median nerve C7, 8, T1). It is tested by holding the other fingers extended and asking the patient to flex the appropriate finger.

5 The metacarpo-phalangeal joints are normally flexed by the lumbrical and interosseous muscles. These also, through the dorsal expansions, extend the interphalangeal joints ('threading a needle' position). When these muscles are paralysed (ulnar nerve C8, T1) the fingers take up the opposite position (provided the remaining muscles are acting), i.e. the 'claw' position. Clawing of the index and middle fingers is less than the ring and little because the lumbricals to these fingers are supplied by the median nerve (Fig. 45.5). The interossei are best tested by asking the patient to spread the fingers or to hold them tightly together. The hands can be compared by pressing the two little fingers together sideways (Fig. 45.6).

6 The metacarpo-phalangeal joints are extended by the extensor digitorum longus which can also extend the interphalangeal joints (posterior interosseous nerve C7, 8).

ULNAR PALSY

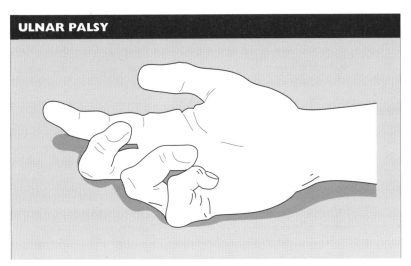

Fig. 45.5

TESTING THE INTEROSSEI

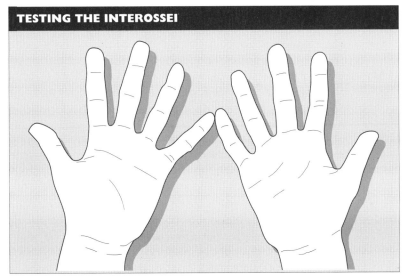

Fig. 45.6

7 The thumb is flexed by the flexor pollicis longus (median nerve C8, TI). The extensor pollicis longus extends the interphalangeal joint, and the extensor pollicis brevis extends the metacarpo-phalangeal joint and the carpo-metacarpal joint (posterior interosseous nerve C7, 8).

8 The thumb is abducted by the abductors pollicis brevis (median nerve C8, TI) and longus (posterior interosseous nerve C7, 8): adduction of the thumb and opposition by the thenar group (median nerve C8, TI) and the adductor pollicis (ulnar nerve C8, TI). All these movements are tested by asking the patient to move the various joints against resistance. 'Trick' movements are common in minor defects of innervation.

9 Wrist extension is produced by the extensor carpi ulnaris (posterior interosseous nerve C7, 8), and extensor carpi radialis longus and brevis (posterior interosseous nerve C6, 7).

SENSATION

The dermatomes are as shown in Fig. A.2 (see Appendix 2). In some individuals the median and ulnar territory divides on the middle instead of the ring finger. Testing with a pin is adequate for most clinical purposes, but finer tests of sensation and hand function are in routine use by specialist hand surgeons. In particular, testing of two-point discrimination using dividers is a helpful test of finger tip sensory function.

Absence of sweating from a finger tip is a useful indication of minimal sensory loss.

CIRCULATION

The radial pulse is easily palpable. Loss of the radial artery interferes with hand circulation in only a small proportion of people who have a deficient palmar anastomosis.

LYMPHATIC SYSTEM

Lymphangitis and lymph gland enlargement are common in hand and finger infections. The gland fields in the axilla should always be palpated in these conditions.

CONDITIONS AFFECTING THE FOREARM, WRIST AND HAND

CONGENITAL

Reduction deformities and hemimelias (pp. 177–8).

DEVELOPMENTAL CONDITIONS

* *Madelung's deformity* (p. 179). A condition in which the radius becomes

bowed and the lower end of the ulna gradually becomes more prominent. It is due to a growth defect in the lower end of the radius.

- *Dyschondroplasia* (p. 206) usually causes multiple swellings in the digits, often with considerable interference with function. Repeated surgery may be necessary over a long period. Achondroplasia produces a hand with short fingers and often a single transverse palmar crease.
- *Trigger thumb* (pp. 178, 289).

TRAUMATIC CONDITIONS
See Chapters 15–16.

INFECTIVE CONDITIONS

Acute infections (pp. 238–41)

1 Acute paronychia—infection under the nail fold.

2 Apical abscess—a small collection of pus under the end of a nail.

3 Intradermal abscess—a collection of pus on the palmar surface of finger or hand, lying between the deep and superficial layers of the dermis, it may communicate with a second collection in the deep tissues—collar stud abscess (Fig. 45.7).

4 Pulp space infection. The pulp space of the finger is divided by septa and becomes very tense and painful if sepsis occurs. The phalanx (usually terminal) may become secondarily infected and an X-ray is essential if infection is well established.

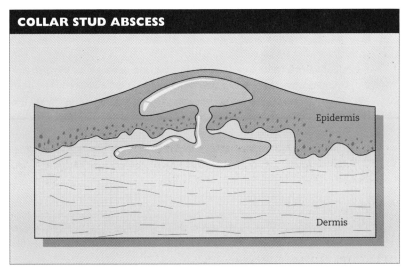

COLLAR STUD ABSCESS

Epidermis

Dermis

Fig. 45.7

Treatment

All the above may respond to antibiotics in the early stages but if pus has formed, surgical drainage is necessary. The acute paronychia is drained by an incision parallel to the nail edge or part of the nail is removed. The other conditions are drained by direct incision, avoiding sensitive areas if possible and conserving skin. Incisions are best made in or parallel to skin creases wherever possible, or along the mid-lateral line of the finger or thumb.

If osteomyelitis has occurred the infected bone may need to be excised.

5 Web space infections. Infection occurs between the fingers and pus may point in the web.

6 Deep palmar space infection. Suppuration in the palmar spaces deep to the palmar fascia is usually localized to one or other of the anatomical palmar spaces.

Both web and palmar space infections cause gross swelling of the hand with oedema of the dorsum. Elevation, usually in hospital, and antibiotic therapy may avoid pus formation, but when pus is present or suspected, incision is necessary, usually at the base of the finger for the web space and preferably through one of the palmar creases for a deep palmar infection.

SUPPURATIVE TENOSYNOVITIS

This is a serious condition usually originating from a penetrating injury which may be minor. The tendon sheath fills with fluid and later pus. Early diagnosis is important as the tendon may become adherent or even slough, and the infection may extend into the deep palm. The digit is swollen, very painful and tender along the whole length of the sheath. All movements are painful.

Treatment is by elevation of the hand and drainage, usually through two incisions, one distally in the finger either in the mid-lateral line or in the distal crease, and a second in the distal palm crease (Fig. 45.8). The sheath is then irrigated with antibiotic—usually penicillin. Primary healing is usual in the early case.

In all hand infections, resting the hand with the fingers and thumb in the functional resting position is important for ultimate function.

Chronic infections

Tuberculosis is now rarely seen in the UK except occasionally in immigrants and old people. The wrist used to be a relatively common site for the development of tuberculous arthritis. Chronic pain and stiffness with marked muscular wasting are usually the symptoms.

INCISIONS FOR DRAINAGE

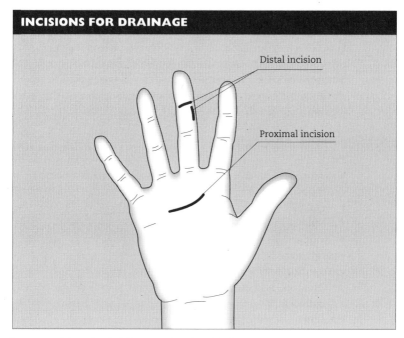

Distal incision

Proximal incision

Fig. 45.8 Incisions for draining a tendon sheath infection.

Tuberculous infection of the flexor sheath can give rise to the classical 'compound palmar ganglion'—a fluctuating swelling extending partly above and partly below the transverse carpal ligament, pressure on one part causing fluctuation through to the other. Nowadays, the commonest cause of a compound palmar ganglion is rheumatoid arthritis. Rarely, tuberculous infection of the metacarpals or phalanges occurs—one of the few sites for tuberculous osteomyelitis as opposed to arthritis.

NEOPLASTIC CONDITIONS

Metastatic tumours are relatively uncommon in the forearm and hand. Pain in this area may be referred from a bronchial neoplasm affecting the apex of the lung and invading the brachial plexus (Pancoast tumour).

Of the primary tumours, enchondromata arising in the fingers and usually expanding the digit are relatively common. Synoviomata occasionally arise in relation to the tendon sheaths. Lipomata and neurofibromata may occur singly or as part of a widespread syndrome. Other neoplasms are uncommon.

METABOLIC DISORDERS

Most of the metabolic disorders produce recognizable radiological abnormalities in the bones of the wrist and hand; indeed, measurement of the density of the metacarpal is sometimes used as an index of the severity of osteoporosis ('Metacarpal Index'). Symptoms are, however, uncommon. Occasionally, the fibrous defects resulting from hyperparathyroidism may cause bone pain. Paget's disease commonly affects the radius, but rarely the ulna, and may cause the bone to become elongated and curved. Bone pain is an occasional complaint. Changes in the hands are rare.

DEGENERATIVE CONDITIONS

Pain in the forearm and hand, occasionally with neurology, may be the presenting feature of a cervical disc prolapse, cervical spondylosis or cervical rib. See also:

- carpal tunnel syndrome (p. 38);
- tenosynovitis (pp. 288–90);
- De Quervain's tenovaginitis (p. 299);
- ganglion (p. 291); and
- Dupuytren's contracture (p. 290).

Osteoarthritis usually only affects joints damaged by disease or injury, e.g. osteoarthritis of the wrist following an un-united fracture of the scaphoid.

Osteoarthritis of the joint between the trapezium and base of the 1st metacarpal occurs occasionally for no obvious reason. It may be treated, if severe enough, by excision of the trapezium, or osteotomy of the base of the metacarpal.

Osteoarthritis of the terminal interphalangeal joints of the fingers (Heberden's nodes) is common and may occur singly or occasionally as a manifestation of generalized osteoarthritis.

RHEUMATIC CONDITIONS

Rheumatoid arthritis

Involvement of the joints and synovial sheaths of the hand is usual in this condition. Stiffness and swelling of the finger joints are frequently the presenting symptoms. As the disease progresses the joints are gradually destroyed. Destruction of the articular surfaces, softening of the ligaments, and muscle spasm combine to produce the characteristic ulnar deviation of the fingers at the metacarpo-phalangeal joints.

Rheumatic involvement of the synovial sheaths, particularly of the extensor tendons, causes painful swelling and in many cases rupture of the tendons, leading to secondary deformities of fingers and thumb. Swan-neck and boutonnière deformities are common (Fig. 45.9), but despite these various deformities and the associated pain and stiffness, function is often preserved for a surprisingly long period.

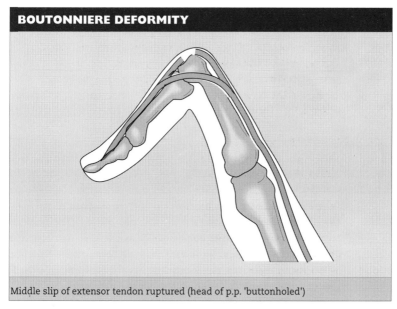

BOUTONNIERE DEFORMITY

Middle slip of extensor tendon ruptured (head of p.p. 'buttonholed')

Fig. 45.9

Treatment

Local measures include rest and splintage during the acute phases, with physiotherapy, active and passive movements using hot wax baths, when symptoms are less acute.

Surgery can offer synovectomy of the tendon sheaths and finger joints to relieve pain, repair of ruptured tendons, and arthroplasties for the various involved joints. Several forms of arthroplasty for the finger joints are available, but a popular one is a flexible silastic implant devised by Swanson which gives stability whilst still allowing movement. Arthrodesis of the wrist can also be helpful in relieving pain and maintaining function in the hand.

Psoriasis

Severe involvement of the hands is unusual, but swelling of the tendon synovial sheaths and moderate involvement of the wrists does occur occasionally. Pitting of the nails may be a useful diagnostic sign.

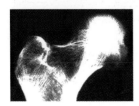

CHAPTER 46

The pelvis, hip and thigh

THE HIP JOINT

Acetabular development appears to depend on the head of the femur being in its normal position, and on the joint moving. The head and acetabulum develop in early embryonic life as a unit, so that congenital dislocation of the hip must occur after this initial development. If the head is persistently dislocated, the acetabulum develops abnormally, indeed a second acetabulum may develop higher up the iliac bone.

The normal femoral neck is anteverted relative to the shaft and the angle of anteversion gradually diminishes after birth. The acetabulum usually points backwards to a variable degree, tending to 'match' the anteversion of the neck. In untreated CDH, the neck usually remains anteverted and the acetabular orientation may also be abnormal.

The epiphysis of the femoral head normally begins to ossify at the age of 4–5 months.

Stability of the hip depends on the shape of the joint, the capsule and ligaments, and the control exerted by the muscles. The iliofemoral ligament is the strongest and most important of the ligaments.

EXAMINATION OF THE HIP AND THIGH

1 INSPECTION

The patient should be seen walking and the gait analysed. In the so-called 'antalgic' or painful hip gait, the patient spends as little time as possible on the hip during the normal stride. A flexion deformity of the hip may reveal itself by the patient tilting the pelvis forwards and arching the lumbar spine to bring his/her trunk upright (Fig. 46.1).

When carrying out Trendelenberg's test, the patient is asked to stand on the leg to be tested. If the hip is normal, the pelvis then tilts up on the other side due to the pull of the glutei. When the pelvis tilts down to the opposite side the test is said to be positive (Fig. 46.2). This occurs in any

PATIENT WITH HIP FLEXION-CONTRACTURE

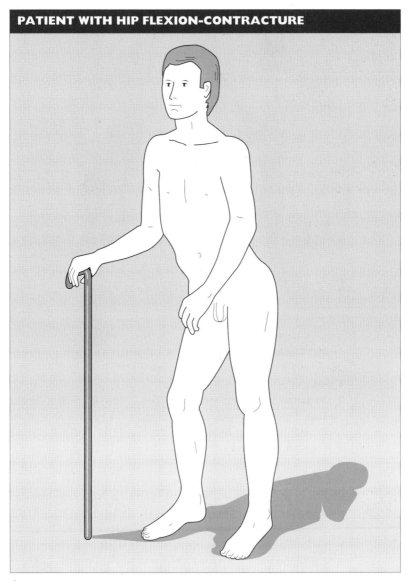

Fig. 46.1

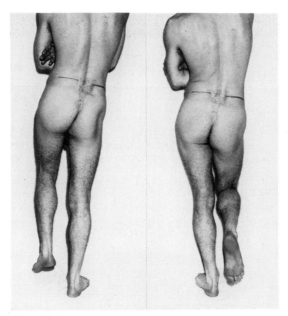

Fig. 46.2 Trendelenberg test.

condition which decreases the mechanical effectiveness of the glutei, i.e. one or more of the conditions listed below.

1 Paralysis or paresis of the glutei.

2 Dislocation of the hip, especially CDH. This shortens the distance between origin and insertion of the glutei, and the stable pivot of the head in the acetabulum is lost.

3 A varus femoral neck.

4 A fracture of the femoral neck.

5 Occasionally, a painful hip causes a Trendelenberg gait. When the glutei contract strongly, the forces across the hip are greatly increased and this makes the pain worse.

The position of the patient in bed should then be noted. The patient should be examined with the legs parallel and in line with the trunk. To achieve this position the pelvis may have to be tilted.

Muscle wasting is common in hip disease and is usually most marked in the buttock and in the adductor region.

A careful search should be made for surface abnormalities—scars, sinuses, etc.

Abnormalities of contour should be noted.

2 PALPATION

The bony *landmarks* around the hip are: anterior superior iliac spine,

NELATON'S LINE

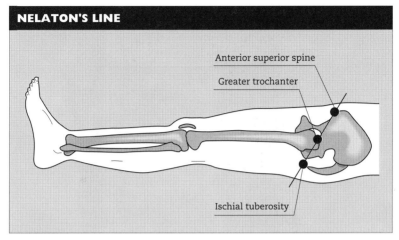

Anterior superior spine

Greater trochanter

Ischial tuberosity

Fig. 46.3

greater trochanter, ischial tuberosity, pubic tubercle. Many methods are described for assessing the normal relationship of these points. The most useful is Nelaton's line—a line joining the anterior superior spine to the ischial tuberosity normally touches the tip of the greater trochanter. A tape measure is useful for testing this. The trochanter will be above this line in dislocation of the hip, fracture of the femoral neck, a varus neck, or a partially destroyed femoral head (Fig. 46.3).

Tenderness is difficult to elicit in hip disease. The head of the femur lies deep to the femoral artery, behind the mid-inguinal point (mid-way between anterior superior spine and symphysis pubis). Tenderness may be felt here, but is more commonly felt over the greater trochanter.

Increase in *temperature* is rarely palpable in hip conditions.

3 MOVEMENTS

The hip has a wide range of movements, these are for convenience classified as:

- flexion–extension
- abduction–adduction
- internal–external rotation.

Extension of the hip may be tested with the patient on his side. The range is only a few degrees and this test is rarely informative. Fixed flexion may be measured by Thomas' test. A patient may conceal a flexion contracture of the hip, even when lying in bed, by arching the lumbar spine. Thomas' test eliminates this by flexing the opposite hip to its full range, then attempting to flex it further. This flattens out the

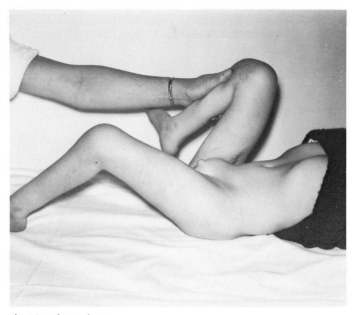

Fig. 46.4 Thomas' test.

lumbar spine, as can be checked by a hand behind the spine, and reveals the flexion deformity of the side being tested (Fig. 46.4). The normal hip will flex until the thigh reaches the chest (140–150 degrees) provided that the lumbar spine can flex normally.

Abduction and adduction are tested by moving the joint while the examiner keeps a hand on the opposite anterior superior spine to detect pelvic movement. Adduction is tested by crossing the leg over the opposite one. Normal range: adduction 40 degrees–50 degrees; abduction 40 degrees–50 degrees.

Rotation can be checked by rolling the leg on the bed and noting the position of the foot or, more accurately, with the patient lying prone and the knee flexed, using the lower leg as a pointer. It can also be tested with the hip in flexion and the patient supine and this gives a slightly different range.

Normal range in extension: internal rotation 20–30 degrees; external rotation 40–50 degrees.

Abnormal movements
Telescoping may rarely be observed if the hip is unstable.

4 NEUROLOGICAL EXAMINATION

The nerves supplying the hip joint are branches of the femoral, sciatic and obturator nerves and hip pain may be felt in the cutaneous distribution of any or all of these nerves.

5 MEASUREMENT

The length of a limb may be measured between any two fixed points depending on the information needed.

True length

This is usually measured from anterior superior spine to medial malleolus. This may be reduced by an abnormality anywhere between these points. A second measurement between the tip of the greater trochanter and medial malleolus may help to localize the pathology.

Apparent length

A fixed adduction or abduction contracture of the hip may be compensated by tilting the pelvis, thus bringing the legs into line with the trunk. A measurement from the mid-line (umbilicus or xyphisternum) will then reveal an apparent difference in leg length. Even though the shortening is only apparent, the patient will still notice that the leg feels short (Fig. 46.5).

CONDITIONS AFFECTING THE HIP AND THIGH

CONGENITAL

Congenital dislocation of the hip (see Chapter 23).

Congenital shortening of the femur and coxa vara (p. 212).

Paralytic conditions, particularly congenital ones such as spina bifida and cerebral palsy, may result in a secondary dislocation of the hip.

DEVELOPMENTAL CONDITIONS

The hip joint is usually affected in epiphyseal dysplasias, most of which result in growth abnormalities, usually producing a varus femoral neck and a distorted and stiff hip (p. 206). The femoral neck is a common site for fibrous dysplasia and pathological fracture may result (p. 211).

- Infantile coxa vara (p. 212).
- Slipped upper femoral epiphysis (p. 212).
- Perthes' disease (p. 232).

Ischaemic necrosis of the femoral head occasionally occurs in a child following a femoral neck fracture or in renal rickets.

TRAUMA

See Chapter 18.

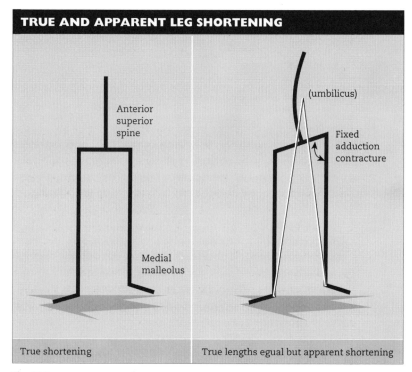

TRUE AND APPARENT LEG SHORTENING

Anterior superior spine

Medial malleolus

(umbilicus)

Fixed adduction contracture

True shortening

True lengths equal but apparent shortening

Fig. 46.5

INFECTIONS

Acute infections

Osteomyelitis and septic arthritis

The metaphysis of the upper end of the femur is inside the capsule so that osteomyelitis starting here quickly spreads to involve the joint. Osteomyelitis occasionally starts on the acetabular side of the hip joint.

Septic arthritis of the hip is not uncommon in neonates (Smith's arthritis). It may be one of several joints involved and is usually secondary to a focus in the lung. The signs may be minimal, the baby being irritable and not feeding. If the condition is neglected, the hip may dislocate and the head may be destroyed, resulting in a stiff joint with disturbance of growth in the limb.

Treatment involves diagnostic aspiration, then open surgical drainage and appropriate antibiotics. The hip is usually splinted in abduction to maintain reduction. A good result can be expected from early treatment.

Septic arthritis in the older child usually presents as an acute fever with extensive pain and spasm in the joint. Differential diagnosis is from 'irritable hip' and acute onset of Perthes' disease. Rheumatic fever and Still's disease occasionally present initially as a mono-arthritis.

Chronic infections

Tuberculosis
The hip is rarely the site of tuberculous infection in the UK, except occasionally in immigrants, but the condition is still a common scourge in under-developed countries. The disease may begin in the metaphysis of the femur or in the synovial membrane and quickly spreads to involve the whole joint. The joint surfaces are gradually destroyed and the capsule becomes distended with pus. Untreated, this eventually breaks through to the surface forming a chronic sinus which becomes secondarily infected.

Clinical features
The child complains of chronic pain in the joint and limps. Loss of weight and local muscle wasting are usual. The hip may become deformed into flexion and adduction by painful muscle spasm.

Radiological appearances
These are initially of porosis of the joint followed by gradual erosion of the joint surfaces and destruction of the femoral head.

Treatment
Management now relies heavily on antibiotic therapy with drainage of chronic abscesses and removal of necrotic debris. The desirable end-point used to be a bony ankylosis of the joint achieved by a long period of plaster immobilization. Nowadays, early treatment may leave the patient with a mobile hip.

NEOPLASTIC CONDITIONS
The upper end of the femur and the pelvis are common sites for the development of metastatic carcinoma. Pathological fracture is common and usually occurs transversely in the sub-trochanteric region. Prophylactic intramedullary nailing may be worthwhile if the condition is spotted before the fracture occurs and the tumour occupies more than 50% of the diameter of the bone. Radiotherapy is used to control the local tumour, and fractures frequently unite.

Primary tumours are much less common, but osteosarcoma, osteoclastoma and chondrosarcoma are all seen in this area. Osteoid osteoma of the femoral neck can be a very difficult condition to diagnose.

METABOLIC DISORDERS

Demineralizing conditions may result in collapse or deformity of the hip joint with stress fractures in the femoral neck. This is particularly noticeable in those conditions arising during growth, i.e. rickets and renal osteodystrophy where the femoral neck may be grossly abnormal with slipping of the epiphysis. In osteomalacia, 'Looser's zones' may be seen in the rami of the pubis and ischium and occasionally in the femoral neck.

Paget's disease commonly affects the pelvis and upper end of the femur. Osteoarthritis of the hip is more common in joints affected by Paget's disease and there may be difficulty in deciding if the pain is due to arthritis or to the underlying bone disease. Pseudo-fractures occur in the varus neck, sometimes leading to true pathological fractures.

DEGENERATIVE CONDITIONS

Osteoarthritis of the hip

The hip is one of the joints most commonly affected by osteoarthritis. In the majority of cases there is no obvious reason for the development of degenerative changes. In a proportion of cases the joint has obviously been damaged by previous disease or injury, notably congenital subluxation, Perthes' disease, slipped epiphysis, infection or rheumatoid arthritis. These cases are known as 'secondary' osteoarthritis.

The peak incidence is in the 6th decade. The disease is frequently bilateral, usually with more advanced pathology or more severe symptoms on one side.

Symptoms

The predominant symptom is pain, usually felt in the groin or buttock, occasionally in the thigh, or over the greater trochanter. The pain is usually worse when weight-bearing and often keeps the patient awake at night when the muscles relax. Stiffness is sometimes a problem and the patients are frequently unable to tie their shoelaces. As time passes, the range of movement diminishes and the pain, which is felt at the ends of the range, becomes more disabling.

Signs

The patient usually limps and often has an antalgic gait. Flexion or adduction deformity may shorten the leg and produce a stooping posture with a hyperextended lumbar spine.

There is wasting of the hip muscles, particularly in the buttock, and usually restriction of movements in all directions. There are frequently contractures in adduction, flexion and external rotation. Thomas' test may reveal fixed flexion deformity. The leg may be truly or apparently short due to flattening of the head and erosion of the acetabulum, coupled with soft-tissue contractures.

Radiological appearances

The typical signs of osteoarthritis are well seen in the hip—distortion and sclerosis of the femoral head and acetabulum, osteophytes around the margin of the joint, with loss of the joint space, which may occur medially, superiorly or anteriorly (Fig. 46.6). The latter may be associated with 'boring in' of the head into the acetabulum—a condition called 'protrusio acetabuli'.

Management

Many patients can be managed conservatively by losing weight, adjusting their activities, using a stick to diminish the forces across the hip, analgesics as necessary and physiotherapy. When mobility is greatly restricted and the pain is interfering with sleep, surgery may be considered.

▌ *Arthrodesis.* Fusion of the joint relieves pain and gives a hip which should remain trouble-free throughout life. It considerably restricts activity and makes sitting uncomfortable. It puts a heavy strain on the back and should be avoided in patients who already have a back complaint. It

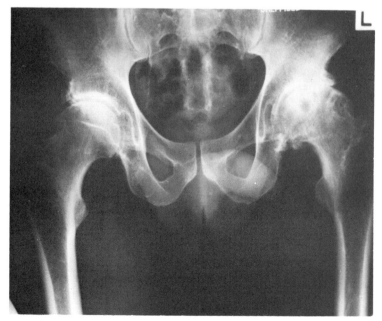

Fig. 46.6 X-ray appearance of osteoarthritic hip.

used to be preferred for the young, fit individual, who had unilateral hip disease, and who was considered to be likely to put considerable demands on the hip. The advent of arthroplasty has made it a much less popular operation.

2 *Osteotomy.* This is a technique, pioneered by McMurray and rarely used now, of dividing the upper end of the femur, usually in the intertrochanteric region and then allowing the osteotomy to unite, either in a plaster-cast or with internal fixation. This was said to give reasonable pain relief in about 70% of patients, but the results are unpredictable and cannot be guaranteed. Its mechanism of action is unknown.

3 *Arthroplasty.* Replacement of the femoral head alone is rarely successful in osteoarthritis since the acetabulum is also abnormal.

Total hip replacement has become almost routine for severe osteoarthritic pain. The patient should be assessed fully in terms of general disability, occupation and overall fitness. Many types of arthroplasty are available. The metal on metal type pioneered by McKee became supplanted by those in which a metal femoral prosthesis articulates with a high density polyethylene cup. Both components are usually fixed in place using acrylic cement. The greatest contribution in the field has been by Charnley, whose prosthesis is widely used. It is designed to give good wear properties whilst minimizing frictional forces which tend to loosen the prosthesis (Fig. 46.7).

Charnley also pioneered the use of a separate operating enclosure to reduce the sepsis hazards. Sepsis, however, remains the principal complication of arthroplasty. Early sepsis has been reduced to low levels but a proportion of patients (approaching 4% in many series although in the best hands, levels of 1% can achieved) develop late sepsis, necessitating removal of the prosthesis. Prophylactic antibiotics, either given systemically or incorporated in the cement, also reduce the sepsis rate. Other complications include breakage of the stem, loosening of either component, dislocation and, rarely, metal sensitivity. Although, taken overall, the complication rate from hip arthroplasty is acceptably low, the large volume of replacement surgery has produced a growing number of patients requiring revision or salvage surgery. This type of surgery is technically difficult and the trend is for such patients to be referred to specialist centres for revision. Sepsis remains the most difficult problem to deal with and many techiques have been tried. There appears to be general agreement that to overcome the sepsis, which usually causes osteomyelitis, all foreign material and dead and infected bone needs to be removed. Opinions then differ as to whether immediate re-replacement should be attempted, with systemic antibiotic cover and antibiotic-impregnated cement, or time should be allowed for the sepsis to subside completely, sometimes aided by the use of removable antibiotic-impreg-

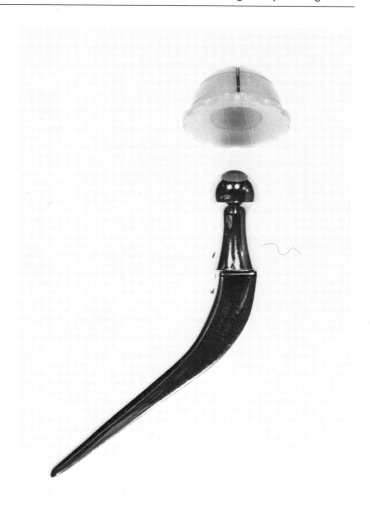

Fig. 46.7 Charnley hip prosthesis.

nated beads, before inserting another prosthesis. The latter regime is becoming more popular.

Results of arthroplasty, at best, are spectacularly good and may restore a totally disabled patient to a relatively normal life. Because of this, and despite the risks, prostheses are now being utilized in much younger patients.

Acrylic cement has many advantages and much effort has been devoted to the improvement of cementing techniques, making loosening less likely. Nevertheless, loosening still does occur and there is suspicion that this may be related to the effects of wear particles and polyethylene debris on the bone cement interface. Cement is also difficult to remove when revision becomes necessary. There has, therefore, been interest in devising new techniques of fixation, such as porous-coated and hydoxyapatite ceramic-coated stems. The latter are interesting in that it is claimed they form a chemical bond with the bone. Similarly, prostheses have been used with an uncemented cup, usually coated with a smooth metal outer surface, the so-called 'bipolar' design. Trials are proceeding of all these devices, particularly for younger patients, but none can, as yet, be said to have demonstrated the survival qualities of a well-cemented Charnley prosthesis.

RHEUMATIC CONDITIONS

Rheumatoid arthritis

The hip is usually involved relatively late in the course of rheumatoid arthritis, but in the severe case, stiffness and pain can be extreme.

Treatment

If surgery becomes necessary, replacement arthroplasty is usually successful, but with steroid therapy healing can be slow and the risk of infection increased. Long-term steroids also have a disadvantage in that they can damage the hip by producing ischaemic necrosis of the femoral head.

Ankylosing spondylitis

In severe cases the large joints, particularly the hip, may be involved with increasing stiffness and pain. Replacement arthroplasty is occasionally indicated.

CHAPTER 47

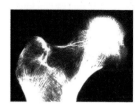

The knee
and lower leg

The knee is not a simple hinge joint. The femoral condyles are of different lengths and flexion occurs by a mixture of gliding and rolling of the condyles on the tibia. Rotation of the tibia about an axis through the cruciate ligaments also occurs and at the end of the extension movement the tibia is screwed into medial rotation relative to the femur—the 'locking-home' mechanism.

The menisci serve to transmit some of the compression forces between femur and tibia into a circumferential force along the length of the meniscus to its attachment at either end. They are avascular stuctures and do not normally heal when torn. Healing may, however, occur if the meniscus is detached from the capsule along its vascular edge. There is currently interest in repairing this type of tear, with the possibility of retaining the meniscus, and in expert hands this can be done arthroscopically.

The cruciate and collateral ligaments are normally tight when the knee is extended. In the flexed position some medial and lateral tilt is possible. The anterior cruciate ligament controls forward movement of the tibia on the femur and the posterior cruciate controls backward movement.

The muscles moving the knee, particularly the quadriceps group, contribute considerably to its stability and can compensate to some extent for ligamentous injuries.

EXAMINATION OF THE KNEE

1 Inspection

Gait. The patient with a painful knee usually walks with the knee held stiffly due to muscle spasm. A patient with an unstable knee may avoid sudden turning movements which cause the knee to 'give way'.

Deformity. Flexion deformities are common. A 'locked' knee is one which will not extend fully, although it may be possible to flex it. The 'locking' may only restrict the last 10–15 degrees of extension.

Abduction and adduction deformities are also common—*bow leg* (*genu varum*) and *knock knee* (*genu valgum*). If these deformities are longstanding, they predispose to arthritis.

Wasting of the quadriceps is almost invariable with organic knee pathology. It is usually most obvious in the fleshy belly of vastus medialis.

Swelling of the whole knee is usually due to an effusion or to synovial thickening, or both. Localized swellings may appear anywhere around the knee, particularly in the popliteal fossa and in relation to the lateral meniscus.

2 Palpation

The useful landmarks are the patella, tibial tubercle, head of the fibula and the medial and lateral joint lines between the femoral and tibial condyles. Some practice is needed to locate these accurately.

An effusion fills up the hollows on either side of the patella. If the effusion is large it 'floats' the patella off the femoral condyles and it can be tapped backwards against the condyles ('patellar tap'). A small effusion can be detected by stroking the fluid out from one of the hollows into the supra-patella pouch and then attempting to fluctuate the remaining fluid across by pressing the opposite hollow.

Synovial thickening has a 'boggy' consistency and the whole synovium is often tender.

Localized swellings should be palpated carefully and an attempt made to determine their attachments; cysts in the popliteal fossa or arising from the meniscus frequently disappear in flexion.

Tenderness is often well localized, e.g. over the medial or lateral joint line or over one or other attachment of the collateral ligaments.

Increased temperature may be felt over an inflamed synovium or over neoplasms or infections around the knee.

3 Movements

Active and passive flexion and extension should be tested. Extension beyond 0 degrees is called 'recurvatum'—it is not uncommon in teenage girls. The normal knee flexes until the calf meets the thigh.

Abnormal movements (p. 146)

To test the collaterals, the knee is held in full extension, then an attempt is made to rock it into varus or valgus. This movement may be painful if it stretches a strained ligament. In the fully extended position the knee will only 'rock' if one of the collaterals and the posterior cruciate is torn. If the test is repeated with the knee in 5–10 degrees of flexion, the cruciates are relaxed and the knee will 'rock' if a collateral ligament alone is torn.

The cruciates are tested by the examiner flexing the knee to 90 degrees (if possible) with the sole of the patient's foot on the couch. He then sits on the foot to stabilize the leg and attempts to draw the tibia forwards or push it backwards relative to its neutral position. If the posterior cruciate is torn, the tibia will fall backwards a little and the knee will look slightly flattened when viewed from the side. Lachmann's test is a variant on the simple draw test and is performed with the knee flexed to 20–30 degrees. In addition to the antero-posterior instability, the tibia may rotate when drawn forwards — so-called *rotatory instability*, in which case, a sudden 'jerk' may be felt on extending the knee with an applied rotational stress — the *pivot-shift* sign.

4 Measurement

The girth of the thigh is a useful measure of quadriceps wasting. The two sides should be compared by measuring up from a fixed point (e.g. the joint line) and noting the circumference. Knock knee may be estimated by measuring the distance between the malleoli with the knees touching in full extension.

5 Neurology

The usual neurological examination should be made if knee pathology is suspected. A grossly arthritic and unstable knee may be due to a neuropathic condition associated with sensory loss (Charcot's joint).

6 Vascularity

Injuries of the popliteal vessels occur commonly in dislocations of the knee. A popliteal aneurysm may masquerade as a popliteal cyst.

7 Lymphatics

The lymph drainage to the groin should be examined in all suspected infective or neoplastic conditions.

CONDITIONS AFFECTING THE KNEE AND LOWER LEG

CONGENITAL

- Congenital dislocation of the knee (p. 179).
- Congenital discoid meniscus (see below and p. 179).

DEVELOPMENTAL CONDITIONS

Cartilaginous dysplasias frequently affect the femur and tibia, and may lead to distorted growth of the knee. Osteochondromata, in particular, are common in the upper tibia and lower femur.

- Recurrent dislocation of the patella (p. 215).
- Genu valgum (p. 217).
- Tibia vara (Blount's disease) (p. 217).
- Osgood–Schlatter disease (p. 235).
- Pseudarthrosis of the tibia (p. 218).

TRAUMA

See Chapter 19.

Meniscus lesions

The menisci are attached firmly at their ends to the tibial eminence (Fig. 47.1). They have a loose attachment to the capsule around their peripheries where vessels enter the meniscus. Tears through this area have the potential for healing.

The medial meniscus forms part of a larger circle than the lateral and is more mobile. It is more frequently damaged.

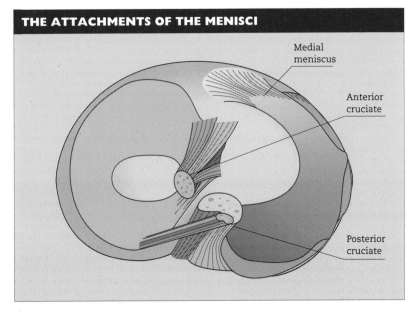

THE ATTACHMENTS OF THE MENISCI

Medial meniscus

Anterior cruciate

Posterior cruciate

Fig. 47.1

Discoid meniscus

In early embryonic life, both menisci form a complete septum between tibia and femur. They normally develop a central opening well before birth. Rarely, one of them remains as a complete disc. This normally affects the lateral meniscus. It is often discovered during childhood or early adult life because of its tendency to 'clunk' loudly as the joint moves. It is more liable to tear than the normal meniscus and the tear may be the cause of symptoms. The condition is frequently asymptomatic and never discovered, but if it causes trouble the meniscus may be excised.

Tears of the menisci

These are some of the commonest of knee injuries. The medial meniscus is torn more frequently than the lateral. It is likely that many menisci which tear are degenerate. This appears to be the case with tears occurring in those patients whose occupations involve crouching and kneeling or repeated trauma to the knee, e.g. miners, electricians and professional footballers.

Typical features

The patient, normally a young male, twists the knee whilst it is flexed and his weight is on that leg. He feels something tear and experiences pain on the side of the knee where the meniscus is torn. The knee may lock, i.e. extension may be impossible. Occasionally, someone may manipulate the knee causing it to 'unlock' suddenly. The injury is a severe one. The footballer is not able to carry on playing and may have to be carried off the field. The knee swells, usually over the next 6–12 hours. Occasionally, swelling occurs within 15–30 minutes. This is due to a haemarthrosis and may mean a cruciate or synovial tear, either of which may be associated with a meniscus tear.

The typical course is then for the swelling and pain to subside over the next few days and for the knee gradually to regain full extension. Occasionally, the joint remains locked and the swelling and pain persist.

After 12–14 days the knee may be back to normal. Symptoms may then recur if the knee is provoked, e.g. by football or a twisting strain at work. It may then lock intermittently, 'give way' due to reflex quadriceps inhibition, and cause episodes of pain and swelling. The pain may move from its original site causing diagnostic difficulties.

The anterior cruciate and medial ligaments are frequently damaged together with the medial meniscus, causing instability of the joint.

The clinical picture is frequently much less classical than that described above, and a tear may occur with minimal violence, particularly in individuals who spend much time crouching. In these cases it is often the persistence of symptoms which leads to the diagnosis.

Signs

At the time of the original injury there may be swelling, tenderness over the meniscus, muscle spasm and perhaps loss of full extension.

In the chronic state, the only signs may be wasting of the quadriceps, perhaps a moderate effusion and usually tenderness over the meniscus itself. The patient rarely tolerates a locked knee for long.

McMurray's sign is a test for a posterior meniscus tear (Fig. 47.2). The examiner flexes the knee fully, asks the patient to relax, grips the heel with one hand and then with the other hand puts his thumb on one knee joint line and his middle finger on the other. He then rotates the tibia on the femur, whilst gradually extending the joint. If the meniscus is torn posteriorly he may feel it 'catch' or 'jump' between the condyles in certain positions of the joint.

Pathology (Fig. 47.3)

1 The commonest tear runs longitudinally along the cartilage, separating a central 'bucket-handle' fragment from a lateral fragment which is still attached peripherally. This bucket-handle varies in thickness and may represent the whole width of the meniscus, when it is called a peripheral detachment.

2 The peripheral detachment may only affect the anterior or posterior horns.

3 Also common is a horizontal cleavage tear which may produce a flap which catches between the condyles ('Parrot beak' tear).

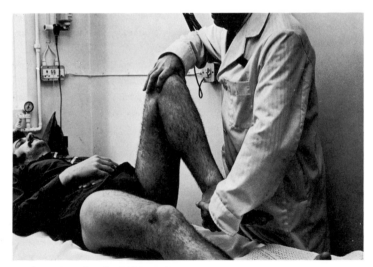

Fig. 47.2 Performing McMurray's test.

PATHOLOGY OF MENISCUS TEARS

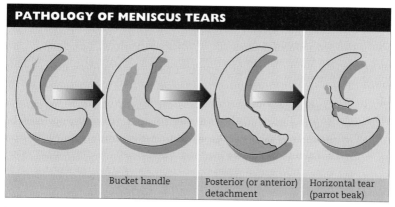

Bucket handle   Posterior (or anterior) detachment   Horizontal tear (parrot beak)

Fig. 47.3

Diagnosis

If an accurate clinical diagnosis of a meniscus tear is to be made, the patient should either have a classical history or classical physical signs or preferably both. Many patients are atypical and can present difficult diagnostic problems. The commonest conditions to be confused with a meniscus tear are ligamentous strains, osteochondritis dissecans, osteoarthritis, acute synovitis. Even at arthroscopy, some patients with a good history and physical signs are found to have no obvious pathology.

Investigations

An ordinary X-ray is only of value in confirming or excluding other conditions. Contrast arthrography using either radio-opaque medium alone or with air can be very helpful in experienced hands but is now being superseded by MRI scanning.

Arthroscopy is a well-established technique which uses an instrument like a cystoscope which is passed into the joint through a small incision (p. 397). It gives an excellent view of most of the structures in the joint, including the posterior half of the menisci which are not visible through an anterior surgical incision.

Meniscectomy

Arthroscopic surgery, which is one example of minimal access therapy (MAT), is now so well-established that almost all meniscus surgery is carried out arthroscopically. Special instruments have been devised to carry out the operative manoeuvres through small puncture wounds and under direct arthroscopic vision. The joint is not opened and recovery from the surgery can be much more rapid than with conventional open techniques. There is some evidence that osteoarthritis may follow excision of a normal meniscus, and it certainly follows a proportion of meniscectomies for a torn meniscus. Current opinion favours trying to preserve as much of the meniscus as possible by trimming away damaged fragments and, wherever possible, repairing longitudinal peripheral tears.

Cyst of the menisci

A cyst usually arises from the lateral meniscus and enlarges under the capsule forming a swelling which is tense in certain positions of flexion. It is accurately located over the meniscus and does not usually reach a large size. It may give rise to pain from tension, and the meniscus, which is usually degenerate and filled with a honeycomb of cysts, is liable to tear, producing acute or chronic symptoms. Removal of the whole meniscus is more likely to produce a lasting cure than simple removal of the cyst.

INFECTIONS

Acute infections

The upper end of the tibia and the lower end of the femur are the commonest sites for acute osteomyelitis in children (p. 242). Spread of infection to the joint is uncommon.

Acute suppurative arthritis is usually seen either in neonates or in adults suffering from rheumatoid arthritis and on steroid therapy. In these latter circumstances the inflammatory response may be considerably masked by the steroids.

An acute arthritis of the knee in a young adult is frequently due to gonorrhoeal infection.

Treatment of all infective conditions around the knee is aided by immobilization of the joint and the Thomas' splint is a convenient way of holding the joint still whilst allowing easy access.

Chronic infections

Tuberculosis of the knee is rare in Europe, but still common in under-developed areas (p. 249). It is characterized by chronic pain and swelling, usually with severe muscle wasting. The condition is usually recognized and treatment instituted before serious destruction occurs, and with modern antibiotic therapy a useful joint may be preserved.

NEOPLASTIC CONDITIONS

Metastatic neoplasms are common in both tibia and femur and may result in pain in the knee.

Primary neoplasms

The upper end of the tibia and fibula and lower end of the femur are the commonest sites for several tumours, notably osteosarcoma and osteoclastoma. They usually present as a painful swelling and may cause a sympathetic effusion in the joint. Diagnosis is usually relatively easy.

METABOLIC DISEASES OF BONE

Few metabolic diseases cause specific problems at the knee. Genu valgum or genu varum may occur as a result of rickets or renal rickets. Scurvy may result in subperiosteal haematoma in the tibia.

Paget's disease typically causes thickening and bowing of the tibia, often with pseudofractures. Pathological fractures are common in the tibia and osteoarthritis may occur in the knee joint affected by Paget's disease.

DEGENERATIVE CONDITIONS

Rupture of the quadriceps mechanism is not uncommon, particularly in middle-aged men (p. 292).

Popliteal cysts

These are common at all ages and usually present as painless swellings in the popliteal fossa, often fluctuating in size. They may arise from one of the anatomical bursae. They tend to be placed medially and rarely reach a large size. They need only be excised if they are giving rise to symptoms. Larger and more diffuse cysts are often associated with pathology in the knee joint, particularly rheumatoid and, less commonly, osteoarthritis. These invariably have a direct connection with the back of the joint through a small defect in the capsule. The rheumatoid cysts are particularly liable to extend and may infiltrate the calf muscles. They are often known as 'Baker's cysts'.

Treatment

The cyst itself is usually of less consequence than the associated arthritis. If a synovectomy is to be carried out this will often cause the cyst to disappear. Extensive cysts may cause pain and interfere with function and may need to be dissected out, but this can be a difficult procedure. The differential diagnosis of popliteal aneurysm should always be considered.

Osteoarthritis (p. 293)

The knee is one of the commonest joints to be affected by osteoarthritis. To a greater degree than in the hip, the condition is usually secondary to some obvious underlying condition. A valgus, and even more so, a varus

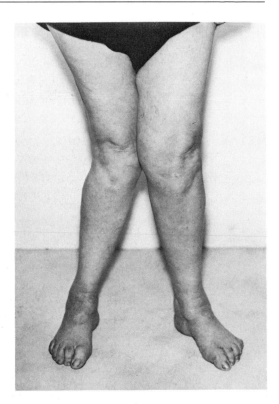

Fig. 47.4 Genu valgum with osteoarthritis.

OSTEOARTHRITIS—CLINICAL FEATURES

- Pain and a limp are the commonest features.
- The knee gradually loses range and varus or valgus angulation may increase.
- There may be an effusion and some synovial thickening or the joint may be dry and crepitant. Acute episodes with synovitis are not uncommon.
- There may be obvious instability, particularly if the knee is very varus or valgus, one tibial condyle usually becoming excavated in these circumstances.
- There is usually much thickening around the joint, with palpable osteophytes and sometimes loose bodies which may cause the joint to lock.

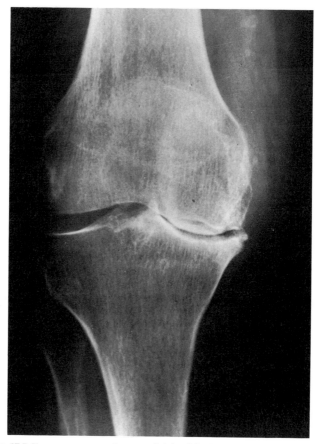

Fig. 47.5 X-ray apearance of osteoarthritis of the knee.

knee, is prone to develop degeneration of the half of the joint bearing the greatest load (Fig. 47.4).

Following chondromalacia of the patella, the arthritis appears to be retropatellar initially, but in all cases, wherever the disease has started, the whole joint eventually degenerates.

Other predisposing conditions are fractures, infective conditions, meniscus and ligamentous injuries, osteochondritis dissecans and rheumatoid arthritis.

Pathology

The knee shows the typical pathological features of extensive wearing away of joint cartilage, with fraying of the menisci, marginal osteophytes and some synovial thickening, but little inflammatory reaction (Fig. 47.5).

Treatment

Many patients can be managed adequately by conservative methods, e.g. by losing weight, using a stick, modifying their work, taking analgesics as necessary, with physiotherapy in the form of heat and exercises in an attempt to maintain range and quadriceps power.

Surgery

A relatively small proportion of patients have symptoms severe enough to warrant surgery. The possibilities are listed below.

1 Arthroscopic lavage—combined with trimming of the articular surfaces and removal of loose bodies and osteophytes, this can give good pain relief for several years.

2 Arthrodesis—this relieves pain, but the stiff leg is a considerable disability. If the operation is contemplated the patient should wear a plaster cylinder for a period to decide if he can accept the permanent stiffness. The Charnley technique is usually used, excising the joint and using compression fixation. This gives reliable results (Fig. 47.6).

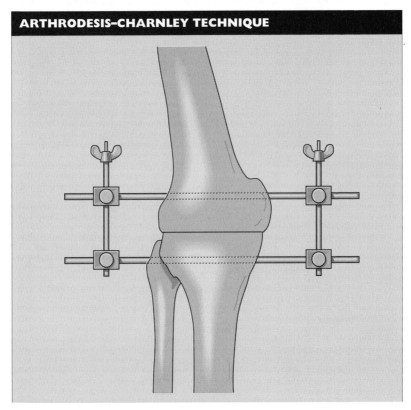

ARTHRODESIS–CHARNLEY TECHNIQUE

Fig. 47.6 Charnley technique for arthrodesis of the knee.

3 Osteotomy—as in the hip, an osteotomy below the joint may give good pain relief and leave the range unchanged. It is usually most successful when used as a corrective procedure for varus or valgus deformity. It unites best when done above the insertion of the patellar tendon.

4 Arthroplasty—many arthroplasties have been designed for the knee. Total replacement is now the procedure of choice and many different types are available. Prostheses designed on the simple hinge principle have been replaced by more complex designs, because it quickly became recognized that some provision was needed to allow for the normal rotational movements.

Present techniques are concentrating on two basic designs:

1 the unconstrained type which is essentially a lining for the condyles (Fig. 47.7) and relies on the joint's own ligaments for stability; and

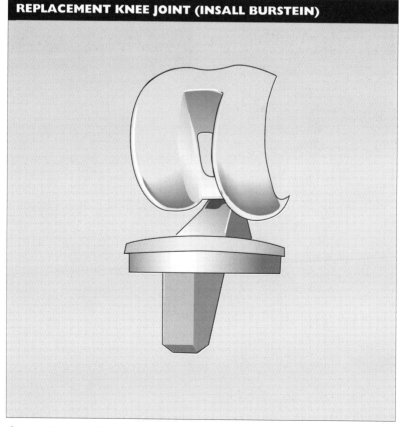

REPLACEMENT KNEE JOINT (INSALL BURSTEIN)

Fig. 47.7 Courtesy of Johnson & Johnson Ltd.

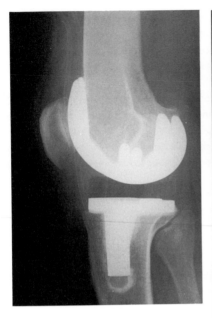
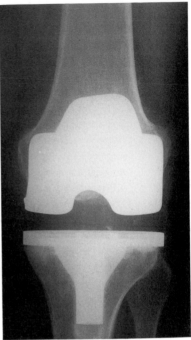

Fig. 47.8 Knee prosthesis *in situ*.

2 the partly constrained type which has some inherent stability, usually dependent on the shape of the articular surfaces.

As with the hip, attempts have been made to rely less on cement fixation and porous-coated and hydroxyapatite-coated designs are available. The most successful current designs are based on the principle of lining the femoral joint surfaces with metal, retaining as much bone as possible in case arthrodesis becomes necessary, and using a polyethylene weight-bearing tibial surface. Designs which incorporate a sliding meniscus principle are also being explored. Reported results of knee replacements for knee arthroplasty are now as good as those for hip replacement.

RHEUMATOID CONDITIONS (See Chapter 41)

Rheumatoid arthritis usually affects the knee, causing pain, stiffness, synovial thickening and effusion. Joint destruction can be very severe and may lead to secondary osteoarthritis.

Treatment

The usual medical and supportive regimes often control the disease in the knee. Every attempt should be made to retain movements. If instability becomes a problem a removable splint may be helpful in maintaining the patient's mobility.

SURGERY

- The knee is the most suitable joint for synovectomy. This can be carried out arthroscopically. The synovium regrows in a matter of weeks but without initially showing signs of disease. The results are best if the operation is done before there is severe joint destruction. The benefits can last many years.
- Arthrodesis. This is usually not suitable for the rheumatoid patient because of the multiple joint involvement and the need to maintain as much movement as possible.
- Arthroplasty. The same procedures as are used for osteoarthritis are suitable for the rheumatoid knee, and the results are often better since the patient makes less demand on the prosthesis.

OTHER ARTHRITIC CONDITIONS

Ankylosing spondylitis (p. 316)

This may cause a similar arthritis to that in rheumatoid.

Gout (p. 319)

This commonly affects the knee, usually on one side only. Severe pain and effusion occurs in attacks and is usually controlled by rest and drug therapy.

Loose bodies tend to cause symptoms by becoming trapped between the joint surfaces. Locking or giving way are usual and the body may be

---

LOOSE BODIES

The knee is the commonest joint to develop loose bodies. These may result from:
- osteochondritis dissecans (p. 236);
- osteochondral fractures;
- detached osteophytes, usually in osteoarthritis;
- soft-tissue fragments, e.g. from a damaged meniscus; and
- synovial chondromatosis—a rare condition where the whole synovium may be studded with cartilaginous nodules. One or more may break free into the joint.

palpable. Loose bodies containing articular cartilage may gradually increase in size.

Treatment

A loose body which is causing symptoms should usually be removed using the arthroscope or if necessary by open operation.

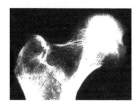

CHAPTER 48

The ankle and foot

The ankle joint is more complex than a simple hinge. Most of the body weight is transmitted from the tibia through the talus, but the fibula also plays a part in weight-bearing. The tibia and fibula are held firmly together by the interosseus membrane and the interosseous ligament, a strong structure which allows a certain amount of 'give' between the bones (see Fig. 20.1).

The medial or deltoid ligament consists of a deep part running from the tip of the medial malleolus to the medial surface of the talus and a wide, superficial part running from the medial malleolus forwards to the navicular, downwards to the sustentaculum tali and backwards to the talus.

The lateral ligament consists of three bands, the anterior talo-fibular, the calcaneo-fibular and the posterior talo-fibular. Strains of the ankle usually affect the anterior talo-fibular ligament but a complete rupture involves all three and allows the ankle to fall open on the lateral side (see Fig. 20.2).

The subtalar joint lies between the talus and the calcaneum. Together with the midtarsal joints between talus and navicular and calcaneum and cuboid, it allows pronation and supination movements of the foot. The head of the talus forms a ball and socket joint with these various articulations. If one of these joints is damaged, all three tend to deteriorate. If arthrodesis is necessary, it is usual to fuse all three rather than to fuse individual joints – 'triple arthrodesis'. The subtalar joint is frequently damaged by fractures of the calcaneum.

The intertarsal joints and the tarso-metatarsal joints, each allow a little gliding movement and, taken together, they contribute to the movements and flexibility of the foot.

The plantar calcaneo-navicular or 'spring' ligament, the long plantar ligament and the plantar aponeurosis all contribute to maintaining the longitudinal arch of the foot.

The height of the arch is very variable. The flatter the foot, the more the forefoot tends to be everted. An abnormally high arch is called pes cavus and an abnormally low arch, pes valgus or flat foot (p. 218). During normal standing and walking, pressure is taken on the heads of all the metatarsals.

The 1st metatarso-phalangeal joint has two important sesamoid bones which take much of the body weight. Dorsiflexion of the metatarso-phalangeal joints is important in the 'push-off' movement of normal walking and the big toe takes much of the weight. The transverse arch of the metatarsal heads is normally concave downwards when non-weight-bearing. In certain conditions it may become convex downwards and the middle metatarsals may then take too much weight during walking, causing pain known as metatarsalgia.

EXAMINATION OF THE ANKLE AND FOOT

1 INSPECTION

Gait. The patient with a painful foot normally walks very gingerly — as if walking barefoot on a pebble beach. Painful conditions of the subtalar joint cause difficulty in walking on uneven ground. Pain in the metatarso-phalangeal joint of the hallux is usually most noticeable in the stepping-off phase of gait when the toe is dorsiflexed.

Deformity. The common deformities of the foot are described on p. 190. Each section of the foot should be considered independently when assessing deformities and movement.

1 The ankle joint itself.
2 The hindfoot in its relationship to the tibia.
  • The long axis of the calcaneum normally inclines upwards and forwards, if this line is inclined more downwards than normal, the position is called *equinus* and if more upwards than normal *calcaneus*.
  • When looked at from behind with the patient weight-bearing, the heel may be in line with the tibia or may be inclined inwards — *varus* (adducted), or outwards — *valgus* (abducted).
3 The forefoot in its relationship to the hindfoot:
  • the forefoot may be normally aligned;
  • dorsiflexed or plantarflexed;
  • adducted or abducted; or
  • rotated (supinated or pronated).
4 The toes — in their relationship to the metatarsals and in the joints within the toes.

Wasting. The muscles of the calf and anterior compartment may show wasting in foot and ankle disease. Wasting of the peronei occurs in several neurological conditions.

Swelling. Swelling of the ankle and foot is often due to oedema which 'pits' on pressure. This may be due to generalized disease or to a local condition. Discrete swellings should be described in the usual way and their relationship to weight-bearing and pressure from the shoe noted.

2 PALPATION

The main landmarks are the two malleoli, the head of the talus, the heel and the 5th metatarsal base. Tenderness and temperature should be accurately assessed. The foot and toes are frequently cold in neurological and circulatory conditions. Increased temperature occurs in infective conditions, neoplasms, gout, rheumatoid arthritis, etc.

3 MOVEMENTS

Ankle movements are tested by flexing the whole foot in the ankle mortice with the heel held in neutral. Fifty degrees of plantarflexion and 20–30 degrees of dorsiflexion are normal. There is normally no adduction or abduction at the ankle joint, but this may occur if the lateral ligament is disrupted.

Subtalar movements are tested by holding the heel and rocking it from side to side on the talus. Inversion and eversion are complex movements involving the subtalar and midtarsal joints. An overall range of 15–20 degrees is usual.

Midtarsal movements are tested by grasping the heel firmly to hold it still and rotating the forefoot around the hindfoot. Movements are usually restricted to a few degrees of rotation which is partly midtarsal and partly intertarsal.

The metatarsals can be moved slightly on the tarsus and the toe movements are tested individually at each joint.

Many of these movements may be painful in pathological conditions.

4 MEASUREMENT

This is rarely of value in the clinical assessment of the foot, but the two feet should be compared for size.

5 NEUROLOGY

A careful neurological assessment is always necessary because of the close relationship between foot pathology and many neurological conditions. It should be remembered that sores on the foot are frequently due to sensory loss, which is often caused by a neuropathy, as in diabetes.

6 CIRCULATION

The assessment of the circulation is always necessary both for diagnosis and in deciding upon treatment. A sore on the tip of the toe or incipient gangrene is a frequent sign of peripheral vascular disease.

7 LYMPHATICS

The principal drainage is to the groin lymph glands.

CONDITIONS AFFECTING THE ANKLE AND FOOT

CONGENITAL

- Talipes (Chapter 24).
- Metatarsus adductus (p. 190).

DEVELOPMENTAL CONDITIONS

Flat foot

Most cases of flat foot in children are physiological (p. 218). The more severe degrees of valgus or pronation of the foot are usually associated with paralytic conditions such as cerebral palsy or with congenital abnormalities of the hindfoot, particularly congenital bars or partial fusions between the hindfoot bones, which can cause the condition known as 'peroneal spasmodic flat foot', so-called because the foot is pulled into severe pronation by spasm of the peronei.

Pes cavus

In the normal foot, the long axis of the calcaneum runs upwards and forwards (Fig. 48.1). The longitudinal arch may be abnormally high with a calcaneus hindfoot, a neutral hindfoot, or even a moderately equinus hindfoot. Severe degrees of pes cavus are usually associated with clawing of the toes (Fig. 48.2) and are often secondary to a neurological condition, with weakness of the interossei. The effects on the foot are rather like the similar condition of interosseus weakness in the hands.

NEUROLOGICAL CONDITIONS

Examples of such neurological conditions are:
- peroneal muscular atrophy;
- Friedreich's ataxia;
- spina bifida;
- spondylolisthesis; and
- poliomyelitis.

In some of these conditions there may be sensory loss and this, coupled with the deformity, may result in pressure sores developing under the metatarsal heads or on the outer border of the foot.

THE POSITION OF THE NORMAL HEEL

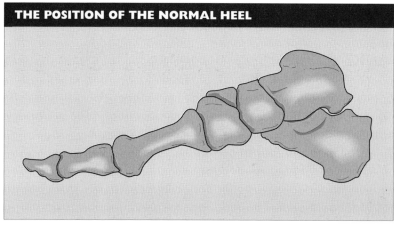

Fig. 48.1

PES CAVUS AND CLAWING OF THE TOES

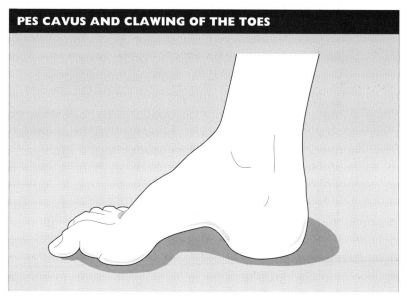

Fig. 48.2

Severe clawing of the toes may result in dislocation of the metatarso-phalangeal joints.

TREATMENT OF CLAW TOES

If the toes are still mobile, transplanting the long flexor tendon around the side of the toe into the extensor tendon may correct the position

HALLUX VALGUS

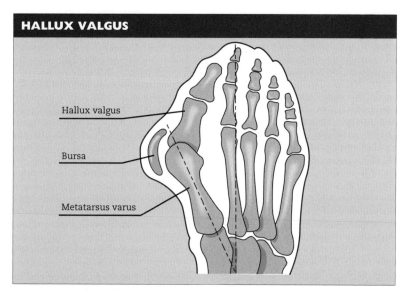

Hallux valgus

Bursa

Metatarsus varus

Fig. 48.3

(Girdlestone), otherwise the proximal interphalangeal joint has to be fused and the extensor tendon divided. The dislocated metatarso-phalangeal joint may require partial excision of the proximal phalanx to produce adequate correction.

The pes cavus may respond to stripping of the plantar fascia from the under surface of the heel (Steindler operation). More severe cases may justify a midtarsal wedge osteotomy.

Calcaneal and navicular exostoses (p. 218).

Osteochondritis of the navicular (p. 236).

Epiphysitis of the calcaneus (Sever's disease) (p. 236).

Osteochondritis dissecans occasionally affects the convex upper surface of the talus.

Hallux valgus

A condition in which the first metatarsal deviates medially to a variable degree (metatarsus primus varus) and the great toe deviates laterally (Fig. 48.3) and may be rotated.

It is often associated with depression of the metatarsals, causing a convex transverse arch. The big toe may over- or under-lap the 2nd toe. Deformity of the other toes is common, e.g. flexion of the proximal interphalangeal joint—'hammer toe' or the terminal interphalangeal joint—'mallet toe'.

Clinical features

The condition is much more common in women. The aetiology is unknown. There is no definite evidence that it is caused by unsuitable footwear, but it may be made worse by badly fitting shoes. It may start in late childhood or early adult life, and usually progresses. It is often associated with metatarsalgia. The metatarso-phalangeal joint usually remains mobile, but the great toe ceases to function during walking.

An adventitious bursa (p. 8) tends to form under the skin overlying the prominent metatarsal head. This may become acutely inflamed and painful—a bunion. Antibiotics may cure the acute episode, but the condition usually recurs.

Treatment

Many patients are asymptomatic but may need to select their shoes carefully. Metatarsalgia may be helped by wearing a metatarsal support which fits in the shoe and supports the metatarsal necks on a cushion, relieving pressure on the heads.

Surgery may be necessary in some patients. Many procedures are available. A few of the more common are listed below (Fig. 48.4).

1 *Metatarsal osteotomy.* A stepped or oblique osteotomy is made through the neck of the metatarsal and the head is displaced inwards and allowed to unite (Mitchell, Wilson). This retains joint movement and is particularly useful in young women.

2 *Keller procedure.* The prominence of the head is trimmed and the base of the phalanx is excised, allowing the toe to drop back into neutral. A fibrous ankylosis is produced. The toe is shortened and usually takes no

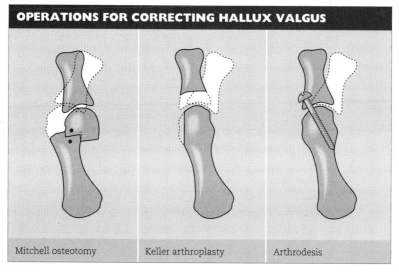

OPERATIONS FOR CORRECTING HALLUX VALGUS

| Mitchell osteotomy | Keller arthroplasty | Arthrodesis |

Fig. 48.4

part in weight-bearing subsequently. Because of this, the operation may increase metatarsal pain and is best avoided if metatarsalgia is complained of pre-operatively. It is usually used in older patients.

3 *Arthrodesis of the metatarso-phalangeal joint.* The joint is fused in slight valgus and about 10–15 degrees of dorsiflexion relative to the metatarsal. It gives good long-term function, but in women may restrict the height of heel which can be worn on the shoe. Occasionally, the 2nd metatarsal head is excised if metatarsalgia is a problem. The great toe still takes part in weight-bearing after a metatarso-phalangeal fusion.

4 *Arthroplasty.* The Keller operation is essentially an excision arthroplasty but the defunctioning of the big toe which it causes is a disadvantage. Flexible silastic implants are available for interposition and can give good function initially, but tend to disintegrate after continued use.

TRAUMA

See Chapter 20.

INFECTIONS

Acute infections

Primary infections are relatively uncommon in the ankle and foot except in relation to the toenails.

Chronic infections

Secondary infections of the joints, especially the metatarso-phalangeal joints, from penetrating ulcers of the foot are common in neurological and ischaemic conditions, particularly in diabetes. The forefoot should be X-rayed if a chronic ulcer fails to heal, in order to detect joint destruction.

In-growing toenail

The big toe is commonly affected. In cross-section, the edges of the nail curve underneath and the nail 'grows' into the soft tissue. Recurrent infections of the nail fold are common and painful.

Treatment

Antibiotics may cure the severe acute episode, but repeated infections are best treated by removal of either the nail edge or the whole nail. The infection then usually clears, but when the nail regrows recurrence is usual. The nail may be prevented from regrowing by excision of the nail bed (Zadek), or by excision of the distal half of the terminal phalanx bearing the nail bed (Jones). Very careful dissection is necessary to excise the whole of the germinal part of the nail bed. A useful technique, if the condition is not too severe, consists of resecting the edge of the nail and cauterizing the nail fold with phenol.

Tuberculosis

This is uncommon in the ankle or joints of the foot. In the ankle joint it can lead to extensive destruction and may necessitate arthrodesis.

NEOPLASTIC CONDITIONS

Primary and secondary neoplasms are relatively uncommon in the ankle and foot. Synoviomata occur in relation to the tendon sheaths and joints and may present as swellings resembling ganglia. All swellings excised should be sent for histology, irrespective of the macroscopic appearance.

DEGENERATIVE CONDITIONS

Osteoarthritis of the ankle

The ankle, despite taking almost the whole of the weight of the body, is not prone to osteoarthrits. Primary osteoarthritis is not common and most cases are secondary to trauma, injuries of the ankle being very common. Other pre-disposing causes are rheumatoid arthritis and osteochondritis dissecans.

Clinical features

Pain on weight-bearing is the main symptom, and the range of movements gradually diminishes. Stiffness of the ankle does not cause significant disability and is rarely a cause for complaint. As the joint space narrows, the talus may tilt within the ankle mortice so that the foot becomes varus or valgus.

Treatment

Disabling pain may require surgery.

1 Arthrodesis is usually not too difficult to achieve, and gives reasonable function. Movement is preserved in the subtalar joint and joints of the foot. The ankle is usually fused in about 5–10 degrees of flexion.

2 Arthroplasty. The fact that arthrodesis gives fairly satisfactory results has delayed development of ankle prostheses. Several designs are now on the market, but these are not yet fully developed or satisfactory. It Is becoming evident that the fibula plays an important role in force transmission and that provision for this needs to be built into the design.

OSTEOARTHRITIS OF THE JOINTS OF THE FOOT

Subtalar osteoarthritis

Osteoarthritis or severe stiffness of the subtalar joint usually follows os calcis fractures. In many cases the joint never becomes painless following the fracture so true osteoarthritis may not be the cause of the pain.

Treatment

It is usual to allow a long period—up to 2 years after the injury—for symptoms to improve, but failing this, it may be necessary to fuse the three joints forming the talo-tarsal articulation: the talo-calcaneal joint, the talo-navicular joint and the calcaneo-cuboid joint—triple arthrodesis. This is not always easy to achieve, but if the fusion is solid and in good position it can give good function. Ankle movement is retained, but the foot is stiff and walking on uneven ground is difficult.

Talo-navicular osteoarthritis

Osteoarthritis of the talo-navicular joint occurs in young people in association with congenital bars or fusions of the hindfoot. It may be associated with a spasmodic flat foot (p. 384). It also occurs in middle age in association with a painful, valgus foot. Triple arthrodesis may be necessary for the severe case.

Hallux rigidus

Osteoarthritis of the first metatarso-phalangeal joint is often called hallux rigidus. This is a common condition, usually occurring in young adults. It is often bilateral and the cause is unknown.

Clinical features

The joint becomes progressively more painful when walking, particularly during the 'push-off' phase. The joint stiffens and, in particular, dorsiflexion is lost, the toe becoming rigid. Some compensatory hyperextension of the interphalangeal joint is usual.

Treatment

Surgery is frequently necessary, and arthrodesis of the joint is the most reliable procedure. In a woman this limits the height of heel which can be worn, but the procedure gives lasting pain relief.

RHEUMATIC CONDITIONS

Rheumatoid arthritis

The joints of the foot and toes and often the ankle are characteristically affected (p. 311).

Clinical features

These joints are often affected early in the disease. At the ankle, synovial thickening and gradual destruction of the joint surfaces lead to pain on weight-bearing. The condition frequently affects the joints of the hindfoot and, again, gradual destruction is usual. The earliest radiological features are a diffuse porosis followed by joint erosions and narrowing. Occasionally, the tarsal joints fuse spontaneously.

The forefoot and toes are often severely deformed, with clawing of the toes or flexion deformities of the interphalangeal joints. The foot frequently develops a cavus or valgus deformity, with prolapse of the metatarsal heads in the sole as the metatarso-phalangeal joints dislocate. The heads come to lie just deep to the skin and cause pain on weight-bearing. Hallux valgus is usual and the toes cease to bear weight during walking. These features are so common in rheumatoid arthritis that any patient who presents with a severely deformed forefoot should be suspected of having the disease and should be fully investigated.

Treatment

Despite severe deformities, many patients can manage to walk surprisingly well, particularly if the disease is controlled and the shoes are suitably modified.

The ankle may require surgical treatment.

• Synovectomy is feasible, but the procedure is less satisfactory than in the knee.

• Fusion may be necessary, but in a generalized joint condition, any procedure which increases stiffness has disadvantages.

• Arthroplasty. Suitable prostheses will undoubtedly be devised to make this a safe and reliable procedure.

Surgery for the hindfoot is not usually necessary. In a severe case with deformity, triple arthrodesis may be helpful.

The forefoot. Many surgical procedures are available for correcting the toes. Clawing of the toes, with pressure from the shoes on the flexed interphalangeal joint, may require either excision of the proximal phalanges or interphalangeal fusions. Symptoms caused by pressure under the metatarsal heads may be treated by excision of all the metatarsal heads including the first, together with an ellipse of skin from the ball of the foot. When this excised wound is closed, the toes are drawn down. This is known as a forefoot arthroplasty and several variants of the operation are available (e.g. Kates–Kessel).

These procedures may make the foot relatively painless if the demands made on it are not too severe.

Gout

This condition characteristically affects the first metatarso-phalangeal joint in men (p. 319). Acute attacks of severe pain with swelling and erythema are usual. The joint is gradually destroyed and develops secondary osteoarthritis.

Treatment
This is by drug therapy (p. 319).

Ischaemia

Arterial disease is common in the ageing population. Lower limb ischaemia may manifest itself as intermittent claudication or by the development of gangrene of the toes, or both.

In the individual with impaired circulation any minor injury may precipitate gangrene and this is particularly likely in the diabetic patient. Although the gangrene may be confined to the toes or forefoot, it is often impossible to obtain healing by peripheral amputation, and it may be necessary to carry out a below-knee or even above-knee amputation. In the diabetic patient who may have small-vessel disease there is a greater chance that a below-knee amputation will be successful, and in some patients an amputation through the forefoot may heal well.

Diabetic neuropathy may also be associated with disintegration of the joints of the foot, with collapse and increasing deformity. Secondary ulceration may then occur. This is a difficult condition to manage, but short periods of cast immobilization may delay progression. Purpose-designed footwear may help to prevent many of these complications.

Orthopaedic techniques

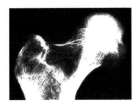

CHAPTER 49

Operative procedures in orthopaedics

JOINT ASPIRATION

Aspiration of a joint is usually carried out for diagnostic purposes. It will distinguish between synovial fluid (effusion), pus (pyarthrosis), or blood (haemarthrosis). An infected joint may contain fluid which is somewhat turbid due to the presence of white cells, or frank pus which is thick and creamy and composed largely of white cells and debris, usually with many organisms. Blood in a joint does not normally clot and may still be aspirated several days after bleeding. In appropriate cases the synovial fluid may be examined for urate or pyrophosphate crystals.

Technique

The risk of introducing organisms is considerable, so that any procedure which involves introducing a needle into a joint should be carried out in the operating theatre with full sterile precautions — with the limb draped and the operator gowned and masked.

General anaesthesia may be used, or local infiltration anaesthesia may be preferred. Lignocaine is a suitable local anaesthetic and after infiltration of the skin, the deep tissues and particularly the synovium should be well infiltrated. Inflamed synovium is very sensitive and difficult to anaesthetize adequately.

For the aspiration a wide bore needle is usually used, attached to a 20–50 ml syringe.

The knee and hip joint require aspiration most frequently.

THE KNEE

This joint will usually be distended and easy to enter. The needle is most easily introduced close to the medial border of the patella near the upper margin. The point should be directed downwards and towards the centre of the joint, with care to avoid the articular cartilage. A definite resistance will be felt as the synovium is entered. After complete aspiration, the joint is wrapped in a Robert Jones pressure bandage of alternate layers of crepe bandage and wool.

THE HIP

Passing a needle into the hip is more difficult because of the depth of the joint. Two techniques are possible. The centre of the head of the femur lies directly under the 'mid-inguinal point' and behind the femoral artery. The needle is inserted 2 cm lateral to the pulsation of the artery and directed backwards and medially.

Alternatively, a long needle may be introduced laterally at the tip of the greater trochanter and passed along the upper surface of the neck into the joint. If the joint is not distended only 2 or 3 ml of fluid may be aspirated.

BIOPSY

Biopsy is used to obtain specimens of tissues for histological examination or culture.

NEEDLE BIOPSY

This is occasionally useful for small specimens of tissue, e.g. from the spine or from bone marrow. The specimen may, however, be inadequate or unrepresentative of the whole lesion.

PUNCH BIOPSY

A more sophisticated technique, using a punch introduced through a cannula. Its main use in orthopaedic work is to take samples of iliac crest bone, usually for the diagnosis of metabolic bone disease. It can give an adequate core of bone with little trauma and without the need for a full exposure. A similar technique is used for bone marrow aspiration, usually from the sternum. With radiological control, specimens can be taken from the spine and paraspinal tissues.

SURGICAL BIOPSY

This is the preferred technique for tumours of soft tissue and bone. With small lesions excision biopsy may be possible, including an adequate margin of normal tissue.

The piece of tissue should be large enough to be representative, should avoid necrotic tissue and should, if possible, contain some normal tissue. This is particularly important with pleomorphic tumours such as osteosarcomata.

ARTHROSCOPY

This procedure has steadily developed over the last 15–20 years with improved optical techniques. The modern instrument is similar in principle to the cystoscope, and uses fibre-optic illumination (Fig. 49.1). The instrument is passed into the joint through a small skin incision under local or general anaesthesia. The telescope fits inside a cannula introduced through the capsule and synovium with a sharp trocar.

The knee has received most attention, but techniques have been developed for examination and surgery of many joints, notably the shoulder, ankle, wrist, hip and small joints of the fingers. There is also increasing interest in performing spinal surgery with similar minimally invasive techniques.

In the knee it is possible to see all the important structures including almost the whole of both menisci, the cruciates and the articular cartilage. Biopsy of the synovial membrane is possible, using special forceps introduced through the trocar and minor operative procedures may be carried out in this way. Techniques have been developed to enable elaborate operations to be carried out. It is possible to excise fragments of damaged tissue, for example from the articular surfaces or menisci, to repair menisci and ligaments and to remove loose bodies and pin osteocartilaginous fragments into position. Extensive synovectomy is possible as is ligament repair and replacement. The operating instruments

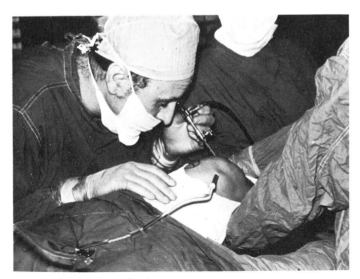

Fig. 49.1 The technique of arthroscopy.

are introduced through small stab incisions or 'portals' and the procedure is viewed through the arthroscope. The use of a small television camera attached to the arthroscope is now almost standard practice and is a valuable teaching aid. The technique requires considerable skill and experience, but results, particularly in terms of rapid rehabilitation, can be very good.

SOFT-TISSUE RELEASE

This is an operative technique designed to correct deformity caused by soft-tissue contracture. It is used for the correction of such conditions as club foot and the deformities associated with paralytic conditions.

The skin may be involved in the contracture and the incision may have to be planned to allow skin elongation.

Tight soft tissues are then released systematically, including fascia, tendons, capsule, etc. Frequently, tendon lengthening alone is sufficient, e.g. the tendo-achilles for an equinus deformity of the ankle. Nerves and vessels may be the ultimate limiting factor. A period in a plaster-cast is usually necessary to maintain correction.

TENOTOMY

This means dividing a tendon—usually to correct a soft-tissue contracture. The procedure may be carried out 'closed', by using a fine knife introduced through the skin. This procedure is dangerous for deeply placed or inaccessible tendons and in these cases the tendon is lengthened by an 'open' operation. If the tendon is to be lengthened and resutured this is usually done by a 'Z' technique (Fig. 49.2).

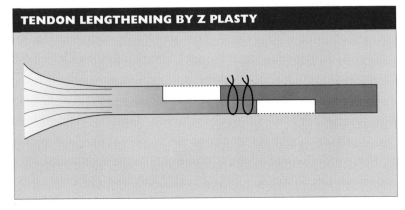

TENDON LENGTHENING BY Z PLASTY

Fig. 49.2

TENDON TRANSPLANTATION

Paralytic muscular imbalance may lead to joint contractures in the growing child. Tendon transplants may be used to restore the balance or occasionally to restore a specific function, for example in the hand.

The best results are obtained when:

1 the muscle whose tendon is to be transplanted has full power and is under voluntary control;

2 the tendon is only transplanted a short distance, e.g. a lateral transplant of the tibialis anterior to correct a varus deformity of the foot (transplants through the interosseous membranes are usually less successful);

3 the muscle works in the same phase as the group it is meant to reinforce, e.g. a flexor tendon to replace a flexor; and

4 the tendon can be implanted firmly into bone under tension.

The wrist flexors can often be spared to replace non-functioning finger or thumb tendons, e.g. flexor carpi ulnaris to replace the long finger flexors. Re-education is quickly achieved.

The tibialis anterior or posterior and the peronei are frequently used to correct inversion or eversion imbalance in the foot.

OSTEOTOMY

This means dividing a bone, usually by open operation (osteoclasis means fracturing a bone).

It is used to correct bone deformity and occasionally persistent joint contracture. In the latter case it should be done as near to the joint as possible. All types of deformity can be corrected, including rotation.

The osteotomy is allowed to unite either with external plaster fixation or by internal fixation. There are many osteotomies for specific purposes, e.g. through the innominate bone to restore acetabular alignment (Salter operation), or through the os calcis to correct inversion of the heel in a club foot (Dwyer).

Osteotomy has also been used to relieve pain in osteoarthritis of the hip and knee. At the hip the bone is divided just above the lesser trochanter (McMurray), and at the knee through the upper tibia. The osteotomies are allowed to unite in the usual way. Pain relief is usually immediate if the procedure has been successful. The mechanism of action is unknown.

ARTHROTOMY

This term simply means opening a joint surgically to secure drainage or to carry out an exploration or surgical procedure.

ARTHRODESIS

Surgical fusion of a joint is known as arthrodesis. (Ankylosis means spontaneous fusion, e.g. following a joint infection.) Arthrodesis is usually performed for one of two reasons:

1 for pain relief in a joint which has been severely damaged by disease; or

2 to stabilize a joint which has lost its stability because of ligamentous damage or paralysis. The joint may be fused either:

(a) by clearing the articular surfaces of cartilage, bringing the raw surfaces together, and holding the position until bony union occurs; or

(b) by an extra-articular technique where the fusion by-passes the joint, e.g. the Britten technique for hip fusion (now rarely used) (Fig. 49.3). Extra-articular fusion used to be popular for fusing tuberculous joints. In many cases, when the disease was cured the joint itself would then fuse by bony ankylosis.

Many techniques are used for fixing the joint until fusion occurs.

1 External fixation, usually Plaster of Paris (e.g. triple fusion of the foot).

2 A combination of external and internal fixation with compression, e.g. the Charnley fusion of the knee, where the condyles are cut off squarely and the cancellous ends held firmly together by Steinmann pins compressed together by clamps (p. 376).

3 Internal fixation by screws, rods, etc., e.g. screw fixation of the metatarso-phalangeal joint or rod fixation of a scoliosis.

4 Fusion may be assisted by bone-grafting, e.g. fusion of the spine may be performed anteriorly by excising the intervertebral disc and putting a graft across the gap, or posteriorly by rawing the posterior bony elements and packing with iliac bone chips or a large cortico-cancellous bone-graft cut to fit around the spinous processes.

Whatever technique is used, protection is necessary for a long period; usually at least three months, and success is more likely if the joint is still before starting.

ARTHROPLASTY

Artificial joint replacement has received much attention over the last two decades, and solutions have been found for many of the engineering and

BRITTEN ARTHRODESIS OF THE HIP

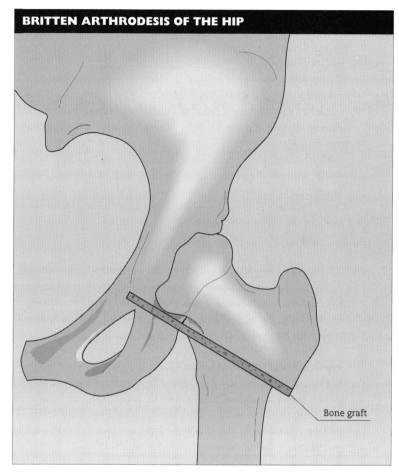

Bone graft

Fig. 49.3

biological problems, only for these to be replaced by other and more subtle problems as experience of the technique grows.

The hip and knee have received most attention and very satisfactory function can be attained with modern techniques.

There are basically three types of arthroplasty.

1 Excision arthroplasty

The joint surfaces are excised completely or partially. Fibrous tissue forms across the gap, giving some stability. Many materials have been interfaced between the joint surfaces to allow better movement, e.g. deep fascia, silastic sheets or flexible connectors, plastic laminae, etc. This type of arthroplasty usually has the disadvantage of incomplete pain relief coupled with instability and is now usually regarded as a 'rescue' procedure following failure of a joint replacement.

2 Partial arthroplasty

Only one of the joint surfaces is replaced, e.g. the Austin Moore arthroplasty for the hip. This is satisfactory if one joint surface is in good condition, e.g. following a fracture, but rarely in osteoarthritis.

3 Total arthroplasty

Both joint surfaces are replaced, either with metal entirely or metal or ceramic bearing against plastic—usually high density polyethylene. These have the advantage of giving good function, but are vulnerable to sepsis or mechanical failure which may loosen or otherwise destroy them.

PRINCIPLES

Current ideas on replacement arthroplasty suggest certain principles.

1 The combination of stainless steel, titanium or cobalt-chrome for one component and high density polyethylene for the other seems to give the best combination of low friction and good wear properties. Ceramic prostheses are also on trial.

2 The articular surface should allow for adequate movement in the required directions whilst restraining movement in unwanted directions, to the extent that this is not prevented by ligaments damaged by disease.

3 The prosthesis should be bonded to bone either by using acrylic cement or, more recently, coated or 'sintered' components into which bone can grow. Hydroxyapatite in ceramic form has also been used as a coating and is claimed to bond chemically with the bone.

4 The operative procedure should be designed to reduce the risk of infection to a minimum.

5 If failure occurs, it should be possible to remove the prosthesis, and, if necessary, perform an arthrodesis.

Replacement of individual joints is considered in the appropriate sections.

LAMINECTOMY

The term strictly means an approach to the spinal canal by removing the laminae of one or more vertebrae with the intervening ligaments. The procedure may be carried out on one side only, or bilaterally, in which case the spinous processes and ligaments are removed. It is often possible to remove a prolapsed intervertebral disc by making an opening through the ligamentum flavum and nibbling away a little of the laminae above and below. This is often called a laminectomy but should strictly be called a 'laminotomy' or 'fenestration'.

AMPUTATION

It may be necessary to amputate part of a limb for one of the reasons listed below.

1 Its retention may threaten life, e.g. neoplasia, 'crush' syndrome, severe infection, etc.

2 It is non-viable, e.g. following trauma, vascular insufficiency, etc.

3 Function or appearance could be improved by replacement of the part with a suitable prosthesis, e.g. congenital or paralytic deformities.

4 Pain which is resistant to other forms of therapy. This is an unusual reason for amputation and if the pain is severe and well established the amputation may fail to relieve the symptoms, with persistence of phantom pain.

The commonest reason for amputation in Western society is ischaemia due to vascular disease.

Whenever amputation is considered, the fullest cooperation with an experienced prosthetist is required, both before and after surgery.

Having decided that amputation is the procedure of choice, the level should be decided to give the best possible function and appearance consistent with removing the pathology. If the amputation is required to eliminate a neoplasm there will usually be little choice of level, this depending on the need to remove the tumour completely. It is usually necessary to amputate through the joint above the pathology or even higher, and this may result in a stump which gives less than optimum function.

Where such considerations do not apply, the level can often be decided on functional grounds, the 'sites of election' for various levels having been worked out from long experience.

The normal considerations, in general terms, are listed below.

1 The more peripheral the amputation, the better, except that for any given level, a stump which is too long may make the fitting of an adequate prosthesis just below it very difficult or impossible.

2 If the elbow or knee joints can be retained, function is very much improved.

3 For most lower limb amputations, very adequate functional prostheses can be provided—the higher the amputation, the more difficult this becomes.

4 Prosthetic function for upper limb amputations is relatively poor because of the complicated demands of hand function and the difficulty of replacing sensibility.

5 The psychological preparation for amputation is very important and, indeed, amputation should usually be regarded as only a stage in a long-term programme of rehabilitation.

LOWER LIMB AMPUTATION

Amputation of toes

This is frequently necessary for trauma and deformity. It is rarely followed by significant functional loss, although the big toe plays a significant part in normal walking.

Occasionally, with penetrating ulcers, particularly in diabetes, it may be necessary to amputate a toe with its associated metatarsal ray. The gap closes and can give a good functional foot.

Amputation through the forefoot

Also usually performed for trauma or occasionally in diabetic ischaemia, it is not suitable for ischaemia due to large vessel disease. It can give good function, the shoe having to be padded.

Amputation through the mid-tarsal region

This is usually better avoided as, depending on the level, the stump may become deformed by the unopposed action of the tibialis muscles, the peronei having been sectioned.

Amputation through the ankle

Symes amputation (Fig. 49.4). In this procedure, the os calcis is shelled out of the heel, the skin of which is then used as a flap to cover tibia and fibula, with the malleoli sawn off level. This gives a satisfactory end-bearing stump. It is usually carried out for deformity or trauma. The prosthesis consists of a hinged foot on a shell which is designed to fit around the prominence of the ankle.

The below-knee amputation

This is one of the commonest amputations – the indications are many. There has been a definite trend in vascular disease to attempt a below-knee rather than the traditional above-knee amputation because of the much better function which can be obtained if the knee is preserved, particularly in old people. The optimal site for tibial section is usually considered to be 17 cm below the knee, but a stump as short as 7 cm can be fitted, albeit with a less satisfactory prosthesis. Traditionally, the fibula is divided 2 cm higher, but the technique of osteomyoplastic amputation divides the fibula at the same level as the tibia, and a periosteal tube is used to form a firm bridge between the two ends.

SYMES AMPUTATION

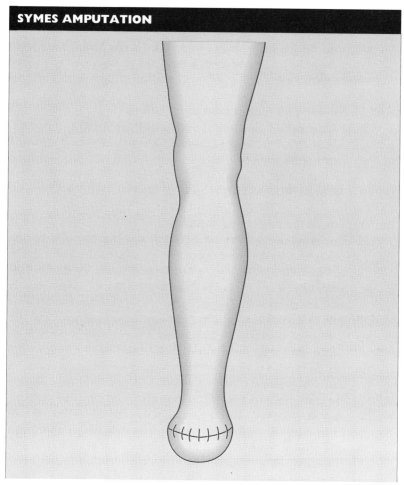

Fig. 49.4

  Equal anterior and posterior flaps are usually used, but in vascular disease a longer posterior flap of skin and muscle is recommended.

  The most satisfactory prosthesis is the patellar-tendon-bearing limb, which fits closely around the upper tibia and takes most weight on the patellar tendon. The end of the stump does not normally bear weight. With this type of prosthesis, if fitted correctly, an above-knee harness is not required. The overall cosmesis can be very satisfactory.

Mid-thigh amputation

  This level of amputation is frequently needed for ischaemia and trauma. Function is less satisfactory than with the below-knee amputation. The stump should be as long as possible, but allowing 12 cm between the end and the position of the knee hinge of a prosthesis. This has a bucket top which fits the stump closely, much of the weight-bearing being taken through the ischial tuberosity. A well-fitted prosthesis can give a very satisfactory gait.

Through-the-hip and hindquarter amputations

These amputations are usually performed for neoplasia. They are mutilating and difficult to fit with a functional prosthesis. This is usually some variant of the tilting table device.

UPPER LIMB AMPUTATION

Amputations of the finger and thumb

These amputations are almost always performed for trauma. Fingers are usually most effectively amputated through the joints. As much length as possible should be preserved, provided that the joints are not stiff. If the whole index is lost it is best to amputate through the 2nd metacarpal to avoid an ugly metacarpal stump. The function of the index is readily taken over by the middle finger. The little finger contributes considerably to the normal power grip. If it is amputated, it may be useful to preserve the head of the metacarpal as this widens the hand.

The thumb is the most important digit and as much length as possible should be preserved, even if it is stiff. The metacarpal alone can give reasonable function. If the whole thumb is lost, it is possible to reconstruct it, either by rotating the 2nd metacarpal to 'pollicise' the index, or by replacing the thumb with a bone-graft and tube pedicle graft. In this case it is necessary to provide an island of sensation, by using an innervated pedicle from another digit. Without sensibility, function of the thumb is greatly reduced.

Amputations through the forearm and upper arm

The elbow should be preserved if possible as its movements may be useful in powering a hand prosthesis, usually a double hook or specialized prosthesis. If the elbow is amputated, the prosthesis is powered by shoulder movements acting through a series of straps and functional capacity is very limited. A cosmetic hand is provided when function is not needed. If the other arm and hand are normal many patients prefer not to bother with a powered prosthesis.

Attempts are now being made to provide external power and some form of sensibility to improve upper limb prostheses.

Amputation through the shoulder and forequarter

As in the lower limb, these are usually needed for neoplasia. If the upper end of the humerus can be preserved this gives a better cosmetic appearance to the shoulder. Even preservation of the scapula alone gives a tolerable appearance, but the forequarter amputation is extremely ugly and very difficult to fit with an adequate prosthesis which is usually only for cosmesis.

AMPUTATIONS IN CHILDREN

These present special problems in that the bones continue to grow if the amputation is through the shafts and the ends may ulcerate through the skin, necessitating re-amputation.

Amputations through the joints avoid this problem and are to be preferred. Children adapt very rapidly to below-knee amputation.

Amputation of the upper limbs for congenital malformation should usually be deferred until the child's function is assessed, as even the most severe deformities can be compatible with good function. If the child has one normal arm, a functional prosthesis on the other side is usually completely ignored.

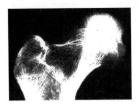

CHAPTER 50

Orthopaedic techniques and appliances

MANIPULATION OF FRACTURES AND DISLOCATIONS

Muscular relaxation is usually necessary for a successful manipulation. This can be achieved by one of the following techniques.

1 Carrying out the manipulation quickly and unexpectedly. This technique is useful for the reduction of finger joints and elbow dislocations. It obviously requires confidence and skill and only one attempt is usually possible.

2 Heavy sedation, e.g. with pethidine or Valium. This has the advantage of avoiding possible complications of a general or local anaesthetic, but rarely allows sufficient relaxation for a difficult manipulation.

3 Local anaesthesia. This may be obtained either by direct infiltration of the site, e.g. the fracture haematoma, or by regional nerve or venous block. The former carries the risk of infecting the fracture site, but both techniques usually relieve muscle spasm as well as pain, and are useful in the unfit patient or where there is a risk of vomiting.

4 General anaesthesia.

The manipulative technique usually consists in working out the mechanism by which the displacement has occurred and reversing this mechanism. It is often necessary to disimpact the fragments by traction and over-riding may need to be corrected by increasing the angulation at the fracture site, then 'hitching' the ends. Difficulties may arise when soft tissues such as muscle or fascia are interposed between the fragments. In these cases there is usually an obvious block to reduction and the skin and soft tissues may be dimpled inwards by the attempt (button-holing). When this happens, open reduction is usually necessary to extract the soft tissues. Forcible manipulation is rarely necessary and may cause serious injury to important soft tissues.

SPLINTAGE

In an emergency, e.g. at the roadside, splints can be improvised from anything available, such as rolled-up newspapers, an umbrella, etc. The upper limb is easily splinted by making up a simple sling. The lower limb can be splinted by tying the legs together. It is usually safe to put the limb gently into a neutral position if it is severely angulated following a fracture.

Types of splint

Splints made from polythene, wire mesh, padded wood, and Plaster of Paris are in widespread use. They are usually bandaged in position, care being taken not to apply them too tightly and to avoid pressure on prominences and superficial nerves. The lateral popliteal nerve at the knee is particularly vulnerable.

Functional splints

These splints may be prescribed to control certain movements whilst still allowing or encouraging function, e.g. various types of springloaded or 'lively' splints are available for the hand, usually to encourage finger movements and avoid contractures (Fig. 50.1).

Slings

Two types of sling are in regular use.
1 The broad sling made from a triangular bandage. This is used when the weight of the whole limb requires support, e.g. a fracture of the clavicle or a dislocation of the shoulder.

LIVELY FINGER SPLINT

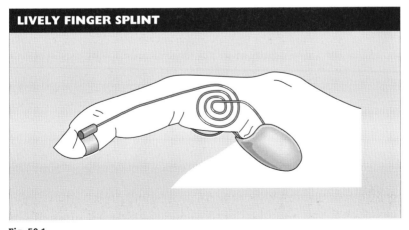

Fig. 50.1

2 The collar and cuff is designed to support the elbow in flexion whilst allowing the weight of the arm to exert traction, for example on a fracture of the humeral shaft. It is usually the most comfortable sling for a severely swollen elbow.

PLASTER OF PARIS TECHNIQUE

Plaster of Paris made from gypsum is the most widely used material for fashioning external splints. It can be used in several ways.

1 As a simple splint. The limbs or joints are placed in the desired position and the splint is fashioned by laying wet plaster in strips to form a half-plaster or 'gutter' splint. A better fit can be obtained by making a complete circumferential plaster and cutting this into two halves longitudinally. Both halves can then be used individually or together.

2 As a complete plaster-cast. The type and extent of the cast will depend on the immobilization required, e.g. half-leg, full-leg, etc.

Plaster-casts which immobilize the hip or shoulder are usually known as 'spicas' and their application requires considerable experience if they are to be comfortable (Fig. 50.2).

HIP SPICA

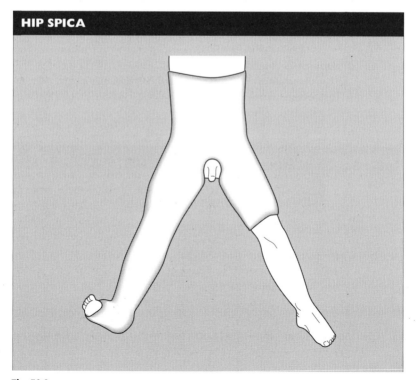

Fig. 50.2

As a general rule, to immobilize a fracture adequately, the joints above and below need to be incorporated in the plaster. This rule may be broken if the fracture is very close to the end of a long bone, e.g. a Colles' fracture.

3 As a functional cast, e.g. by the incorporation of hinges or springs. This technique allows greater function in the joints with less stiffness.

4 As a plaster bed in which the patient can lie for long periods without developing pressure sores, the plaster being made to conform to his/her contours. These are now rarely used.

Application of Plaster of Paris

The routine use of Plaster of Paris requires considerable skill and attention to detail, but every doctor should be capable of applying a simple cast to immobilize a fracture.

It is usual nowadays to use ready prepared plaster bandages which are reliable and predictable in their setting. Everything should be assembled before starting to apply the plaster, as the setting time is short.

1 The amount of protection for the limb depends on the circumstances. If swelling is present or expected, some padding is necessary, usually a single layer of plaster wool wrapped evenly round the limb, paying particular attention to pressure points and prominences. If swelling is unlikely to be a problem, the plaster may be applied unpadded and skin-tight. This gives good immobilization, but is dangerous if applied incorrectly and is difficult to remove. This problem may be partly overcome by applying a stretch stockinette sleeve to the limb before applying the plaster.

2 The roll of plaster is soaked in lukewarm water in a bucket until bubbles begin to emerge from the ends of the roll. Surplus water is then gently squeezed out and the bandage rolled onto the limb, without applying any tension and carefully avoiding folds and wrinkles. The plaster is rubbed to distribute the material evenly between layers and finally smoothed off. An assistant may be needed to hold the limb in the correct position, but he should be careful to avoid pressure with his fingers on the cast until it is set. The plaster wool or stockinette may be folded over the ends of the cast to give a neat comfortable finish.

3 The cast dries within 5–10 minutes, but is not fully hard until 24 hours later. At that time a heel or iron may be incorporated in the plaster to allow the patient to walk if this is considered appropriate.

4 The patient should be given printed instructions to watch for changes in the circulation and sensation in the limb, and to return if the cast is uncomfortable, tight or rubbing the skin.

412 Chapter 50: Orthopaedic techniques and appliances

COMPLICATIONS

- Occlusion of the circulation. If the limb is likely to swell considerably, the patient is best kept under observation.
- Nerve palsies due to pressure.
- Pressure sores – often signalled by staining of the cast or by smell.
- Occasionally, patients in a hip spica develop paralytic ileus, with vomiting and collapse. This can usually be cured by splitting or removing the plaster.

If there is any suggestion that a plaster is too tight, it should be split with a plaster saw and the opening spread. If this is done, the split should be made down to the skin throughout the whole length of the plaster.

A fracture which is not in correct alignment may be improved by wedging the plaster. This involves making a cut around half the circumference and wedging the opening with a wooden block. If the X-ray is then satisfactory, the plaster may be completed again (Fig. 50.3).

SYNTHETIC CASTING MATERIALS (p. 58)

TRACTION (pp. 59–64)

BRACES AND SUPPORTS

The design of splints, braces and other appliances has received a good deal of attention recently and the subject is now known as orthotics and the appliances as orthoses.

An orthopaedic appliance is usually used to hold a joint or a limb:
1 to relieve pain;
2 to allow a fracture to unite by relieving stresses; and
3 to compensate for weakness of muscles, ligaments or bones during weight-bearing or other functions.

COMMON TYPES OF APPLIANCE IN THE MANAGEMENT OF FRACTURES AND DISLOCATIONS

THE THOMAS SPLINT (pp. 60, 63)

This was devised by Hugh Owen Thomas as a knee splint. It is now mainly used for femoral shaft fractures and has the advantage that the patient can be moved with the splint in position. Its application is straightforward, but attention to detail is necessary if complications are to be avoided.

WEDGING A PLASTER CAST

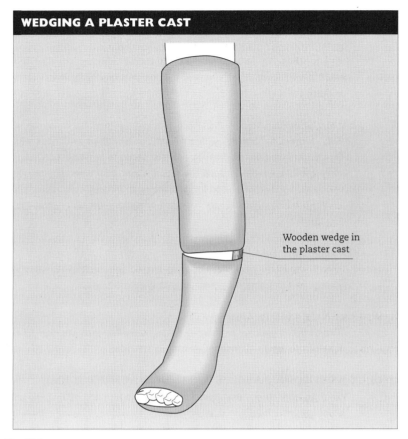

Wooden wedge in the plaster cast

Fig. 50.3

1 The splint is selected by measuring the circumference of the upper thigh at groin level to give the ring size. The length should be that of the good leg from crotch to sole of foot, plus 15–23 cm.

2 The splint is prepared by covering it with three slings made from non-stretch bandage or commercially available Velcro slings, one under the thigh, one under the knee and one just above the tendo-calcaneus.

3 The limb is shaved, the fracture manipulated, and the skin traction applied on each side, with felt pads over the malleoli to prevent pressure. A crepe bandage then holds the extensions in place.

4 The tapes are tied over the end of the splint, the outer one going over the lateral bar and the inner one under it to counteract the tendency of the limb to rotate externally. Pads and small aluminium 'gutter' splints may be used under the thigh to secure the correct position of the fracture.

5 If the splint is to be on for a long period, it may be suspended by overhead slings and a weight may be attached to the end to relieve the groin pressure.

6 The splint may be used with skeletal traction through the tibia, but a knee flexion piece is then needed and the principle of fixed traction no longer applies.

THE THOMAS WALKING CALIPER

This is the same device, with the end connected to two rods which fit into either side of the heel of the shoe. It is fitted so that the patient bears weight through the ischial tuberosity when standing and walking. This is usually used for protecting an incompletely united fracture of the femur but has now been largely susperseded by the cast-brace (Fig. 50.4).

THE CORSET TOP CALIPER

This is similar in principle, but does not achieve weight-bearing completely, and protects the femur against angulation.

THE BRAUN FRAME (p. 66)

This device is used for supporting the leg in the elevated position. Its use is self-explanatory. The leg is usually on traction.

THE CONTINUOUS PASSIVE MOTION MACHINE (CPM)

This device incorporates an electric motor to flex and extend the joint to be moved. Movement is achieved passively with a slow and controlled rhythm and the range can be adjusted as the movement improves. It is particularly useful following knee arthroplasty (Fig. 50.5).

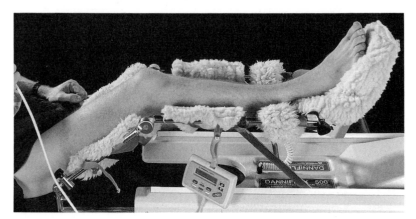

Fig. 50.5 Continuous passive motion machine.

THOMAS WALKING CALIPER

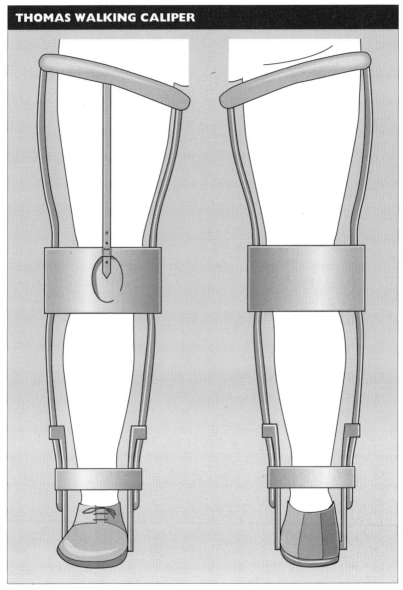

Fig. 50.4

LUMBO-SACRAL SUPPORT

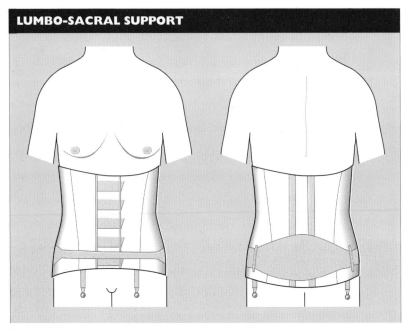

Fig. 50.6

TYPES OF CERVICAL COLLAR

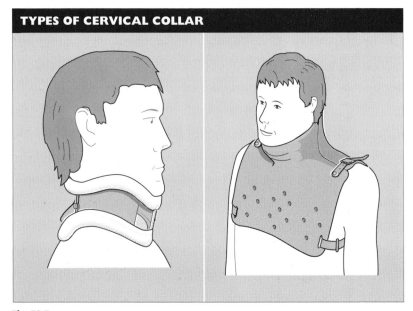

Fig. 50.7

THE LUMBO-SACRAL SUPPORT OR CORSET

Many types are available. They are usually made of canvas with steel inserts or of block leather and aluminium, or more recently of polythene and plastazote. They are made either by moulding directly on to the patient (Fig. 50.6) or on to a plaster-cast.

THE CERVICAL COLLAR

This is useful for the relief of pain in acute conditions or spondylosis, or for immobilization of injuries. Many types are available.

1 The polystyrene type which can be cut to size and held with Velcro. It is valuable and reliable for short-term use.

2 The fully-shaped collar made from polythene and foam-lined. This may be made adjustable (Fig. 50.7).

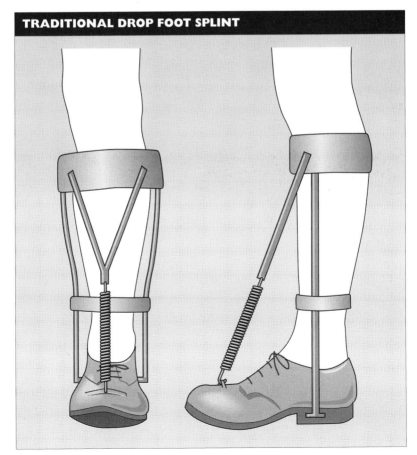

TRADITIONAL DROP FOOT SPLINT

Fig. 50.8

INSIDE IRON AND T-STRAP

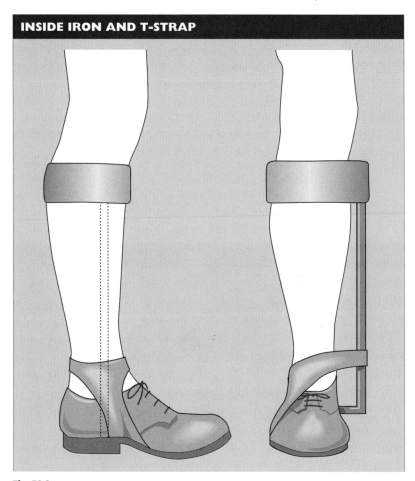

Fig. 50.9

Splints can be used to control joints in paralytic conditions or following ligamentous or bony damage.

1 The full leg caliper to control knee, ankle and foot, with stops entering the heel of the shoe. This may be supplied with a lockable knee hinge to allow sitting.

2 Below-knee calipers to control ankle or foot movements. These may have a single iron on one side or a double iron. Examples are the drop foot splint or spring (Fig. 50.8), and the iron with T-strap around the ankle, usually to control varus or valgus instability (Fig. 50.9). The trend

ORTHOLENE DROP FOOT SPLINT

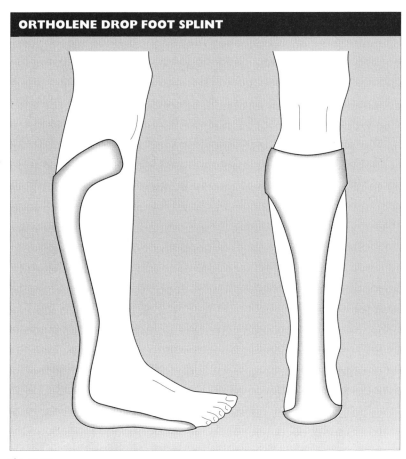

Fig. 50.10

is towards calipers which are more cosmetically acceptable, and fibreglass and moulded polythene ('Ortholene') splints can be used for many conditions (Fig. 50.10).

3 Arch supports and metatarsal supports. These are moulded to suit the condition to be treated, e.g. a metatarsal support provides for weight-bearing behind the metatarsal heads.

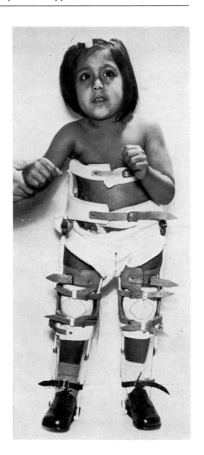

Fig. 50.11 Extensive calipers used in severe paralysis from spina bifida.

4 Specialized braces such as the Milwaukee and the extensive sets used in certain cases of spina bifida (Fig. 50.11).

5 Walking appliances. Many types are in use, axillary and elbow crutches, walking frames, rollators etc. (Fig. 50.12).

WALKING APPLIANCES

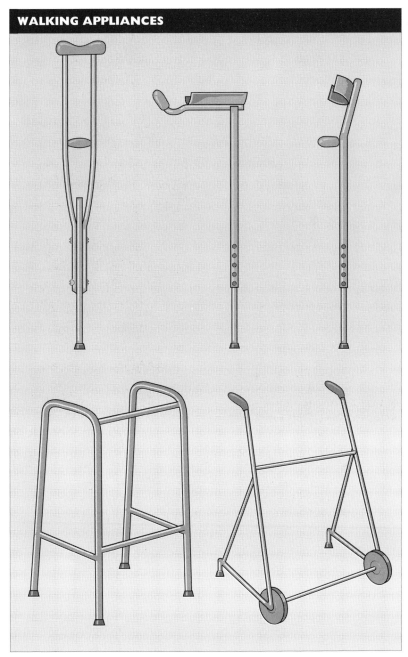

Fig. 50.12 Axillary, gutter and elbow crutches, walking frame and rollator.

Useful pathological values

	Normal ranges
Haematological	
Haemoglobin (g/dl)	♀14 ♂15.5 ± 2.5
Red blood cells (10^{12}/l)	3.5–5.5
White blood cells (10^9/l)	3.5–9.5
Platelets (10^9/l)	140–370
Mean corpuscular haemoglobin concentration (g/dl)	27–34
Erythrocyte sedimentation rate (Seditainer) (mm/h)	♀1–20 ♂1–10
Packed cell volume	% ♀42 ♂47 ± 6
Biochemical (serum values)	
Sodium (mmol/l)	130–147
Potassium (mmol/l)	3.3–5.5
Urea (mmol/l)	1.7–8.3
Creatinine (mmol/l)	50–120
Calcium (mmol/l)	2.12–2.63
Phosphate (mmol/l)	0.6–1.5
Globulin (g/l)	16–33
Albumen (g/l)	35–53
Total protein (g/l)	66–87
Bicarbonate (mmol/l)	22–32
Chloride (mmol/l)	95–107
Alkaline phosphatase (iu/l)	60–306
Acid phosphatase (iu/l)	0–4.0
Uric acid (mmol/l)	140–420

These values are currently in use in the laboratories of the Sheffield University Hospitals Trust. Minor variations may be found in other laboratories.

The muscles of principal importance supplied by the major nerves

Accessory nerve and	C3, 4	Trapezius
Thoraco-dorsal nerve	C5, 7, 8	Latissimus dorsi
Dorsal scapular nerve	C4, 5	Rhomboids
Lateral pectoral nerve	C5, 6, 7	Pectoralis major
Medial pectoral nerve	C8, T1	Pectoralis minor
Long thoracic nerve	C5, 6, 7	Serratus anterior
Axillary nerve	C5, 6	Deltoid. Teres minor
Subscapular nerves	C5, 6, 7	Subscapularis, Teres major
Suprascapular nerve	C4, 5, 6	Supraspinatus, infraspinatus
Musculo-cutaneous nerve	C5, 6, 7	Coraco-brachialis, biceps, brachialis (C6, 7)
Median nerve	C5, 6, 7, 8, T1	Pronator teres (C6)
		Flexor carpi radialis (C6, 7)
		Palmaris longus (C7, 8)
		Flexor carpi ulnaris (C7, 8)
		Flexor digitorum superficialis (C7, 8, T1)
		Flexor pollicis longus (C8, T1)
		Flexor digitorum profundus (C8, T1)
		Pronator quadratus (C8, T1)
		Abd. pollicis brevis, Opponens pollicis, Flexor pollicis brevis, Lateral 2 lumbricals (C8, T1)
Ulnar nerve		Flexor carpi ulnaris (C7, 8)
		Flexor digitorum profundus (C8, T1)
	C7, 8, T1	Flexor pollicis brevis
		Adductor pollicis (C8, T1)
		Palmaris brevis
		Hypothenar muscles, interossei, medial two lumbricals (C8, T1)

continued on p. 424

Radial nerve	C5, 6, 7, 8, T1	Triceps (C6, 7, 8)
		Brachio-radialis (C5, 6)
		Extensor carpi radialis longus and brevis (C6, 7)
		Extensor digitorum (C7, 8)
		Ext. dig. minimi (C7)
		Extensor carpi ulnaris (C7, 8)
		Supinator (C5, 6)
		Abd. pollicis longus (C7, 8)
		Ext. pollicis brevis (C7, 8)
		Ext. pollicis longus (C7, 8)
		Ext. indicis (C7, 8)
1st lumbar nerve	L1	Psoas minor
2nd and 3rd lumbar nerves	L1, 2 (3)	Psoas, major, iliacus
Obturator nerve	L2, 3, 4	Gracilis (L2, 3)
		Adductor longus (L2, 3, 4)
		Adductor brevis (L2, 3, 4)
		Adductor magnus (L3, 4 + sciatic)
		Obturator externus (L3, 4)
Femoral nerve	L2, 3, 4	Sartorius (L2,3)
		Quadriceps (L2, 3, 4)
		Pectineus (L2, 3)
Superior gluteal nerve	L4, 5, S1	Gluteus medius, gluteus minimus, Tensor, fasciae latae
Inferior gluteal nerve	L5, S1, 2	Gluteus maximus
Sciatic nerve	L4, 5, S1, 2, 3	Add. magnus (L4, 5 + obturator)
		Biceps femoris (L5, S1, 2, 3)
Sciatic tibial division		Semitendinosus (L5, S1, 2)
		Semimembranosus (L5, S1, 2)
		Biceps (S1, 2, 3)
		Gastrocnemius (S1, 2)
		Soleus (S1, 2)
		Plantaris (S1, 2)
		Popliteus (L4, 5, S1)
		Flexor hallucis longus (S2, 3)
		Flexor digitorum longus (S2, 3)
		Tibialis posterior (L4, 5)
		Plantar muscles (S2, 3)
Sciatic, common peroneal		Biceps (L5, S1)
		Tibialis anterior (L4, 5)
		Extensor hallucis longus (L5, S1)
		Extensor digitorum longus, peroneus tertius (L5, S1)
		Peroneus longus, peroneus brevis (L5, S1)
		Extensor digitorum brevis (S1, 2)

BRACHIAL PLEXUS

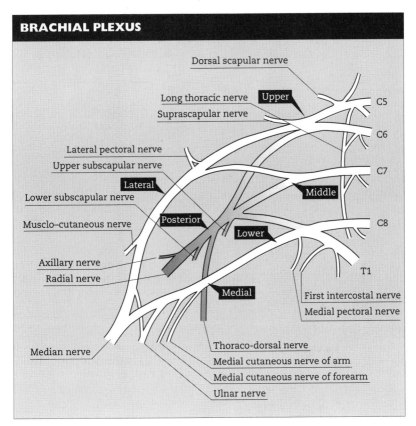

Fig. A.1

SENSORY DERMATOMES

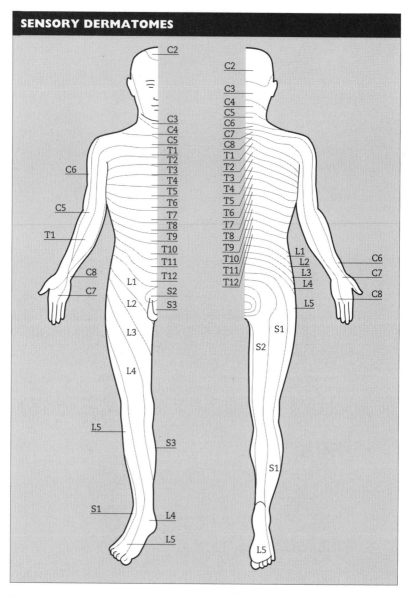

Fig. A.2

Index